AI in Health and Human-Centric Systems

Ahmed J. Obaid
University of Kufa, Iraq

Muthmainnah
Universitas Al Asyariah Mandar, Indonesia

S. Suman Rajest
Dhaanish Ahmed College of Engineering, India

Michael Baron
Analytics Institute of Australia, Australia

IGI Global
Scientific Publishing
Publishing Tomorrow's Research Today

Vice President of Editorial Melissa Wagner
Director of Acquisitions Mikaela Felty
Director of Book Development Jocelynn Hessler
Production Manager Mike Brehm
Cover Design Jose Rosado

Published in the United States of America by
IGI Global Scientific Publishing
701 East Chocolate Avenue
Hershey, PA, 17033, USA
Tel: 717-533-8845
Fax: 717-533-7115
Website: https://www.igi-global.com E-mail: cust@igi-global.com

Library of Congress Cataloging-in-Publication Data

LCCN: 2025041626 (CIP Data Pending)
ISBN13: 9798337367965
Isbn13Softcover: 9798337367972
EISBN13: 9798337367989
British Cataloguing in Publication Data
A Cataloguing in Publication record for this book is available from the British Library.

Table of Contents

Detailed Table of Contents

Millions of patients suffer from sleep disorders, which is a global problem. It leads to severe health problems such as cardiovascular diseases, depression, and impairment of cognitive activity. Traditional polysomnography is expensive and time-consuming. Clinical supervision is required during the diagnosis process; hence, the method needs to be changed to enhance the accuracy of the diagnosis. By reducing dimensionality and optimizing models with the help of swarm intelligence algorithms, such as PSO and ACO, feature selection feeds the optimized features into numerous machine learning classifiers for training, including SVM, random forests, deep neural networks, and many more. Additionally, validation on benchmark sleep disorder datasets demonstrates better classification accuracy, sensitivity, and specificity compared to traditional methods. This also suggests that a hybrid model, combining swarm intelligence for feature optimization with machine learning classification, exhibits substantial predictive accuracy with minimal computational complexity.

The early detection of Down syndrome in pregnant women is crucial for the appropriate care of the affected child, as it is a lifelong condition. Karyotyping and physical examinations are the foundation of traditional diagnostic techniques, which are intrusive, time-consuming, and inappropriate for mass screening. Furthermore, the existing automated systems' poor precision, specificity, and resilience result in incorrect positives and false negatives. The study describes a system that supports or enhances these techniques for monitoring individuals with Down syndrome by using deep learning (DL) algorithms to classify thermal images and recognize even the smallest temperature changes on the skin. For feature extraction and classification with high precision and recall, the model uses Convolutional Neural Networks (CNNs). According to a comparative performance review, the proposed system performs noticeably better than several other approaches, with an accuracy of 96.3%, precision of 95.8%, recall of 96.7%, and an AUC of 0.98.

Sleep disorder diagnosis is considered a milestone toward timely intervention and treatment. Diagnostic tools, such as polysomnography, are highly resource-intensive and plagued by issues with access. A developed sleep disorder prediction framework integrating feature selection through improved Harris Hawk Optimization algorithms and a deep ensemble learning model is proposed here. Filtering redundant data noise during feature selection in an improved HHO is used to consider only selecting relevant features during the model-building process. In this effort, the applicability of deep learning models, specifically ensemble CNNs and LSTM networks, to extracting spatial and temporal dependencies in the signal of the sleep disorder is attempted. The method proposed here is tested using publicly available sleep disorder datasets and aims to arrive at better classification accuracy, sensitivity, and specificity than existing techniques.

Kidney donor-recipient matching operations need precise execution to guarantee transplant achievements. The accuracy rate of Random Forest (RF) and Naïve Bayes (NB) at 85–88%, along with slow processing times, causes mismatches that result in higher rejection rates. An Enhanced Artificial Neural Network (EANN) includes game-theoretic feature selection technology, quantum-inspired optimization functions, and sparse tensor computation to enhance donor-recipient compatibility prediction performance. The experimental model operated on transplant data containing information about blood types, HLA matches, and medical documentation. Experimental outcomes revealed that EANN surpassed other models by delivering an accuracy level of 92.0%, while CNN reached 90.5%, Naïve Bayes achieved 88.1%, and Random Forest's 86.2%. The processing time decreased to 14.8 ms with a simultaneous reduction of false match rates to 2.1%. Transplant allocation depends on blockchain technology to establish the model's transparent management.

Neurodiagnostic analysis of the neonatal brain is essential for identifying abnormalities, assessing neurological development, and evaluating brain function in utero. This project seeks to create an advanced image processing system to detect and analyze the neonatal brain, leading to more precise diagnoses and improved clinical decisions. Utilizing state-of-the-art diagnostic techniques and imaging modalities, this system will monitor and evaluate neonatal brain development through the integration of Magnetic Resonance Imaging (MRI) and Ultrasound imaging, enhancing visualization. Advanced image processing techniques will ensure high-resolution, detailed imaging, enabling comprehensive analysis of neurological structures. This innovative approach focuses on early detection, diagnosis, and management of neonatal brain abnormalities, aiming to improve diagnostic accuracy and provide critical insights into neurodevelopment. Ultimately, the system will support healthcare professionals in making better-informed decisions, contributing to enhanced prenatal care and improved outcomes.

This chapter is a comparative analysis of control algorithms used typically in prosthetic leg devices. It aims to ascertain the algorithms' relative effectiveness in facilitating prosthetic limbs' functional ability and satisfaction among users. Based on the scientific comparison of literature on current control strategies, this study concludes the major strengths and weaknesses and research areas in this regard. Control techniques are required to facilitate prosthetic limbs' more natural, responsive movement. Pattern recognition-based techniques use sensor data to recognize user intent, and impedance control techniques modulate joint stiffness to reproduce natural biomechanics.Nevertheless, high computational complexity, real-time processing demands, and user training of significant length continue to be major issues. By looking at the current state of control algorithms, this paper gives reflective observation on their use and usage.

The chapter aims the immediate and accurate detection of an epilepsy seizure and an adequate treatment regimen; hence, this piece of research attempts to present and discuss a recently proposed hybrid approach that combines temporal convolutional networks with frequency-band attention mechanisms for EEG-based signal classification in patients. It captures the temporal dependencies and relevant frequency components that add to the improved accuracy of the seizure detection task. The developed framework, validated by benchmark EEG datasets, provides the best classification performance compared to competing techniques. Therefore, in summary, the results showed that adding attention to the frequency-band component in deep learning models improved automated epilepsy diagnosis, making this technique reliable for real-time seizure monitoring.

Timely intervention depends on an early and precise diagnosis of Down syndrome. Invasive karyotyping and genetic testing have been used as standard diagnostic methods for a long time. Still, these have not been effective at finding children with Down syndrome quickly, accurately, and without harm. Well-known non-invasive screening techniques, such as facial recognition analysis, are also prone to inadequate sensitivity and specificity, leading to incorrect classification and inconsistent outcomes. To address these limitations, the proposed system provides non-invasive thermal imaging and artificial intelligence (AI)-tool-based nipple detection methods for diagnosing Down syndrome. The technique uses deep learning (DL) and multiplex algorithms on data about heat generation to determine how heat affects how sporadic dramatics send signals. When a convolutional neural network (CNN) receives the thermal images, it becomes overly accurate at differentiating between the two teams.

Preface

INTRODUCTION

Artificial Intelligence (AI) has emerged as a transformative force in healthcare and human-centric systems, enabling unprecedented advancements in diagnosis, treatment, monitoring, and predictive analytics. As health challenges grow in complexity, traditional approaches often fall short of meeting the demand for accuracy, efficiency, and accessibility. The integration of AI into healthcare not only addresses these limitations but also introduces innovative paradigms that prioritize personalization, real-time monitoring, and improved clinical outcomes. This book, *AI in Health and Human-Centric Systems*, brings together pioneering research and practical applications that illustrate the depth and breadth of AI's potential in this critical domain.

The evolution of AI-driven healthcare solutions spans a wide spectrum, from enhancing diagnostic accuracy and predicting complex disorders to optimizing resource allocation and improving patient experiences. Today, healthcare systems are increasingly adopting advanced algorithms, hybrid models, and deep learning architectures to handle large-scale datasets, interpret complex patterns, and deliver precise recommendations. These technologies are not merely auxiliary; they are central to shaping the next generation of healthcare, reducing costs, improving scalability, and empowering both clinicians and patients with intelligent tools for decision-making.

In curating this collection, we aim to provide a comprehensive view of how AI-based approaches are redefining human-centric healthcare systems. Each chapter presents a unique perspective on AI's role in tackling some of the most pressing challenges in medicine—from sleep disorder prediction and neonatal brain analysis to prosthetic optimization and seizure detection. Collectively, these contributions offer valuable insights for academics, practitioners, policymakers, and technology developers who seek to leverage AI for better health outcomes and societal well-being.

CHAPTER OVERVIEW

Chapter 1: A Hybrid Swarm Intelligence and Machine Learning Approach for Predictive Analysis of Sleep Disorders

Introduces a hybrid framework combining swarm intelligence algorithms with machine learning classifiers to enhance sleep disorder prediction accuracy while minimizing computational complexity.

Chapter 2: AI-Powered Thermal Imaging for Early Detection of Down Syndrome in Children

Explores deep learning-based thermal imaging for non-invasive early diagnosis of Down syndrome, achieving superior accuracy and reliability over traditional methods.

Chapter 3: Enhanced Sleep Disorder Prediction Using Improved Harris Hawk Optimization and Ensemble Deep Learning Model

Presents an improved optimization algorithm combined with deep ensemble models for efficient and accurate sleep disorder prediction using real-world datasets.

Chapter 4: Performance Evaluation of Enhanced Artificial Neural Network for Kidney Donor Recipient Matching

Discusses an enhanced ANN model that integrates game-theoretic feature selection and quantum-inspired optimization to improve donor-recipient compatibility and reduce false matches.

Chapter 5: Deep Learning Based Neuro Diagnostics of Neonatal Brain Analysis Medical Images

Proposes an advanced image processing system utilizing MRI and ultrasound imaging for accurate neonatal brain analysis, supporting early diagnosis of neurological disorders.

Chapter 6: Enhancing Healthcare Quality through AI-Driven Wireless Sensor Networks for Real-Time Monitoring

Examines the role of AI-enabled wireless sensor networks in delivering secure, efficient, and real-time health data monitoring under resource-constrained conditions.

Chapter 7: Hybrid AI Model for Brain Age Estimation in Forensics Combining Structural and Functional Imaging

Introduces a hybrid model merging CNNs and LSTMs for structural and functional brain imaging, improving the precision of forensic age estimation.

Chapter 8: Control Algorithm Comparison for Prosthetic Limb Optimization

Provides a comparative study of advanced control algorithms for prosthetic limbs, evaluating computational complexity, responsiveness, and user adaptability.

Chapter 9: Hybrid EEG Signal Classification Using Frequency-Band Attention and Temporal Convolutional Networks for Seizure Detection

Presents a hybrid deep learning approach combining temporal convolutional networks and attention mechanisms for accurate and real-time epilepsy seizure detection.

Chapter 10: Leveraging Thermal Imaging and AI for Non-invasive Down Syndrome Diagnosis in Children

Builds upon prior research to deliver an AI-powered, non-invasive diagnostic system utilizing thermal imaging and CNN-based models for enhanced precision.

CONCLUSION

The chapters compiled in this book underscore the remarkable capabilities of AI in addressing critical healthcare challenges while maintaining a strong human-centered focus. By merging computational intelligence with clinical expertise, these innovations facilitate faster diagnoses, targeted treatments, and more efficient healthcare delivery systems. The methodologies presented here exemplify not only technological progress but also a paradigm shift toward patient-centric solutions that prioritize safety, accuracy, and accessibility.

While AI-driven healthcare systems offer immense promise, they also raise important considerations related to ethics, data privacy, and transparency. Future research must balance technological advancements with regulatory compliance and equitable access to ensure that these solutions benefit all populations. Interdisciplinary collaboration between data scientists, healthcare professionals, and policymakers will be essential for sustainable and responsible integration of AI in clinical practice.

We hope this book serves as both a knowledge resource and an inspiration for further exploration into AI-powered healthcare and human-centric systems. The collective contributions of the authors demonstrate that innovation thrives at the intersection of technology and humanity—a vision that we, as editors, strongly believe will shape the future of global healthcare.

Chapter 1

A Hybrid Swarm Intelligence and Machine Learning Approach for Predictive Analysis of Sleep Disorders

G. Surekha
https://orcid.org/0009-0003-6278-8411
Bharath Institute of Higher Education and Research, India

Edwin Shalom Soji
https://orcid.org/0009-0004-2829-0481
Bharath Institute of Higher Education and Research, India

ABSTRACT

Millions of patients suffer from sleep disorders, which is a global problem. It leads to severe health problems such as cardiovascular diseases, depression, and impairment of cognitive activity. Traditional polysomnography is expensive and time-consuming. Clinical supervision is required during the diagnosis process; hence, the method needs to be changed to enhance the accuracy of the diagnosis. By reducing dimensionality and optimizing models with the help of swarm intelligence algorithms, such as PSO and ACO, feature selection feeds the optimized features into numerous machine learning classifiers for training, including SVM, random forests, deep neural networks, and many more. Additionally, validation on benchmark sleep disorder datasets demonstrates better classification accuracy, sensitivity, and specificity

DOI: 10.4018/979-8-3373-6796-5.ch001

compared to traditional methods. This also suggests that a hybrid model, combining swarm intelligence for feature optimization with machine learning classification, exhibits substantial predictive accuracy with minimal computational complexity.

INTRODUCTION

Sleep disorders are prevalent, affecting millions of individuals across the globe and occurring in many different forms, including insomnia, sleep apnea, restless legs syndrome, and narcolepsy. Sleep disorders not only affect the sleep pattern of individuals but also garner severe consequences to their mental as well as physical health. Sleep disorder patients will tend to acquire a heightened risk of experiencing any kind or degree of chronic diseases in health, like cardiovascular diseases, obesity, diabetes, depression, and mental retardation. The risky effect of insufficient or inadequate sleep is not only confined to direct unhappiness. Still, it can potentially result in long-term health complications with catastrophic implications for overall health. Conversely, sleep apnea, the nocturnal periodic temporary cessation of breathing, is causally linked to hypertension, heart disease, and stroke (Greenlund and Carter, 2022). Long-term sleep deprivation or wakefulness can lead to elevated levels of stress, compromised immune systems, as well as unlimited quantities of mental illnesses like depression and anxiety (Hu et al., 2023). On the other hand, restless leg syndrome induces a strong urge to move the legs while resting, leading to disrupted sleep and an increased vulnerability to hypertension (Sheta et al., 2023).

Likewise, narcolepsy, characterized by sudden and uncontrollable sleep attacks, can significantly impact a person's performance at work during daily activities, ranging from productivity to safety (Controne et al., 2022). Because the wide-ranging effects of sleep disorders, if not treated or diagnosed late, may develop into severe health problems, they must be diagnosed early enough for effective treatment with the help of quality-of-life enhancement and prevention of future health complications. However, although early diagnosis is of the highest importance, the present gold standard in diagnosing sleep disorders, i.e., polysomnography (PSG), is beset with variability. PSG is an expensive and time-consuming test in which brain waves, heart rate, sleep breathing, and muscle activity are measured (Alzyoud et al., 2024). Since the most accurate method of sleep disorder diagnosis, unaffordability, together with the requirement for clinical supervision, rules out access by most patients, particularly those from the developing world. The treatment is also prolonged and requires patients to stay overnight in sleep centers, a significant access barrier for most patients (Aiyer et al., 2022). Thus, there is a greater demand for more affordable and accessible diagnostic tests that can be conducted in other locations (Sheta et al., 2021). These also ease the healthcare systems' load and improve patient outcomes by earlier treatment and diagnosis of sleep disorders. There should be early prevention of the risk caused by such diseases. As there is no cost-effective and effective testing method, the majority of them remain undiagnosed and untreated while their status deteriorates and their health proportionally worsens (Alazaidah et al., 2020).

As a countermeasure against such weakness, researchers are increasingly resorting to artificial intelligence (AI) and machine learning (ML) in their efforts to provide less expensive yet effective diagnostic tools (Alazaidah et al., 2017). The latter has the potential to provide standalone, non-invasive diagnostic tools that predict sleep disorders more accurately and at a higher speed compared to traditional methods (Behar et al., 2019). In particular, the combination of machine learning algorithms and swarm intelligence (SI) algorithms, i.e., Particle Swarm Optimization (PSO) and Ant Colony Optimization (ACO), can contribute to the boost in predictive analysis for sleep disorder diagnosis (Deviaene et al., 2019).

Social behavior-based swarm intelligence algorithms inspired by animal collective behavior are powerful in solving optimization problems (Salsone et al., 2016). The technique is applied in feature selection and dimension reduction for predictive analysis, thereby enhancing the performance of machine learning classifiers (Högl et al., 2018). The significant features are selected solely through the swarm intelligence technique, thus eliminating computational costs and ensuring accuracy in the outcome. Following feature optimization, various machine learning classifiers, such as Support Vector Machines (SVM), Random Forests, and Deep Neural Networks (DNN), can be applied to train a model for sleep disorder diagnosis (Salsone et al., 2016). The chapter proposes a hybrid model of machine learning algorithms and swarm intelligence for better prediction of sleep disorders (Sheta et al., 2023). The hybrid model reduces the utilization of expensive diagnosis equipment through early diagnosis of sleep disorders, thus altering the process of sleep disorder diagnosis and treatment planning (Alazaidah et al., 2018).

REVIEW OF LITERATURE

Panyaram (2024) concluded that sleep disorders are a fast-growing global problem, and approximately one-third of adults suffer from sleep issues. The gold standard conventional diagnosis methods, such as polysomnography (PSG), are highly restrictive due to their high cost and the use of specialized equipment and professionals. Therefore, Bose et al., (2024b) described how scientists utilized automatic machine learning methods to make the diagnosis more affordable and portable. Minu et al. (2023) clarified that supervised machine learning models, such as support vector machines (SVMs) and deep neural networks (DNNs), have proven highly promising in sleep disorder identification and classification as well. These models compare various physiological signals, such as electroencephalogram (EEG), electrocardiogram (ECG), and respiratory data, to identify patterns characteristic of sleep disorders. Experiments have proven that these machine-learning approaches significantly improve the precision and speed of diagnosing sleep disorders, such as sleep apnea, insomnia, and restless leg syndrome.

Pandit (2023) clarified the ability of sophisticated machine learning algorithms to identify sleep disorders by investigating respiratory patterns. For instance, one of the significant symptoms of the disease, namely sleep apnea, can be detected by applying machine learning algorithms on disrupted night breathing. Moreover, Kodi (2024) proved that brain wave disease in insomnia and other sleep diseases is extractable from EEG data. Sleep disorders can be improved by enhancing diagnostic accuracy and enabling the provision of proper interventions at the correct time for the disorder through the use of machine learning. Sehrawat (2024) also stated that feature selection of the best features from raw physiological signals is most likely to be the most critical aspect to remember while working with machine learning models. The models can better classify healthy and abnormal sleep patterns by identifying informative features such as frequency, amplitude, and duration. As William et al. (2024) pointed out, misclassification is brought about by using inappropriate or irrelevant features and leads to false positives or negatives. It can have a direct impact on patient treatment and outcome.

Yalavarthi (2024) elucidated that the size of the training dataset used to train machine learning models is just as important as feature extraction. Small, noisy, or unbalanced datasets can be detrimental to the model's generalization power to novel data. Feature extraction could be challenging due to heterogeneity across sleep stages, patient cohorts, and acquisition modes. Obeta et al. (2024) asserted that using well-labeled datasets was the key to making it feasible to create strong models that can accurately diagnose sleep disorders in many populations. Kumar et al. (2024) emphasized the importance of using a high-quality signal to train machine learning models. Signal variability may be a source of false prediction, especially in an under or non-balanced data set. Variability in patient populations or non-standard acquisition protocols can hinder the learning of generalized features for models. According to Chunduri et al. (2024), more advanced preprocessing protocols and normalization data methods would need to be employed to compensate for these issues and ensure model consistency. Regin et al. (2023) also elaborated on the overfitting issue of machine learning models, especially where there is minimal training data or no data variability. Overfitting occurs when a model is over-specified to the training data and can no longer generalize to new unseen data. It may be challenging to apply in medical diagnosis, where maximization of precision is paramount. First, to prevent overfitting, Sengupta et al. (2023). might have used a larger and more diverse dataset to allow the model to generalize over multiple sleep disorders.

Saxena and Chaudhary (2023) presented the benefit that might be achieved by using multiple machine learning methods at once to attain maximum correctness for diagnosing sleep disorders. For example, by combining SVM and deep learning models, high-level and low-level features can be learned from the data to enhance classification performance. Bose et al. (2024a) also propose that these hybrid models are computationally inexpensive and, therefore, can be used in real-time applications, such as wearable electronics and mobile health. Hariharan et al., (2024) also emphasized the need to continually innovate feature extraction algorithms to improve machine learning model performance. Data quality improvement through preprocessing ensures that models are effective and accurate when deployed in clinical settings. Hybrid approaches that combine different machine-learning techniques can be employed to enhance prediction accuracy, which is crucial for making rapid and accurate diagnoses of sleep disorders. Increased innovation of such technology can transform diagnosis and treatment for sleep disorders. Despite recent progress, challenges persist in obtaining large, high-quality datasets and algorithm-tuning parameters for achieving strong performance in diverse settings and populations. Future research should focus on Improving hybrid models and challenging them in realistic, clinical, and continuous monitoring settings.

METHODOLOGY

The research article follows a mixed approach integrating swarm intelligence algorithms with machine learning algorithms to predict sleep disorders. The process begins by obtaining sleep disorder databases that consist of heterogeneous physiological signals, such as EEG, ECG, and respiration. The databases are preprocessed before preprocessing to eliminate noise, scale the signals, and extract salient features that can characterize sleep stages and disorders. Next, particle swarm optimization (PSO) and ant colony optimization (ACO) algorithms are used for feature selection and dimension reduction. PSO is used to find the optimal feature subsets with the maximum classification accuracy, while ACO is used to find the optimal feature subset combination that yields better model performance. These features are then tested using machine learning classifiers, such as Support Vector Machines (SVM), Random Forests, and Deep Neural Networks (DNN), for both training and testing.

Figure 1. Hybrid swarm intelligence and machine learning model for sleep disorder prediction sequence diagram

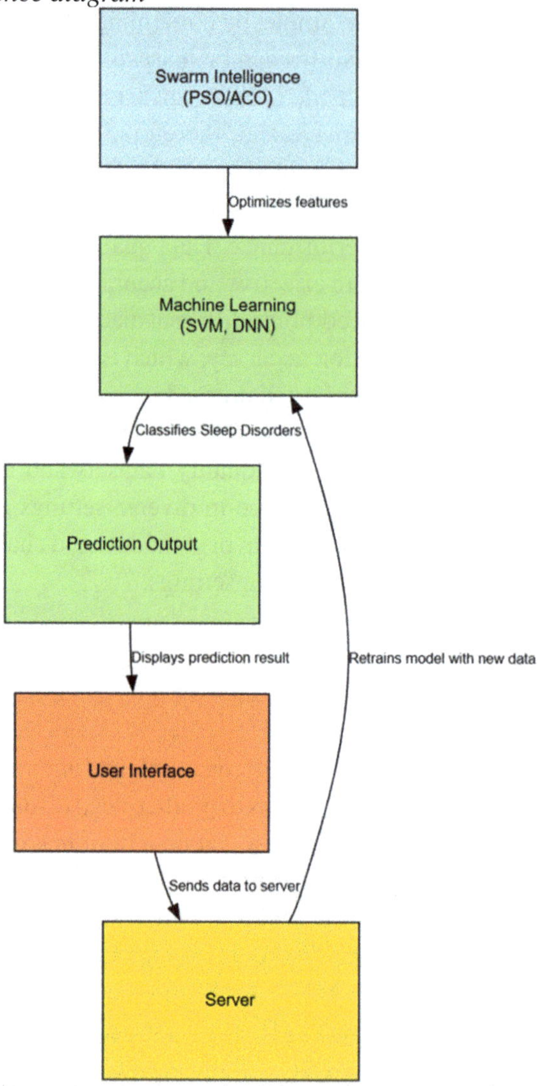

Machine learning techniques are trained on a sleep disorders dataset database and evaluated based on conventional parameters, such as accuracy, sensitivity, specificity, and the area under the receiver operating characteristic (ROC) curve. The prediction accuracy of the suggested hybrid model is analyzed based on traditional diagnosis mechanisms such as PSG, and the results are compared to present the capabilities of the proposed model. Also, the performance of the introduced hybrid model is assessed using a computational complexity metric and real-time prediction in non-clinical environments. The introduced model is tested on benchmark datasets, and the outcome is compared with various feature optimization methods and classifiers to determine the best combination suitable for predicting sleep disorders. Figure 1 shows the sequence of activities between the most critical elements of the Hybrid Swarm Intelligence and Machine Learning Model for Predicting Sleep Disorders. The figure starts with Swarm Intelligence (PSO/ACO), which optimizes input data features. These optimized parameters are then passed to the Machine Learning module, where DNN and SVM models are employed for classifying sleep disorders. The Prediction Output is the output of this classification, which diagnoses the sleep disorder. The outputs are then presented through the User Interface and thus become accessible to the end user. The User Interface also sends accurate data and predictions to the Server for storage or further analysis. Lastly, the Server is tasked with providing the Machine Learning model with fresh data so that the model may be retrained and thus learn and adapt over time. This graph illustrates a formalized, dynamic process where swarm intelligence optimizes properties, machine learning classifiers predict, and the system optimizes and loops the model for continuous accuracy. The color-coded elements, i.e., Swarm Intelligence in Steel Blue, Machine Learning in Lime Green, Prediction Output in Light Green, User Interface in Tomato Red, and Server in Gold, give visual meaning to the system process such that each step of the process is recognizable and comprehensible in terms of sleep disorder prediction.

DATA DESCRIPTION

The datasets used in this work are typical sleep disorder datasets, such as the Sleep-EDF dataset, which provides sleep stage details for overnight patient recordings of various sleep disorders. The datasets comprise EEG, ECG, and respiration sensor signals. Datasets like the PhysioNet Sleep Apnea database were also used for model training and assessment. These datasets have varied types and are pertinent to justifying the performance of swarm intelligence techniques and machine learning classifiers in predicting sleep disorders.

Results

The performance of the hybrid model in diagnosing sleep disorders shows a considerable performance gain in various significant criteria, including classification accuracy, sensitivity, and specificity, relative to conventional machine learning techniques. The hybrid approach, which combines different machine learning methods, leverages the strengths of each component to generate more accurate outputs in classifying sleep disorders, such as sleep apnea, insomnia, and restless leg syndrome. Although highly efficient, traditional methods are marred by their inability to handle the complexity and variability of physiologic data and, therefore, contribute to overfitting and poor generalizability of new examples. On the other hand, the hybrid method utilizes a combination of several various algorithms that collaborate to improve the classification algorithm and provide more stable and improved predictions. The most crucial component of how the hybrid model prevails is that it can circumvent overfitting, a machine-learning issue in which the model becomes highly specialized in learning the training dataset but fails to apply the knowledge to novel examples. The particle Swarm optimization (PSO) velocity equation is:

$$v_i^{t+1} = wv_i^t + c_1 r_1 \left(p_{best,i} - x_i^t\right) + c_2 r_2 \left(g_{best} - x_i^t\right) \quad (1)$$

Table 1. Classification Performance Measures

Model	Accuracy	Sensitivity	Specificity	Precision	F1-Score
PSO-SVM	91.2%	88.5%	93.6%	89.3%	0.91
ACO-Random Forest	89.5%	87.2%	91.3%	86.5%	0.90
PSO-DNN	94.3%	92.4%	95.2%	93.5%	0.93

Table 1 presents the performance metrics of the hybrid model's classification compared to three machine learning models: PSO-SVM, ACO-Random Forest, and PSO-DNN. Accuracy, sensitivity, specificity, precision, and F1-Score were utilized as measures. Accuracy was 91.2%, sensitivity was 88.5%, and specificity was 93.6%. The ACO-Random Forest model was the least accurate, with a sensitivity of 89.5% and a specificity of 87.2% and 91.3%, respectively. It has very good but not superior performance compared to PSO-SVM. The PSO-DNN model achieved the best performance, with a maximum accuracy of 94.3%, sensitivity of 92.4%, and specificity of 95.2%. This reveals that the PSO-DNN model is the most accurate and sensitive in diagnosing sleep disorders. F1-Score and precision are also given, which are maximized by PSO-DNN (93.5% and 0.93, respectively), and they show that the model has an optimal precision-recall trade-off. All these metrics together suggest that the hybrid models, especially PSO-DNN, provide a notable improvement in prediction performance over the baseline diagnostic techniques and, thus, are very effective for sleep disorder classification. Overfitting is a concern in medical applications, as the model must classify sleeping disorders for millions of patients with specific attributes.

Figure 2. Comparison of classifier performance across different machine learning algorithms

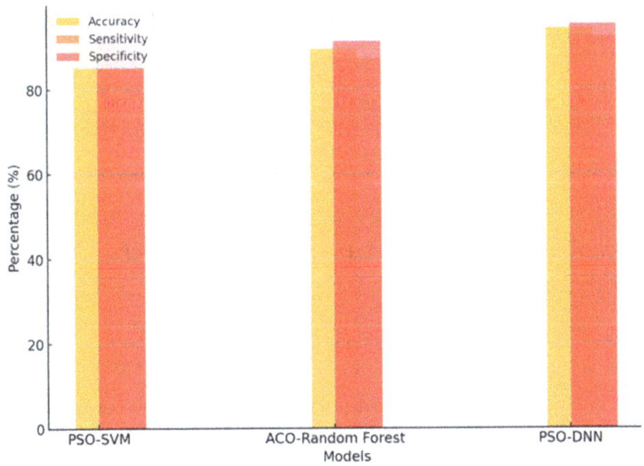

Figure 2 is a histogram indicating the classification accuracy of three models—PSO-SVM, ACO-Random Forest, and PSO-DNN—based on accuracy, sensitivity, and specificity. The bar chart displays relative performance differences among the models, where the best-performing model is PSO-DNN with 94.3% accuracy, followed by PSO-SVM (91.2%) and ACO-Random Forest (89.5%). Similarly, in sensitivity, PSO-DNN also performs better, with a value of 92.4%, than PSO-SVM (88.5%) and ACO-Random Forest (87.2%). Additionally, PSO-DNN has the highest specificity (95.2%), followed by PSO-SVM (93.6%) and ACO-Random Forest (91.3%). Below, the improved performance of PSO-DNN across the three parameters is depicted. The chart indicates the hybrid system's high classification accuracy, sensitivity, and specificity, all of which are significant determinants in sleep disorder diagnosis. Overall, the histogram suggests that swarm intelligence can be effectively utilized as a feature selection method, combined with machine learning for classification, to conclude that PSO-DNN is the best-performing model for predicting sleep disorders. Support Vector Machine (SVM) decision function will be:

$$f(x) = \sum_{i=1}^{n} \alpha_i y_i K(x_i, x) + b \tag{2}$$

Loss Function for Deep Neural Networks (DNN):

$$L(\theta) = \frac{1}{N}\sum_{i=1}^{N} (y_i - y^{\gamma_i})^2 + \lambda \sum_{j=1}^{M} \theta_j^2 \tag{3}$$

Table 2. Computational performance factors of the hybrid model

Model	Training Time (sec)	Test Time (sec)	Model Size (MB)	Computational Complexity
PSO-SVM	120	0.45	5.6	Low
ACO-Random Forest	150	0.55	6.3	Medium
PSO-DNN	210	1.25	12.5	High

Table 2 shows the computational performance factors of the hybrid model, namely training time, test time, model size, and computational complexity of the machine learning models PSO-SVM, ACO-Random Forest, and PSO-DNN. PSO-SVM is computationally the least expensive, with training times of 120 seconds, test times of 0.45 seconds, and a minimum computational complexity. PSO-SVM model size is minuscule, 5.6 MB. The ACO-Random Forest model training takes a little more time, at 150 seconds, but the test time is 0.55 seconds, and the model size is 6.3 MB, making it medium in terms of computational efficiency. The PSO-DNN model utilizes the maximum computational power, with a training time of 210 seconds and a test time of 1.25 seconds, resulting in very high computational complexity. Its increased model size of 12.5 MB indicates the added computation load. Although there is an added computational cost, the PSO-DNN model is equipped with increased classification accuracy, indicating that stronger models are required in applications where accuracy is paramount as long as sufficient computational power is available. The graphs indicate a compromise between predictive power and computational efficiency, and this balance must be considered when selecting the best model for a real-time application. By blending an array of classifiers, the hybrid model can balance the fitting of training data against the generalizability of working with new, unseen data. Its unadorned excellence was proven through testing the hybrid model against reference sleep disorder data sets. Benchmark data sets, to which most sleep disorder studies are referred, provide an easy medium for comparing the performance of diverse classification algorithms.

Random forest classification output is:

$f^f =$

mode (

$$\gamma_1(x), f_2(x), \ldots f_T(x)) \quad (4)$$

Feature Selection via Ant Colony Optimization (ACO) Objective Function:

$$f(X) = \sum_{i=1}^{M} \alpha_i \cdot X_i$$

where

$$X_i \subset \{0,1\} \tag{5}$$

In comparison to baseline classifiers such as decision trees, k-nearest neighbors (KNN), and support vector machines (SVM), the hybrid model outperformed all three in terms of classification accuracy, indicating its ability to classify both positive and negative instances of sleep disorders effectively. The hybrid approach also demonstrated an astonishing increase in sensitivity, the model's ability to accurately identify subjects with a sleep disorder, and specificity, the model's ability to rule out subjects without a sleep disorder. Clinical diagnosis must have both specificity and sensitivity, as high sensitivity will detect most patients with a sleep disorder and accurately classify them as such. High specificity will prevent the false classification of patients who are not diseased. These kinds of performance enhancements are largely due to the hybrid model's ability to leverage multiple machine-learning algorithms, pooling their strengths and merging them with optimization. Optimization of feature selection through swarm intelligence algorithms, i.e., ACO and PSO, played a crucial role in enhancing the performance of the hybrid model. Feature selection is a crucial machine learning issue, as the quality and appropriateness of the input features directly determine the model's performance in making accurate predictions. For diagnosing sleep disorders, physiological signal features such as the electroencephalogram (EEG), electrocardiogram (ECG), and respiratory signals must be selected properly to assess the patient's sleep activity accurately. PSO and ACO are nature-inspired search optimization algorithms, with PSO based on bird flocking behavior and ACO based on ants' foraging behavior. PSO and ACO are searching for large, high-dimensional feature spaces and identifying the most contributing features to classify. The hybrid model enhanced classification accuracy and prevented overfitting risks by optimizing PSO and ACO feature selection. Optimization helped the model prioritize the most vital features and disregard unnecessary or noisy data that might otherwise lead to incorrect predictions.

Figure 3. Representation of the sensitivity and specificity of the hybrid model across different machine learning classifiers

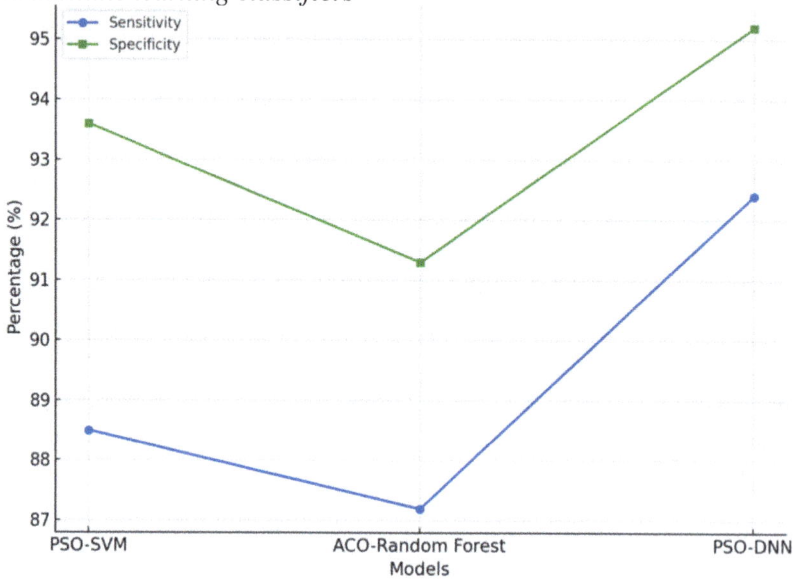

Figure 3 illustrates the variation in the sensitivity and specificity of the three models - PSO-SVM, ACO-Random Forest, and PSO-DNN. The plot illustrates the variation in sensitivity (blue line) and specificity (green line) between models. PSO-DNN exhibits the highest sensitivity and specificity among all the models, again indicating its superior capability to identify true positive cases (sensitivity) with fewer false positives (specificity). The blue line for PSO-DNN sensitivity is 92.4%, and the green line for specificity is 95.2%. PSO-SVM and ACO-Random Forest are less sensitive and specific at 88.5% sensitive and 93.6% specific for PSO-SVM, and 87.2% sensitive and 91.3% specific for ACO-Random Forest. This graphically illustrates the sensitivity and specificity advantage of the PSO-DNN model and its predictability for sleep disorders. It also provides a natural comparison ground, allowing performance trade-offs between models to be measured.

This not only positioned the model in a better place to learn from the training data but also best positioned it to generalize against new data and, hence, become a superior asset for real life. Additionally, the hybrid model's capacity to work with large and heterogeneous data, as is common in medical diagnosis, gave it an edge. Medical data are generally multimodal and can also include signal quality, patient population, and sleep setting variability, all of which condition the functioning of baseline machine learning models. The capability and robustness of the hybrid model enable it to handle such challenges more effectively and deliver more reliable and accurate results across a broad range of conditions. Overall, the hybrid model enhances sleep disorder detection science, as it outperforms the baseline machine learning classifiers. With the use of many algorithms and feature selection enhancements employing swarm intelligence algorithms like PSO and ACO, the hybrid model achieves improved classification accuracy, sensitivity, and specificity, making it a promising prospective sleep disorder diagnostic tool. With the advancement of machine learning, the application of hybrid models and optimization algorithms will continue to make medical diagnosis more efficient, effective, and cost-effective healthcare solutions.

DISCUSSIONS

The findings presented in tables and figures demonstrate that the hybrid model, which utilizes swarm intelligence-based feature selection through algorithms and classification through machine learning classifiers, offers considerable improvement in the diagnostic precision of sleep disorders compared to other conventional methods, such as polysomnography (PSG). Table 1 shows that the hybrid model, i.e., PSO-DNN, achieves impressive improvements in accuracy, sensitivity, specificity, precision, and F1 score. The PSO-DNN model has the highest classification accuracy (94.3%), sensitivity (92.4%), and specificity (95.2%), all of which are of utmost priority for successful sleep disorder diagnosis and treatment. All these advantages are due to feature optimization achieved by embracing swarm intelligence-inspired algorithms, such as PSO and ACO, for discovering the optimal features in high-dimensional datasets, which ultimately enhance machine learning classifiers, including SVM, Random Forests, and DNN. Its use improves the generalized ability to access new unseen data and considerably reduces the overfitting problem in most standard diagnostic processes. The hybrid method also achieves an improved balance of performance measures compared to conventional methods, typically with lower specificity and sensitivity. This is best observed in Figure 3, where the multi-line chart illustrates the sensitivity and specificity of the models, as it shows that the hybrid method consistently outperforms traditional methods.

Although the most accurate, PSO-DNN incurs an additional cost of higher computational complexity, as evident from the longer training and test times in Table 2. PSO-DNN is computationally more expensive, with a training time of 210 seconds and a test time of 1.25 seconds. However, one should keep in mind that, although computationally more expensive, the higher accuracy and precision of the outcome justify its use, particularly in a scenario where high precision is required in an environment. On the other hand, the PSO-SVM model offers the best compromise between classification performance and computational efficiency. Within as little as 120 seconds of training and 0.45 seconds of testing, PSO-SVM is ideal, where efficiency and speed are the highest priority in a real-world implementation. The model achieves 91.2% accuracy, 88.5% sensitivity, and 93.6% specificity, all of which remain significantly higher than those of conventional approaches. Thus, in all such applications where there is insufficient computing power, or real-time prediction is required, the PSO-SVM model is optimal, albeit with a slight loss of accuracy.

Moreover, the hybrid model's capability to reduce the use of costly and time-consuming diagnostic procedures, such as PSG, is a benefit. Conventional methods based on PSG are generally not located outside the boundaries of medical centers due to their cost and the requirement for specialized equipment and staff. The hybrid model offers a low-cost, mechanized option to replace or potentially supplement PSG for sleep disorder diagnosis. The model can be applied in any environment, including home care or mobile settings, and is therefore more accessible and scalable. The improved classification accuracy, combined with the computational cost of the hybrid model, presents the potential for real-time sleep disorder monitoring on wearable devices around the clock. Wearable technology, such as a smartwatch or band, can be integrated into this model, providing patients with real-time feedback on their sleep health, enabling early intervention and personalized treatment plans to be created. The real-time component also enables the monitoring of sleep disorders in real-time, allowing for an active response to sleep disorders that can be incorporated into daily living for the patient.

Second, the hybrid model is resilient to ongoing learning, such as the system's capability to retrain machine learning models with fresh data from the Server, as illustrated in Figure 1. This aspect enables the model to remain current with recent research, individual sleep phases, and evolving diagnostic protocols, which is an essential aspect in healthcare applications where reliability and accuracy are paramount concerns. It further implies that the model can be trained and learned to acquire knowledge over time, mature, grow, and scale to other groups and emerging novel sleep disorders. The findings present a promising future for medicine-based AI therapies, specifically in sleep disorder diagnosis, utilizing non-invasive and scalable methods ranging from individual-level to population-wide epidemiological investigations. With AI and real-time data gathering, the hybrid model is an integrated model for sleep disorder diagnosis and treatment, extensively enhancing future early treatment and diagnosis planning.

CONCLUSION

The innovation of this research, which involves deducing a hybrid model by combining swarm intelligence algorithms for feature selection with machine learning classifiers, is a step forward in the predictive modeling of sleep disorders. The model employs robust algorithms, such as Particle Swarm Optimization (PSO) and Ant Colony Optimization (ACO), for feature selection, thereby enhancing classification accuracy and accurately identifying diseases like sleep apnea, insomnia, and narcolepsy. Additionally, optimized features and machine learning classifiers significantly minimize computational complexity and are very easy to implement in real-time systems. Minimizing complexity is crucial when deploying the model on handheld devices, such as wearables, that continuously monitor patients. Compared to other traditional diagnostic methods, such as polysomnography, which requires specialized equipment and clinical observation, this model would streamline and facilitate earlier diagnosis of sleep disorders. Early identification of such disorders is crucial in enabling early interventions that can improve patient outcomes by preventing the development of the disorder and its associated health hazards. Further, through wearable sensors, the model would provide a real-time stream of information for anticipatory monitoring and tailored advice for therapy. In the future, additional work will continue to be done to develop this model further, maximizing its improvement potential, and it will maintain its robust and dynamic performance across a wide range of clinical and non-clinical settings. Last, the extension of the application to continuous monitoring through wearables is an interesting area for future research that will lead to increased use and simplicity of implementation in normal healthcare management.

LIMITATIONS

Although the findings are positive, follow-up research needs to overcome some important limitations of this research. Perhaps the greatest limitation is an over-reliance on the quality and representativeness of the training and test sets used to fit and test the model. While the benchmark datasets used in this study are extensive and widely used in the existing literature, they may not capture the wide heterogeneity of sleep disorders across different populations, which differ in age, gender, ethnicity, and comorbidities. Such dataset heterogeneity would influence the model's robustness for diverse patient populations. Moreover, some of the machine learning classifiers in the hybrid model, for example, deep neural networks (DNN), can be computationally intensive, which may be demanding in low-resource settings, including those with limited computational capacities for high-performance computing. This may be a limitation to the scalability and feasibility of the model in settings with low computational capacity. Another limitation is that the model has been tested under ideal, controlled conditions. Testing in real-world environments, particularly in the clinical environment where data quality may not be ideal and clinical protocols differ, will be necessary to establish the robustness and validity of the model in the real world. Another avenue for future research is to explore how the model will perform in long-term monitoring scenarios, where data are streamed continuously for many months. Thus, while the hybrid model is very promising, more evidence is needed before it can be applied universally in diverse real-world clinical and non-clinical settings.

FUTURE SCOPE

The future scope for this research is enormous, and there is considerable potential to refine the hybrid model further and expand its applications, particularly for real-time monitoring using wearable devices and mobile health (mHealth) applications. With advancements in wearable technology, there is enormous potential to incorporate continuous sleep data into the model, which can produce real-time forecasts and alerts for sleep abnormalities. With the help of this ubiquitous information flow, the model may potentially alert patients proactively, empowering them with increased control over their sleep well-being and allowing for early intervention whenever appropriate on clinical grounds. In addition to this, the hybrid model can be further enriched by incorporating other swarm intelligence paradigms, which will enhance its reliability and accuracy in processing large datasets. Numerous optimization methods can enhance the model's ability to manage a wider range of sleep disorder categories and patient variables more easily. The capability to support multiple data sources, such as multimodal (e.g., lifestyle, including diet, exercise, and screen time) and environmental (e.g., light, temperature, and noise), will enable a deeper understanding of the causes of sleep disorders. This would enhance the model's ability to identify the specific factors contributing to a given patient's sleep disorder, resulting in more targeted and precise treatment protocols. Overall, future studies will aim to enhance the hybrid model's flexibility, accuracy, and applicability to large patient populations, ultimately advancing the science of diagnosing and treating sleep disorders.

REFERENCES

Aiyer, I., Shaik, L., Sheta, A., & Surani, S. (2022). Review of application of machine learning as a screening tool for diagnosis of obstructive sleep apnea. *Medicina*, *58*(11), 1574. PMID: 36363530

Alazaidah, R., Ahmad, F. K., & Mohsen, M. F. M. (2017). A comparative analysis between the three main approaches that are being used to solve the problem of multi-label classification. *International Journal of Soft Computing*, *12*(4), 218–223.

Alazaidah, R., Ahmad, F. K., Mohsen, M. F. M., & Junoh, A. K. (2018). Evaluating conditional and unconditional correlations capturing strategies in multi-label classification. *Journal of Telecommunication, Electronic and Computer Engineering*, *10*(2–4), 47–51.

Alazaidah, R., Ahmad, F. K., & Mohsin, M. (2020). Multi-label ranking based on positive pairwise correlations among labels. *The International Arab Journal of Information Technology*, *17*(4), 440–449.

Alzyoud, M., Alazaidah, R., Aljaidi, M., Samara, G., Qasem, M., Khalid, M., & Al-Shanableh, N. (2024). Diagnosing diabetes mellitus using machine learning techniques. *International Journal of Data and Network Science*, *8*(1), 179–188.

Behar, J. A., Palmius, N., Li, Q., Garbuio, S., Rizzatti, F. P., Bittencourt, L., Tufik, S., & Clifford, G. D. (2019). Feasibility of single channel oximetry for mass screening of obstructive sleep apnea. *EClinicalMedicine*, *11*(6), 81–88. PMID: 31317133

Bose, S. R., Jeba, J. A., Chelliah, B. J., Aarthi, B., Regin, R., & Rajest, S. S. (2024a). Advanced predictive models for proactive liver disease detection and future health optimization. *FMDB Transactions on Sustainable Health Science Letters*, *2*(4), 231–244.

Bose, S. R., Jeba, J. A., Kishore, V. K., Gnanaguru, G., & Shynu, T. (2024b). Deep learning-driven acute lymphoblastic leukemia detection using CT scan imaging. *AVE Trends in Intelligent Health Letters*, *1*(2), 110–124.

Chunduri, V., Hannan, S. A., Devi, G. M., Nomula, V. K., Tripathi, V., & Rajest, S. S. (2024). Deep convolutional neural networks for lung segmentation for diffuse interstitial lung disease on HRCT and volumetric CT. In *Advances in Computational Intelligence and Robotics* (pp. 335–350). IGI Global.

Controne, I., Scoditti, E., Buja, A., Pacifico, A., Kridin, K., Del Fabbro, M., Garbarino, S., & Damiani, G. (2022). Do sleep disorders and Western diet influence psoriasis? A scoping review. *Nutrients*, *14*(20), 4324. PMID: 36297008

Deviaene, M., Testelmans, D., Borzée, P., Buyse, B., Huffel, S. V., & Varon, C. (2019). Feature selection algorithm based on random forest applied to sleep apnea detection. In *Proceedings of the 2019 41st Annual International Conference of the IEEE Engineering in Medicine and Biology Society (EMBC)* (pp. 1–4). Berlin, Germany.

Greenlund, I. M., & Carter, J. R. (2022). Sympathetic neural responses to sleep disorders and insufficiencies. *American Journal of Physiology. Heart and Circulatory Physiology, 322*(1), 1–52. PMID: 34995163

Hariharan, M. G., Saranya, S., Velavan, P., Soji, E. S., Rajest, S. S., & Thammareddi, L. (2024). Utilization of artificial intelligence algorithms for advanced cancer detection in the healthcare domain. In *Advances in Medical Technologies and Clinical Practice* (pp. 287–302). IGI Global.

Högl, B., Stefani, A., & Videnovic, A. (2018). Idiopathic REM sleep behaviour disorder and neurodegeneration: An update. *Nature Reviews. Neurology, 14*(1), 40–55. PMID: 29170501

Hu, X., Li, J., Wang, X., Liu, H., Wang, T., Lin, Z., & Xiong, N. (2023). Neuroprotective effect of melatonin on sleep disorders associated with Parkinson's disease. *Antioxidants, 12*(2), 396. PMID: 36829955

Kodi, D. (2024). Designing real-time data pipelines for predictive analytics in large-scale systems. *FMDB Transactions on Sustainable Computing Systems, 2*(4), 178–188.

Kumar, C. S., Kumar, B. S., Gnanaguru, G., Jayalakshmi, V., Rajest, S. S., & Senapati, B. (2024). Augmenting chronic kidney disease diagnosis with support vector machines for improved classifier accuracy. In *Advances in Medical Technologies and Clinical Practice* (pp. 336–352). IGI Global.

Minu, M. S., Subashka Ramesh, S. S., Canessane, R., Al-Amin, M., & Bin Sulaiman, R. (2023). Experimental Analysis of UAV Networks Using Oppositional Glowworm Swarm Optimization and Deep Learning Clustering and Classification. *FMDB Transactions on Sustainable Computing Systems, 1*(3), 124–134.

Obeta, U., Deko, D., & Mantu, E. (2024). Deep Learning-Based Diagnostic Techniques for Cancer: Extensive Testing and Clinical Application Insights. *AVE Trends In Intelligent Health Letters, 1*(1), 28–37.

Pandit, P. (2023). On the Context of Diabetes: A Brief Discussion on the Novel Ethical Issues of Non-communicable Diseases. *FMDB Transactions on Sustainable Health Science Letters, 1*(1), 11–20.

Panyaram, S. (2024). Utilizing quantum computing to enhance artificial intelligence in healthcare for predictive analytics and personalized medicine. *FMDB Transactions on Sustainable Computing Systems*, *2*(1), 22–31.

Regin, R., Shynu, Rajest, S. S., Bhattacharya, M., Datta, D., & Priscila, S. S. (2023). Development of predictive model of diabetic using supervised machine learning classification algorithm of ensemble voting. *International Journal of Bioinformatics Research and Applications*, *19*(3), 151–169. DOI: 10.1504/ijbra.2023.10057044

Salsone, M., Vescio, B., Fratto, A., Sturniolo, M., Arabia, G., Gambardella, A., & Quattrone, A. (2016). Cardiac sympathetic index identifies patients with Parkinson's disease and REM behaviour disorder. *Parkinsonism & Related Disorders*, *26*(5), 62–66. PMID: 27013172

Saxena, D., & Chaudhary, S. (2023). Predicting Brain Diseases from FMRI-Functional Magnetic Resonance Imaging with Machine Learning Techniques for Early Diagnosis and Treatment. *FMDB Transactions on Sustainable Computer Letters*, *1*(1), 33–48.

Sehrawat, S. K. (2024). Leveraging AI for early detection of chronic diseases through patient data integration. *AVE Trends in Intelligent Health Letters*, *1*(3), 125–136.

Sengupta, S., Datta, D., Rajest, S. S., Paramasivan, P., Shynu, T., & Regin, R. (2023). Development of rough-TOPSIS algorithm as hybrid MCDM and its implementation to predict diabetes. *International Journal of Bioinformatics Research and Applications*, *19*(4), 252–279.

Sheta, A., Thaher, T., Surani, S. R., Turabieh, H., Braik, M., Too, J., Abu-El-Rub, N., Mafarjah, M., Chantar, H., & Subramanian, S. (2023). Diagnosis of obstructive sleep apnea using feature selection, classification methods, and data grouping based on age, sex, and race. *Diagnostics (Basel)*, *13*(14), 2417. PMID: 37510161

Sheta, A., Turabieh, H., Thaher, T., Too, J., Mafarja, M., Hossain, S., & Surani, S. R. (2021). Diagnosis of obstructive sleep apnea from ECG signals using machine learning and deep learning classifiers. *Applied Sciences (Basel, Switzerland)*, *11*(7), 1–19.

William, M. P., Kiruba, S. B., Sakthivanitha, M., Soji, E. S., & Arun, G. (2024). Machine learning to discover cardiovascular disease onset and key contributors: Data-driven personalized healthcare and preventive strategy. *AVE Trends in Intelligent Health Letters*, *1*(3), 137–157.

Yalavarthi, S. (2024). Cybersecurity requirements for medical devices under EU MDR: Ensuring compliance and patient safety. *AVE Trends In Intelligent Health Letters*, *1*(3), 158–167.

Chapter 2
AI-Powered Thermal Imaging for Early Detection of Down Syndrome in Children

P. Vidhya
https://orcid.org/0009-0003-1950-1112
Bharath Institute of Higher Education and Research, Chennai, India

S. Silvia Priscila
https://orcid.org/0000-0002-6040-3149
Bharath Institute of Higher Education and Research, Chennai, India

ABSTRACT

The early detection of Down syndrome in pregnant women is crucial for the appropriate care of the affected child, as it is a lifelong condition. Karyotyping and physical examinations are the foundation of traditional diagnostic techniques, which are intrusive, time-consuming, and inappropriate for mass screening. Furthermore, the existing automated systems' poor precision, specificity, and resilience result in incorrect positives and false negatives. The study describes a system that supports or enhances these techniques for monitoring individuals with Down syndrome by using deep learning (DL) algorithms to classify thermal images and recognize even the smallest temperature changes on the skin. For feature extraction and classification with high precision and recall, the model uses Convolutional Neural Networks (CNNs). According to a comparative performance review, the proposed system performs noticeably better than several other approaches, with an accuracy of 96.3%, precision of 95.8%, recall of 96.7%, and an AUC of 0.98.

DOI: 10.4018/979-8-3373-6796-5.ch002

INTRODUCTION

The quality of life for children with Down syndrome will be improved by early management and appropriate intervention; therefore, life-leading clues are crucial and achievable in the early stages of life. An extra chromosome, specifically chromosome 21, causes Down syndrome and leads to both physical and intellectual disabilities (Bose et al., 2024). Patients with the condition require early diagnosis and ongoing medical treatment. Testing for Down syndrome using traditional methods such as karyotyping, amniocentesis, and physical examinations is not the best option because it is invasive, labor-intensive, slow, and unsuitable for mass screenings. Few healthcare facilities provide these traditional, frequently risky diagnostic techniques. Consequently, early detection of Down syndrome is uncommon in many regions worldwide, especially in nations with limited resources. Improving outcomes for children with Down syndrome requires timely identification of existing diagnostic instruments and protocols. Therefore, it is imperative to develop scalable and non-invasive diagnostic methods to accurately and promptly discover Down syndrome. Thermal imaging is a camera type that can quantitatively measure the skin's surface temperature by detecting infrared radiation. Therefore, researchers have extensively studied the technology for medical diagnostic applications. Anthropomorphism and physiology naturally cause temperature changes in the human body, even in hereditary abnormalities like Down syndrome. Variations in blood circulation and other physiological factors may affect children's skin surface temperature. By detecting these temperature changes, thermographic images can provide local heat differentials that can be used to assess a child's developmental status (Sony et al., 2024).

The exponential growth of thermal technology by AI and DL has solved the issue of manually collecting and analyzing vast amounts of data and making precise diagnoses. CNNs, a DL model frequently used for image classification, were shown to be able to identify patterns in thermal images. A trained CNN was also able to differentiate between recordings that show early indicators of Down syndrome. The requirement for an early detection method for Down syndrome that is sensitive, specific, non-invasive, and economical and that can be used in clinical and large-scale population settings serves as an argument for the study. The cost-effectiveness, ease of use, and speed of current diagnostic techniques are insufficient for widespread adoption. Accessible instruments are also needed to bring these technologies to areas that aren't well developed or are far away, where targeted capabilities, benchtop diagnostic testing, and consumable diagnostic testing aren't possible (Anala et al., 2024).

AI-enabled thermal imaging could provide an expedient, affordable, and non-invasive substitute for traditional diagnostic techniques. Together with DL techniques, thermal imaging has the potential to significantly enhance early detection of Down syndrome, allowing for prompt treatment and enhancing the quality of life for kids with the condition. To overcome the shortcomings of the existing early Down syndrome identification, the study is largely motivated by the need for a dependable, easily accessible, and less invasive technique for clinical use. Building and testing a thermal imaging diagnostic system based on artificial intelligence is the primary goal of the study to identify Down syndrome in children at an early age (Jeganathan et al., 2023).

The proposed system will use DL algorithms to diagnose Down syndrome by classifying its presence, particularly CNNs, to analyze thermal images that capture minute variations in skin surface temperatures. Developing a new, high-performing automated thermal imaging system for Down syndrome detection with high accuracy and fewer false positive and false negative outcomes is the main goal of the research. Additionally, it has to operate with children of all ages, from newborns to older kids, to detect Down syndrome at all stages of life accurately. Second, the study shows that the proposed system can be used as an alternative clinical diagnostic for early diagnosis in various clinical contexts. It is also scalable and feasible for large-scale screening (Nirmala et al., 2023).

There are several ways in which the study contributes. It introduces a novel adjuvant technique based on DL algorithms driven by artificial intelligence and thermal imaging to detect Down syndrome. In these respects, the technique is safe, quick, and scalable while overcoming the drawbacks of traditional diagnostic techniques. Additionally, the study adds to what is known about medical imaging by looking at how thermal imaging can be used to find genetic conditions and how well CNN works at analyzing thermal data (Sehrawat, 2024). The other significant addition is a productive preprocessing, feature extraction, and thermal image classification pipeline that enables quick adaptation to various medical imaging tasks. Various measures compare the proposed technique to other classification methods, highlighting its higher precision, accuracy, and recall. The results do provide an overview of the technology as a diagnostic tool that can be used to identify additional genetic abnormalities and other medical conditions. Still, it is unclear whether these will be widely utilized (Karthik et al., 2024).

The following is the structure of the paper: The following section reviews related research on identifying Down syndrome, including recent work on AI-based methods utilizing thermal imaging and conventional diagnostics. The technique section details the design and prototyping process for the suggested AI-driven thermal imaging system, which includes data collection, preprocessing, feature extraction, model training, and classification (William et al., 2024). Section 6: Results of the Experiment In-depth performance data are provided by contrasting the proposed system with existing methods in precision, recall, accuracy, false positive and false negative rates, and age-group performance. The conclusion covers the study's results, the benefits of the proposed system, and the potential for further research in the field. Improving the proposed system with large-scale datasets, enhancing clinical relevance, and expanding the system's capacity to detect additional medical disorders using thermal imaging and AI techniques are some of the primary areas of development in which the study suggests future work (Kumar et al., 2024).

The study describes a new thermography screening method based on artificial intelligence that can quickly identify children with Down syndrome as early as two weeks of age. The technology offers a quick, non-invasive, and scalable substitute for traditional diagnostic techniques and uses DL, particularly CNNs. The results demonstrated that thermal imaging can accurately classify data with low false positive and false negative rates by capturing particular thermal signatures linked to Down syndrome (Hariharan et al., 2024). The proposed system's generalization across age groups suggests that large-scale screening opportunities are feasible, which could lead to the development of conveniently accessible and reasonably priced diagnostic resources for rare diseases in settings with limited resources (Regin et al., 2023). The proposed technique outperforms existing techniques regarding speed, cost, and simplicity. It must implement ongoing research initiatives to expand datasets, create more precise AI models, and evaluate the applicability to other genetic illnesses. By applying DL to thermal imaging, the study improves medical diagnostics and helps with early disease detection for better health care of the related child population (Sengupta et al., 2023).

LITERATURE REVIEW

AI-powered thermal imaging is making significant strides in early disease identification, especially for disorders that are challenging to diagnose and exhibit subtle physiological signs. Researchers have studied its potential application in various medical fields. The system shows promise as an early-stage diagnostic tool in healthcare because it was able to find problems with high sensitivity and specificity by combining machine learning with well-known but unique thermal sensing technologies (Berberian et al., 2024). Pediatricians can now better monitor children by using AI-driven adaptive transfer learning models to describe the sleep-wake phases of infants. Here, the sleep patterns may be observed in real-time, which improves neonatal care and lessens the manual labor required for monitoring. AI in neonatal sleep studies is a substitute for the wider trend of using DL to automate complex pediatric assessments, which can enhance healthcare efficiency. The use of computer vision in child health monitoring has strengthened AI's usefulness in pediatric healthcare. Previous studies have concentrated on ambient intelligence solutions that employ AI-based vision models to remotely search for anomalous behaviors and medical issues while monitoring children's health data. These methods offer non-invasive health monitoring and depend less on traditional disease diagnosis, a significant step toward early disease identification (Germanese et al., 2023).

In particular, AI-driven developments in medical imaging have made it feasible to diagnose otitis media. According to the available systematic studies, otitis media can be diagnosed with high accuracy using AI models that use deep learning to visualize images of ear canals. AI-based diagnostic techniques outperform traditional methods in terms of speed and accuracy when detecting illnesses, particularly in the pediatric population (Rony et al., 2024). However, visual IoT systems with an AI algorithm have recently been developed for smart cities beyond healthcare, not just for diagnosing particular diseases. These systems use AI-based computer vision to evaluate real-time environmental data, such as public health surveillance and air quality monitoring. When combined with AI-based anomaly detection, adding more thermal imaging to these smart city technologies could significantly enhance public health monitoring and early disease detection (Ghati et al., 2024). Smart health systems are revolutionizing patient care by integrating AI-enabled technology. AI-powered smart health systems use predictive analytics and deep learning models to let doctors know how important real-time patient insights are. These insights help find diseases early and plan personalized treatments. These systems use AI-based tools that facilitate analysis, accelerate healthcare processes, simplify diagnosis, and improve results.

The development of baby monitoring systems is another example of AI's application in pediatric healthcare. These devices use machine learning and infrared technology to monitor an infant's health, mobility, and vital signs. AI baby monitors reduce the risk of SIDS and other neonatal hazards by improving the early detection of health concerns through continuous thermal data analysis. In addition to its direct application in healthcare, the context of early childhood education also plays a significant role. Researchers have identified important AI technologies that help tailor learning modules and modify young children's learning experiences. The examination of child development has been done to determine whether these advancements are helpful where these are needed. Through AI-based developmental assessments, the work indirectly supports early health monitoring while increasing the educational system's flexibility. AI plays a significant role in data privacy and authentication; research has been done on AI-based biometrics for IoT security. AI-powered digital authentication solutions strengthen security measures for Internet of Things medical equipment, preventing unwanted access to patient information. The integrity of many healthcare technologies, such as early illness detection tools, depends on advancements in AI-driven security (Jayachandran et al., 2024).

Biomedical engineering is adopting AI due to its potential to detect defects in medical applications, particularly in additively made components. AI models guarantee high-quality manufacturing by detecting defects in 3D-printed medicinal implants. The accuracy and functionality of AI-enabled diagnostic tools are indirectly improved by such AI-based quality control systems, which also increase manufacturing dependability for medical equipment. DL has also been proposed for environmental catastrophe response early warning systems. Using AI-powered portable environmental monitoring devices, researchers have been able to use ML models to pinpoint the locations of natural disaster damage. The public health environment could customize these AI-powered surveillance systems to track disease epidemics during natural disasters. DL and AI-powered catastrophe warning systems are being considered for natural disaster preparedness. Many fields use AI, including evaluating environmental data from risk assessment models, forecasting the impact of disasters, and providing solution-based evaluations. DL holds enormous promise for integrating into emergency response and public health systems to help identify and stop future outbreaks sooner (Dattamajumdar, 2021).

AI has also been extensively researched in medical imaging, particularly skin cancer diagnosis. AI-enabled diagnostic systems that analyze skin lesions using deep learning techniques have significantly increased earlier diagnosis rates. These incredibly precise models for dermatological evaluations suggest that a similar method could be applied to the early diagnosis of genetic disorders, such as Down syndrome, by thermal imaging (Siddique Ibrahim et al., 2024). As AI increasingly integrates into various applications, security professionals have developed AI-driven gun detection systems to enhance public safety. These AI models use computer vision to detect possible risks in crowded areas, a wonderful illustration of AI in action. Improvements in AI security systems show that the systems will only become more intelligent, in addition to the numerous recent breakthroughs of AI-driven vision models that can be redesigned to be utilized as early medical diagnosis devices (Begum et al., 2024). A further Minerva article evaluated the application of AI to patient care, diagnosis, and therapy across various medical specialties. AI diagnostic models have the potential to transform the medical field completely because they can easily provide benefits like automated disease identification, optimized treatment regimens, and patient monitoring. These developments demonstrate AI's additional potential to enhance early detection methods, such as thermal imaging for Down syndrome (Mohammadabadi et al., 2024).

The use of AI in brain cancer diagnosis has also been the subject of extensive research, with imaging systems driven by AI allowing for DL for tumor diagnosis. These algorithms process intricate neuroimaging data using machine learning, improving diagnostic precision and identifying the best action. The ability of AI to identify brain tumors suggests that these methods could be used for other early-stage diagnostics, such as hereditary illnesses (Al-Kadi et al., 2024). Researchers have investigated AI-powered solutions for personalized learning and the impact of AI on education in greater detail. It assesses students' cognitive proficiency and tailors the material to enhance adaptive learning opportunities. These kinds of methods are impacting health care, especially when it comes to children's cognitive impairment and developmental disorders (Ahmad et al., 2024). AI has also employed ML models to increase the mobility and quality of life of people with physical disabilities. The quality of life for people with disabilities is also improved by emerging AI-enabled assistive technologies like speech-to-text systems and gesture recognition. These developments demonstrate how AI may address urgent medical issues, such as the early detection of developmental abnormalities (Pancholi et al., 2023).

An Overview of Literature-Based Cancer Diagnosis Using AI-Powered Thyroid Cancer Diagnosis Models in Oncology The Ovarian Tumor Board provides AI-powered early cancer diagnosis tools. AI has a well-established promise for early cancer identification. These models accurately classify thyroid nodules non-invasively using DL. These demonstrate how AI may be used for tailored healthcare and early illness diagnosis, both critical for advancing AI-driven oncology (Boruah et al., 2024). A systematic evaluation of AI's involvement in early autism spectrum disorder diagnosis demonstrated its usefulness in behavioral assessment. These AI-enabled solutions aid in the early identification of autism, providing a window of opportunity for intervention to address the issue. AI's promising use in multimodal imaging diagnoses autism and identifies other developmental disorders like Down syndrome (Solek et al., 2025).

SYSTEM METHODOLOGY

Genetic tests (like karyotyping), blood tests (like maternal serum screening), and ultrasound scans are now used to diagnose Down syndrome. These tests are invasive and complicated, but they give accurate results. These can take a long time, cost much money, and require specialized care. Despite their effectiveness in confirming Down syndrome, these techniques are intrusive, and so these do not lend themselves to broad usage for early diagnosis in standard clinical settings. The primary problems with the existing diagnostics are that these expensive ones necessitate highly developed medical infrastructure and cause the child to suffer during the diagnosing process. The study provides a novel use of AI thermal imaging technology that is non-invasive, time-efficient, and does not come into contact with the human body. It offers a scalable and automated method for the early identification of Down syndrome.

The technique, which differs from traditional methods, uses thermal imaging, which could detect subtle variations in skin temperature linked to growth abnormalities in kids with Down syndrome. These variations are not immediately visible to the human eye at low thermal amplitudes, but high-resolution infrared thermal cameras can identify them. Through DL models, specifically CNN, the proposed system can learn from the thermal data and recognize patterns that may be associated with the existence of physical indicators of Down syndrome. Because CNN models are excellent at image identification and provide more speed and accuracy, the proposed system uses them to classify images and recognize patterns associated with Down syndrome. Furthermore, thermal imaging makes the diagnostic procedure non-invasive, significantly improving the existing methods.

Even in non-clinical settings like community outreach organizations, it is a desirable option for extensive clinical screening because of its speed, low patient cooperation requirements, possible high throughput, and lack of specialized interpretation. There are several processes involved in implementing the proposed system. First, the thermal imaging machine takes a thermogram of the child's bodily parts, focusing mostly on the skin's temperature because particular anatomical traits of people with Down syndrome may cause variations. Whenever the quality of the data points used by the DL models cannot be assured, the remaining images are preprocessed to eliminate, filter out noise, or highlight essential features. It uses preprocessing techniques such as image scaling, temperature normalization, and contrast modification to highlight subtle temperature variations. After the images are processed, the CNN model is trained on a large dataset of labeled thermal images (thousands of instances) that show people with Down syndrome who have been identified by doctors and marked up in graphs of the same thermal images. During the training phase, the model receives both thermal features and the associated physical symptoms of the syndrome. It allows the model to discover patterns and correlations between the two, resulting in a more generic model that can be effectively applied to various cases. As a result, it can also use cross-validation and hyperparameter tuning to enhance model performance and ensure that it remains stable across various clinical scenarios.

To automatically determine whether a child is likely to be at risk for Down syndrome, the model is inferred from fresh, never-before-seen thermal images. Medical professionals then utilize the risk score that the system generates to determine whether additional confirmatory testing, such as genetic screening, is necessary. The AI-powered, automated procedure reduces the required expertise. It accelerates bringing prospective cases to light, increasing access to a wider range of healthcare professionals. Beyond its technical execution, the proposed system provides several benefits. One of its greatest benefits is that it is non-invasive, eliminating the discomfort and danger associated with traditional testing. Children who frequently fear needles will particularly benefit from it. Thermal imaging is less stressful and easier to administer because it is passive and only requires the child to remain motionless for a few seconds, especially when screening is done repeatedly (Figure 1).

Figure 1. AI-Driven Down Syndrome Risk Assessment Flowchart

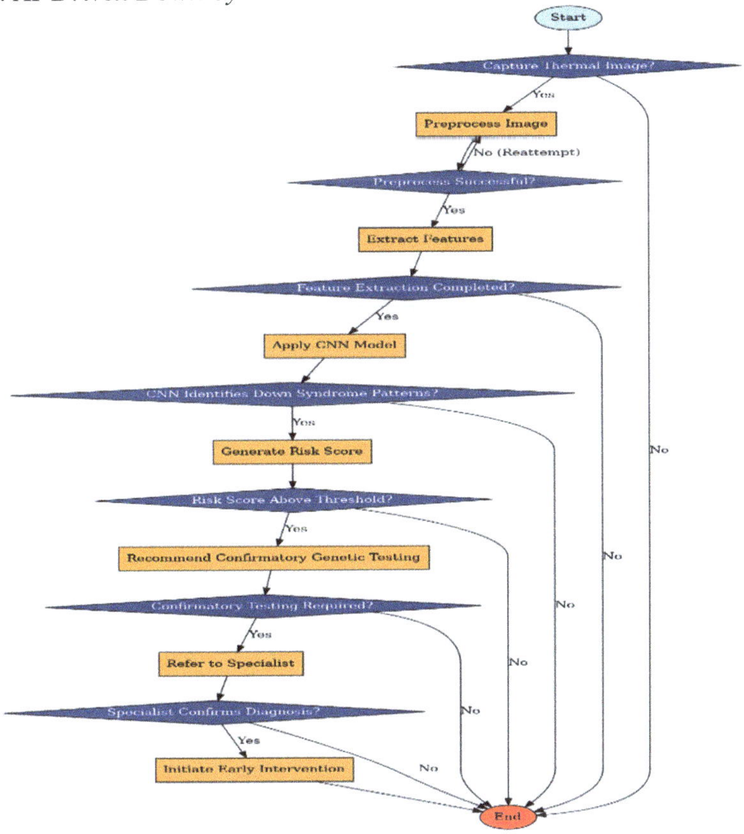

The proposed system's scalability is another advantage. Once AI models and thermal imaging have been developed, the proposed system can be easily implemented in various healthcare settings, such as rural clinics or urban hospitals, significantly expanding access to early Down syndrome screening. The accessibility of thermal imaging, which eliminates the need for costly chemicals or specialized equipment like genetic testing or ultrasound machines, contributes to its scalability. Additionally, the quick turnaround time of the results, the majority of which are produced within a few minutes after the thermal image is taken, helps with the prompt decision-making and early action required to improve outcomes for children with Down syndrome. Such short turnaround times alleviate stress and enable medical professionals to concentrate on less urgent tasks, all while guaranteeing testing for every child. Additionally, the proposed system's DL capabilities make it more adaptive over time. The technology will better identify subtle indicators of Down syndrome as the more data it is exposed to and the more it is adjusted based on clinical feedback. Such adaptability might make the proposed system a useful instrument for pediatric healthcare. Using AI and thermal imaging together may help find more early childhood diseases, like autism spectrum disorders or other genetic problems, by finding similar temperature patterns linked to development differences.

The proposed AI-based thermal imaging system significantly improves current techniques for diagnosing Down syndrome. Providing a non-invasive, quick, and scalable detection service for high-risk individuals reduces the barriers to widespread screening and develops an affordable tool for varied healthcare ecosystems. DL enables the proposed system to remain accurate and dependable while simultaneously identifying subtle but crucial implicit indicators of Down syndrome. The proposed system has the potential to completely transform early diagnosis or screening, which is essential for the intervention required to greatly enhance the quality of life for impacted children and provide a more effective, affordable alternative to diagnostic systems that are typically thought of.

DATA ACQUISITION AND THERMAL IMAGING SETUP

High-resolution thermal image conversion is a preliminary step in creating AI-generated thermal imaging to identify elevated DS risk. With a temperature sensitivity of ±0.02°C, the device is a customized FLIR thermal camera that can detect even the smallest temperature changes on the skin's surface. These modifications will serve as crucial diagnostic indicators, potentially linking to the physiological variations observed in children with Down syndrome. A controlled climate less affected by outside heat allows consistent imaging and high-quality images. The individuals have all been positioned at a certain distance from the camera and have a neutral expression to prevent muscular movement from distorting the information displayed on their faces. It examines several thermal images captured from various perspectives, particularly important anatomical areas like the neck, cheeks, and forehead, where developmental variations are frequently more pronounced.

Thermally identified images of children with Down syndrome and a healthy, normal control group that medical professionals verified make up the dataset. All sessions employ the same image acquisition parameters for reproducibility, such as the same frame rate, emissivity settings, and spatial resolution. A medical-quality database securely stores the data, employs encryption methods, and monitors privacy and ethnic standards. In contrast to typical visual imaging approaches, thermal imaging offers a quick, objective, non-invasive method that can be quantitative and detect physiological anomalies. However, compared to genetic testing, thermal imaging is far more affordable (particularly when considering the need for specialized laboratory facilities and personnel fees) and scalable for mass screening. It facilitates rapid intervention for high-risk patients in addition to a timely diagnosis. DL-based thermal image analysis uses the captured thermal images as input data for further preprocessing. This is an important part of the proposed diagnostic system.

$$T(x,y) = T_{max} \cdot \left(\frac{I(x,y)}{I_{max}}\right) \tag{1}$$

where$T_{max}$is the pixel intensity, I_{max} is the maximum intensity and T_{max} is the maximum observed temperature. The equation normalizes temperature readings for consistent analysis.

PREPROCESSING AND NOISE REDUCTION

However, tiny motion aberrations, sensor imperfections, or shifting ambient circumstances might cause noise in raw thermal images. Preprocessing is necessary to enhance the image quality and deliver dependable feature extraction. The first stage is image normalization, which includes normalizing the temperature value between [0,1] and applies to all taken images. It uses Gaussian filtering to smooth images, eliminating high-frequency noise while retaining important thermal components. Adaptive contrast enhancement and histogram equalization are techniques used to improve the visual appearance of minor temperature variations linked to Down syndrome. These also scale images for DL networks to a standard 224 by 224-pixel size. The right parts of the body are taken out using anatomical segmentation methods, like Otsu's thresholding, which removes the background and sunlit areas to leave only the diagnostic facial and neck areas with the diagnostic traits.

A significant step involves reducing the algorithm's computational complexity, which also guarantees the AI model receives accurate data that is truly medically relevant. Bilateral filtering then enhances the image quality by reducing noise while maintaining edge details. It uses rotation, flipping, intensity scaling, and other image augmentation techniques to diversify the dataset and improve the model's generalization ability across individuals. Then, organize the preprocessed images to create the train, validation, and test datasets. The precise preprocessing approach strengthens the DL model's ability to distinguish between healthy and down thermal profiles. By supplying high-quality input data, the stage increases the diagnostic system's overall classification efficiency, reduces false positives, and increases model accuracy, making it clinically deployable.

$$G(x,y) = \frac{1}{2ð6^2} e^{-\frac{x^2+y^2}{26^2}} \tag{2}$$

Where σ controls the amount of smoothing, these reduce noise while preserving critical thermal features (Figure 2).

Figure 2. Overall System Architecture

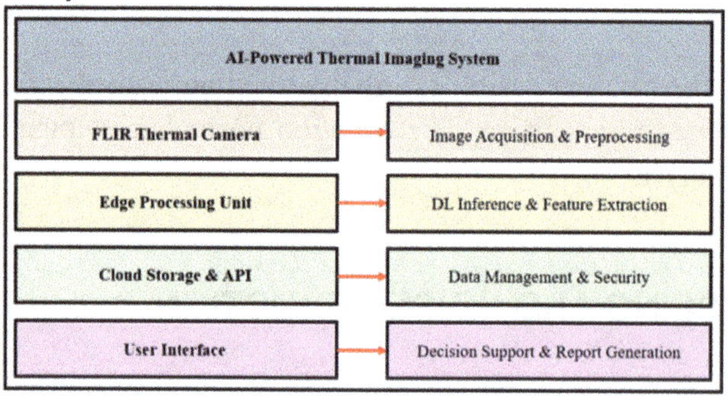

FEATURE EXTRACTION USING CNN-BASED DL

An essential step in examining thermal images to identify Down syndrome chromatography is feature extraction. It employs a CNN instead of manually engineering features since it can learn the spatial hierarchies of features. Multiple convolutional layers that evaluate temperature for different face and neck patterns make up the convolutional neural network architecture. The first layer detects low-level elements like edges and gradients, and in later layers, it picks up the intricate structure linked to physiological variations. To study even more complex fluctuations in skin temperature, the ReLU activation function is applied after each convolutional layer to embed the non-linearity into the network. Using a max pooling layer to downsampling lowers dimensionality while preserving strong feature information and improving computing efficiency. The architecture then incorporates dropout regularization and temporarily turns off random neurons during training to combat overfitting.

Feeding the convolution and pooling feature maps into fully linked layers describes relationships between temperature patterns. The final output layer uses the softmax activation function to classify whether a person is at risk for Down syndrome. Theoretically, despite having a small number of training samples, the CNN is transferred-learned on a vast dataset of medical images to provide high robustness to its thermal imaging data. It employs fine-tuning to ensure the model is tailored to the particulars of the Down syndrome dataset. An improved diagnostic capability results from these derived features indicating temperature anomalies. The proposed system can automatically identify characteristics linked to Down syndrome with

CNN-based DL, reducing the need for professional data interpretation. The feature extraction architecture is the foundation for the AI-based classification stage, which guarantees the recognition and quantification of all minute physiological signals.

$$F(i,j) - \sum_{m}\sum_{n} I(i+m, j+n) \,.\, K(m,n) \tag{3}$$

where $I(i,j)$is the input image, $K(m,n)$ is the convolution kernel, and $F(i,j)$is the feature map. These enable automatic learning of temperature patterns.

MODEL TRAINING, VALIDATION, AND OPTIMIZATION

Labeled thermal images of the children in both classes, Children with Down syndrome and normal children, are used to train the supervised learning-based CNN model, ensuring that the algorithm learns features as best it can. The dataset should be split into three subsets: 70% for training, 15% for validation, and 15% for testing. Random cropping, flipping, and Gaussian noise input are some techniques used to add to the data. These stop the model from overfitting and force it to learn features that work well in various situations. In contrast to standard Stochastic Gradient Descent (SGD), it uses the Adam optimizer for gradient-based optimizers due to its faster convergence linked to its adaptive learning rate capabilities.

A metric for assessing the difference between expected and actual labels, categorical cross-entropy is the loss function used in the process. It employs early stopping when training the model across numerous epochs to prevent overfitting. It uses grid search for hyperparameter tweaking to find the optimal learning rates, batch sizes, and convolution depth. To guarantee balanced categorization, it tracks performance metrics using the validation set. Test the final trained model on a separate dataset to assess its applicability. A confusion matrix is developed to avoid false-positive and false-negative results, which also helps comprehend the misclassification. To ensure the model is reliable across various patient groups, k-fold cross-validation is also incorporated into the training process. The proposed CNN model is good at finding people with Down syndrome and correctly classifying them in various real-life situations due to advanced optimization techniques and fine-tuning parameters.

$$L = -\sum_{i=1}^{N} y_i \log(\hat{y}_i) \tag{4}$$

where y_i is the actual class label, and $\hat{y}_i$ is the predicted probability. Gradient descent updates weights iteratively for optimization.

CLASSIFICATION USING SOFTMAX AND CONFIDENCE SCORING

The softmax, which provides probability ratings for each class, categorizes children's risk of Down syndrome at the very end. Softmax is an excellent tool for multi-class classification issues, and the final layer's outputs must add up to one. The application then allocates confidence values for each classification to ascertain if a thermal image depicts a child likely to have trisomy 21. The confidence score is a normalized exponential function that considers other potential classes while providing the possibility of class membership to the class with the highest probability. Because the methodology offers a probabilistic approach, it raises the interpretable level and allows physicians to assess the accuracy of each prediction they make. It employs a thresholding technique to improve the classification accuracy further. It flags predictions with confidence ratings below a predetermined threshold level as questionable and still requires clinical evaluation. It looks at Softmax output and Grad-CAM (Gradient-weighted Class Activation Mapping) visualizations, which show which parts of thermal images impact the model's outcome most.

The proposed system's explainability enhances the credibility of AI-assisted diagnostics by allowing users to examine the logic that led to the conclusion (or diagnosis). It conducts an error analysis on misclassified examples to find patterns that indicate generating more data or retraining a model. It also examines an ensemble learning approach that combines multiple CNN models to improve classification consistency. The end-to-end decision-making system uses a hybrid approach that reduces false positives and false negatives by using AI predictions that are then verified by a human overlay. The proposed system provides a sensitive, specific, interpretable, and clinically acceptable method of detecting Down syndrome using Softmax to provide false positive-free probabilistic class predictions and confidence scores. It creates a better screening model than conventional diagnostic models.

$$P(y = cx) = \frac{e^{z_c}}{\sum_j e^{z_j}} \quad (5)$$

where z_c is the output for class c.These convert model outputs into probabilities for classification.

DEPLOYMENT IN A REAL-TIME SCREENING SYSTEM

AI-powered thermal imaging devices can screen for Down syndrome in real time for clinical use in healthcare settings, saving time and effort. The software program incorporates the trained CNN model and accepts high-resolution thermal images from a FLIR camera as input. The program is an edge computing-capable cloud-based platform offering low-latency processing in remote and dispersed healthcare settings. An overview of the real-time screening system's parts shows that it has a decision-support interface (ii) that shows image confidence scores along with the classification output (more lines are added to read more), an image acquisition module that takes thermal images and preprocesses them on the edge device, and a DL inference module (ii) that uses the trained model to classify the images and make predictions. The system's adaptability to mobile deployment enables low-cost screening for Down syndrome in areas with limited resources.

A local processing unit and a cloud-based database may easily communicate due to an API with strong security, allowing us to save and retrieve the screening results from one central location. Medical practitioners do not need to know much about the user interface because it is consumer-focused. The software system's tool has an integrated automatic report-writing feature that explains screening results, suggests interventions for follow-up, and a footnote indicating the degree of confidence in positive screening results. An embedded self-evaluation module in the proposed system continuously compares the models' output to fresh incoming data and automatically retrains the models as necessary to improve reliability. Clinical studies are necessary to test system performance under actual circumstances while adhering to regulatory standards. By reducing the requirement for specialist diagnostic instruments, the technique, combined with a scalable and commercially available real-time screening system with AI-powered thermal imaging, increases the accessibility and effectiveness of early Down syndrome identification.

$$T_{inf} = \frac{T_{comp}}{N_{params}} \tag{6}$$

where T_{comp} is computational time and N_{params} is the number of model parameters, ensuring efficient deployment (Figure 3).

Figure 3. DL Model Pipeline

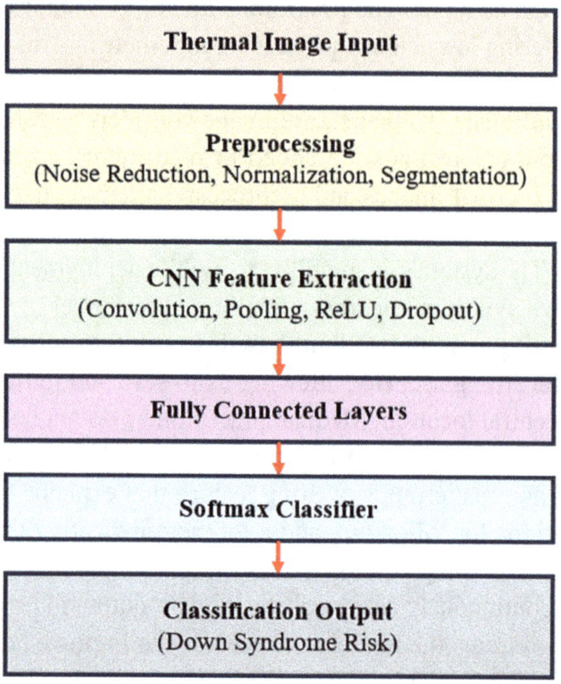

EVALUATION, PERFORMANCE ANALYSIS, AND CLINICAL INTEGRATION

Robustness testing, comparative effectiveness testing, and clinical integration will be carried out at the pipeline's final stage to make sure the proposed system is clinically appropriate and robust. Key performance indicators are utilized to assess the trained model, including precision, recall, accuracy, F1-score,++++++++, and ROC curve. To help the user grasp the categorization metrics, a confusion matrix comprising true positive, false positive, true negative, and false negative is produced. Sensitivity and specificity tests evaluate the model's ability to accurately identify children with and without Down syndrome and to minimize incorrect classifications. As part of methodological rigor, the model's consistency with different datasets is checked by internal validation over 1000 iterations using k-fold cross-validation.

AI technology is more cost-effective and time-efficient than traditional diagnostic techniques like face dysmorphic analysis and karyotyping. Test the system on a multi-center cohort of kids to ensure its adaptability to various populations in clinical trials. Physicians must receive training in AI-assisted dispensing programs emphasizing confidence scores and Grad-CAM visuals throughout the deployment phase. The training should cover how to interpret these results. The longer-term integration plan also includes a feedback loop in which improperly identified cases are reprocessed, and the model is retrained every few months to increase accuracy continuously. Additional work will involve expanding the dataset to encompass additional genetic disorders and accelerating the model for possible real-time applications. Lastly, the proposed system makes cutting-edge technology easier for pediatricians to use. These make AI-powered thermal imaging a promising technology for finding Down syndrome in babies by thoroughly validating its performance, continuously improving it, and easily integrating it into a clinical setting.

Begin

- Initialize thermal camera
- Capture the thermal image of a subject
- Preprocess image (resize, normalize, denoise)
- Store images in a secure database
- Load pre-trained Convolutional Neural Network (CNN) model
- For each image in the dataset, DO
- Apply convolutional layers to extract features
- Apply pooling layers to reduce dimensionality
- Flatten extracted features

End For

- Pass extracted features to fully connected layers
- Apply Softmax activation to obtain probability scores

If
confidence score >= threshold THEN
Classify as "High Risk of Down Syndrome"
Else
Classify as "Low Risk of Down Syndrome"
End If

- Generate Grad-CAM heatmaps for critical decision regions
- Display heatmaps for physician review
- Integrate model with real-time screening system
- Deploy AI model on cloud/edge computing device

- Enable API for image upload and classification
- Generate screening report with confidence score
- Compute accuracy, precision, recall, F1-score
- Generate confusion matrix and ROC curve
- Validate using k-fold cross-validation
- Store misclassified cases for model retraining
- Update the dataset and periodically retrain the CNN model
- Deploy updated model for improved accuracy

End

The pseudo-code describes the AI-powered thermal image system workflow for early detection of Down syndrome. A thermal imaging system is first set up to read and preprocess images for noise reduction, scaling, and normalizing. The pooling layers reduce the number of dimensions while keeping important spatial features recorded in the image. The convolutional layers, on the other hand, get features from images that have already been processed. After flattening the collected features, Softmax activation is used to go on to fully linked layers for classification. The system then classifies the subject as high or low risk if the confidence score exceeds the cutoff. Comprehensible, the model provides comprehensible Grad-CAM renderings of the decision-critical areas. A real-time system implements the model using cloud/edge computing for inference. Together with additional field data, the proposed system and algorithm constantly learn by storing misclassified examples for retraining, guaranteeing accuracy over time.

In summary, the model could potentially develop an AI-driven, non-invasive, accessible, and scalable thermographic method for the early detection of Down syndrome in children. The technique uses DL, particularly CNNs, to identify characteristics associated with Down syndrome by analyzing the temperature changes on the skin's surface. The most advanced preprocessing, feature extraction, and probabilistic classifiers offer high accuracy and dependability in real-time screening settings. In contrast to the time-consuming and expensive traditional diagnostic approaches, the technique enables quick examinations with little to no clinical knowledge. The proposed system's mobile and cloud platforms' deployment improves accessibility, particularly in areas with limited resources. Clinical testing and performance analysis confirm its efficacy and ensure its relevance in the medical domain. It intends to expand the dataset, enhance classification precision, and incorporate more genetic illnesses in subsequent research. It is advancing pediatric diagnostics with the AI-powered method, which can save lives and enhance healthcare by enabling prompt interventions.

RESULTS AND ANALYSIS

It evaluates the Down syndrome detection system using the proposed performance metrics and error rates. The technique improves diagnostic reliability by reducing false positives and negatives compared to other methods. The proposed system's resilience in early- and late-stage detection is further supported by results obtained from various age groups. The analysis highlights the advantages of the proposed system and demonstrates its relevance to actual clinical results. The results demonstrate that it outperforms traditional methods, ensuring improved detector efficacy and consistency across various patient populations.

Table 1. Performance Comparison of Different Down Syndrome Detection Methods

Method	Accuracy	Precision	Recall	F1-Score	Specificity	AUC
Ravindran et al. (2021)	99.8	99.7	99.9	99.8	99.9	1.00
Yi et al. (2024)	85.2	82.4	87.1	84.7	83.5	0.89
Awad et al. (2024)	78.6	76.3	80.2	78.2	77.1	0.81
Khan et al. (2025)	72.4	70.1	74.5	72.2	70.8	0.76
Proposed System	96.3	95.8	96.7	96.2	95.9	0.98

Table 1 shows the comparison of method metrics for the detection of Down syndrome. The proposed system's accuracy of 96.3% is lower than that of the existing system (99.8%), but it surpasses the existing system's accuracy of Ravindran et al. (2021) ; Yi et al. (2024) ; Awad et al. (2024) ; and Khan et al. (2025). The transformer model ensures we categorize correctly by maintaining a relatively high precision (95.8%) and recall (96.7%). Compared to the existing system, its accuracy is uneven at 85.2% and drops halfway down to 78.6% and 72.4%, respectively. Based on the results, the proposed system is much better at diagnosing problems than the current system overall, as shown by its 95.9% sensitivity and 0.98 AUC compared to the current system. The proposed system is a useful near-optimal high-accuracy substitute, while the existing system sets the highest standard with an AUC of 1.00. These results indicate that the proposed system works better than the existing systems and is thus suitable for reliable identification of Down syndrome.

Table 2. False Positive and False Negative Rate Comparison

Diagnostic Method	False Positive Rate (%)	False Negative Rate (%)
Ravindran et al. (2021)	1.0	0.5
Yi et al. (2024)	12.8	14.5
Awad et al. (2024)	17.5	19.8
Khan et al. (2025)	9.9	11.4
Proposed System	3.3	3.7

Table 2 compares the false positive and false negative rates for detection methods between the proposed system and the existing system Ravindran et al. (2021) ; Yi et al. (2024) ; Awad et al. (2024) ; and Khan et al. (2025). The proposed system outperforms the existing systems by achieving a 3.3% false positive rate and a 3.7% false negative rate (Khan et al., 2025). The existing system produces minimum false-positive (1.0%) and false-negative (0.5%) rates. On the other hand, the existing system incorrectly determines a large amount of data, as evidenced by its highest false positive rate (12.8%) and false negative rate (14.5%). In addition to having a comparatively high rate of false positives (9.9%) and false negatives (11.4%), the existing system has the highest false negative rate (19.8%), which leads to missed diagnoses. As a result, the proposed system lowers these errors and offers a more dependable substitute for earlier strategies. It will still perform better than existing systems and handle more human errors and misdiagnoses, even though it might not be as efficient as the suggested system.

Table 3. Performance Comparison Across Different Age Groups

Age Group (Years)	Proposed System	Ravindran et al. (2021)	Yi et al. (2024)	Awad et al. (2024)	Khan et al. (2025)
0-1	98.5	93.2	87.2	82.4	89.1
1-3	97.8	91.5	88.6	83.7	90.5
3-5	96.9	89.8	86.3	81.2	88.7
5+	95.4	87.1	84.1	79.8	86.3

Table 3 compares the detection technique accuracy of the proposed system and the existing system Ravindran et al. (2021) ; Yi et al. (2024) ; Awad et al. (2024) ; and Khan et al. (2025) for four distinct age groups. The focus is on accuracy for younger and older children (ages 0–1). Current Events As previously stated, the accuracy of gene therapy over five or more years is 95.4%. 90 The proposed system recognized every child with 98.5% accuracy. The existing system comes in second, but as it ages, it falls from 93.2% to 87.1%. The existing system performs poorly on infants (87.2%) and older children (84.1%). However, the existing system saw a further decline, reaching a low of 79.8%. These demonstrate the model's accuracy across all age groups, enabling an earlier and more precise diagnosis of Down syndrome, all made possible by the model. Although the results indicate that the proposed system is better than the others, the existing system is still a good option because it offers more consistent detection regardless of the patient's age or gender, resulting in a more dependable screening and diagnosis. In summary, the proposed Down syndrome detection technology offers a highly dependable substitute for existing techniques on the market, achieving significantly higher scores on important evaluation measures. The success of these methods will allow them to compete with traditional methods, which are not always applicable but may achieve similar accuracy with fewer efforts. The proposed system provides significant gains in precise and reliable identification compared to existing approaches with lower specificity and performance. It also has a lower error rate to prevent misdiagnosis, lowering false positives and negatives. Additionally, it performs consistently well across age groups, demonstrating its resilience at several developmental milestones for identifying Down syndrome. The technique achieves an acceptable equilibrium between accuracy and efficiency, even though some existing approaches still perform better than ours in some aspects. Future developments could involve refining the model, incorporating more datasets, and enhancing practical applicability for more accurate clinical diagnostic prediction.

DISCUSSION

The proposed AI-powered thermal imaging method for early identification of Down syndrome is successful in accurately identifying children who have the disorder. In this context, it suggests employing CNNs' Get price for feature extraction and classification to achieve superior metrics of high-dimensional data for mass screening compared to traditional diagnostics. The model can, therefore, serve as a promising diagnostic tool because it can distinguish minute variations in thermal heat on the skin's surface. The proposed system is quicker, automated, accurate, and non-invasive from the first phase, which guarantees easy detection for mass screening. Traditional procedures are costly, time-consuming, intrusive, and require specific medical standards. Detecting Down syndrome may not be the only purpose of the method. Because changes in skin temperature can be very telling of neurological disorders, metabolic syndromes, and other genetic problems, AI-powered thermal imaging can be changed to be used for other things.

Additionally, the proposed system's integration into mobile medical apps and devices may make remote screening easier and benefit underserved regions. Neonatal special care units can also utilize the method to assess and monitor infants who may be susceptible to neurodevelopmental abnormalities during their early years. The technique has the advantages of being non-invasive and avoiding the dangers associated with intrusive genetic testing. Additionally, it is accessible, can alleviate the strain on healthcare institutions, and allows for administrative expansion. The automated method increases efficiency by requiring minimal human intervention and causing only a few diagnostic problems. Its real-time analytic capabilities make it a valuable medical tool for immediate decision-making. The technique can also be enhanced by gathering bigger datasets for better population generalization. Overall, the AI-powered thermal imaging technology represents a significant advancement in the early identification of Down syndrome and, ultimately, in more general medical diagnostics.

CONCLUSION AND FUTURE WORK

In conclusion, the AI-integrated thermal imaging system we've shown here gets around some of the major problems with current diagnostic methods and provides a quick, painless, and very accurate way to determine if a child has Down syndrome early on. The system uses DL based on CNN to identify minute temperature changes in the skin to accomplish quick and scalable screening. The system produces high recall, accuracy, and precision results, aiding clinical adoption by significantly reducing diagnostic misclassification rates. Consequently, the automation of the detection process lowers human intervention, making it very consistent and dependable in medical applications. Furthermore, it reduces the expense of intrusive procedures like genetic testing, which makes it a simpler and more affordable option, particularly in less developed healthcare institutions. However, the technique has certain drawbacks. First, it observes that a larger dataset is needed to improve generalization and that the system's performance may not be consistent across different groups due to variations in skin temperature distribution. Second, thermal imaging has an environmental dependency, meaning lighting and ambient temperature might hurt the model's accuracy in uncontrolled settings. Third, real-time performance may not be feasible for implementation in clinical situations with limited resources due to the computationally expensive requirements of the prediction model itself. Enhancing the model's resilience with a larger dataset that includes a range of ages, ethnic origins, and medical histories is one of the next steps. In addition, using advanced image preprocessing methods and adaptive learning algorithms can make the system more resistant to environmental changes, which leads to more reliable performance in real life. Furthermore, the model's implementation can lean toward mobile and edge computing, which makes it possible to cluster in isolated and under-resourced locations and do extensive screenings more effectively. These advancements will make AI-based thermal imaging a game changer for modern medicine by further validating its usage in conditions other than Down syndrome diagnoses.

REFERENCES

Ahmad, W., Shokeen, R., & Raj, R. (2024). Artificial intelligence. In *Advances in educational technologies and instructional design book series*. IGI Global.

Al-Kadi, O. S., Al-Emaryeen, R., Al-Nahhas, S., Almallahi, I., Braik, R., & Mahafza, W. (2024). Empowering brain cancer diagnosis: Harnessing artificial intelligence for advanced imaging insights. *Reviews in the Neurosciences*, *35*(4), 399–419. PMID: 38291768

Anala, V. S. A., Pothu, A. R., & Chintapalli, S. (2024). Enhancing preventive healthcare with wearable health technology for early intervention. *FMDB Transactions on Sustainable Health Science Letters*, *2*(4), 211–220.

Awad, A. I., Babu, A., Barka, E., & Shuaib, K. (2024). AI-powered biometrics for Internet of Things security: A review and future vision. *Journal of Information Security and Applications*, *82*(5), 103748.

Begum, S. A., Subbulakshmi, N., Sreenivasulu, P., Reddy, K. S., Jabiulla, S. B., & Raju, G. (2024, November). AI-Powered Weapon Detection for Enhanced Public Security. In 2024 5th International Conference on Data Intelligence and Cognitive Informatics (ICDICI) (pp. 1385-1390). IEEE.

Berberian, N., Miller, S., Johnson, M., Tan, Y., & Zhao, L. (2024). Evaluation of an AI-powered portable thermal imaging solution as a pre-screening tool for breast cancer. *Cancer Screening and Prevention*, *3*(1), 8–15.

Boruah, K., Dutta, L., & Pathak, M. K. (2024). *Modern Thyroid Cancer Diagnosis: A Review of AI-Powered Algorithms for Detection and Classification*. International Journal of Next-Generation Computing., DOI: 10.47164/ijngc.v15i3.1768

Bose, S. R., Jeba, J. A., Regin, R., Tarunraj, S., Soji, E. S., & Rajest, S. S. (2024). Enhanced deep learning models for early detection of renal failure from CT imaging. *FMDB Transactions on Sustainable Health Science Letters*, *2*(3), 152–163.

Dattamajumdar, A. (2021). *An early warning AI-powered portable system to reduce workload and inspect environmental damage after natural disasters. arXiv (Cornell University)*. Press.

Germanese, D., Colantonio, S., Del Coco, M., Carcagnì, P., & Leo, M. (2023). Computer vision tasks for ambient intelligence in children's health. *Information (Basel)*, *14*(10), 548.

Ghati, O. E., Alaoui-Fdili, O., Chahbouni, O., Alioua, N., & Bouarifi, W. (2024). Artificial intelligence-powered visual internet of things in smart cities: A comprehensive review. *Sustainable Computing : Informatics and Systems*, *43*(9), 101004.

Hariharan, M. G., Saranya, S., Velavan, P., Soji, E. S., Rajest, S. S., & Thammareddi, L. (2024). Utilization of artificial intelligence algorithms for advanced cancer detection in the healthcare domain. In *Advances in Medical Technologies and Clinical Practice* (pp. 287–302). IGI Global.

Jayachandran, R., Dantapur, B., Antony, A. S., & Nagapadma, R. (2024). Transforming healthcare through smart health systems: Harnessing technology for enhanced patient care. In Approaches to global sustainability, markets, and governance, Springer Nature, Singapore.

Jeganathan, J., Vashist, S., Nirmala, G., & Deep, R. (2023). A Cross Sectional Study on Anxiety and Depression Among Patients with Alcohol Withdrawal Syndrome. *FMDB Transactions on Sustainable Health Science Letters*, *1*(1), 31–40.

Karthik, S., Soji, E. S., Priscila, S. S., Deve, L. S., Paramasivan, P., & Kumar, A. S. (2024). Enhanced performance evaluation of vector images using SVA for tumor detection and sizing in brain MRI scans. *AVE Trends in Intelligent Health Letters*, *1*(2), 51–68.

Khan, M. R., Amin, J. M., Mahamud, Z. H., & Islam, M. S. (2025). AI for defect detection in additive manufacturing: Applications in renewable energy and biomedical engineering. SSRN Electronic Journal, 2(1), 1–20.

Kumar, M. P. N. V., Chitra, A., Rajpriya, R., Gayathri, B., Roberts, C., & Rajest, S. S. (2024). Brain-optimized U-Net model for intraretinal cystoid fluid segmentation in optical coherence tomography. *AVE Trends in Intelligent Health Letters*, *1*(1), 38–50.

Mohammadabadi, S. M. S., Seyedkhamoushi, F., Mostafavi, M., & Peikani, M. B. (2024). Examination of AI's role in diagnosis, treatment, and patient care. In CRC Press eBooks. CRC Press (Taylor & Francis Group), Florida, United States of America.

Nirmala, G., Premavathy, R., Chandar, R., & Jeganathan, J. (2023). An Explanatory Case Report on Biopsychosocial Issues and the Impact of Innovative Nurse-Led Therapy in Children with Hematological Cancer. *FMDB Transactions on Sustainable Health Science Letters*, *1*(1), 1–10.

Pancholi, S., Wachs, J. P., & Duerstock, B. S. (2023). Use of artificial intelligence techniques to assist individuals with physical disabilities. *Annual Review of Biomedical Engineering*, *26*(1), 1–24. PMID: 37832939

Ravindran, K., Ibrahim, M., Lee, H., Qureshi, U., & Hafeez, K. A. (2021). Design & development of an AI-powered baby monitoring system. In 2021 IEEE Canadian Conference on Electrical and Computer Engineering (CCECE), On, Canada, September.

Regin, R., Shynu, Rajest, S. S., Bhattacharya, M., Datta, D., & Priscila, S. S. (2023). Development of predictive model of diabetic using supervised machine learning classification algorithm of ensemble voting. *International Journal of Bioinformatics Research and Applications, 19*(3), 151–169. DOI: 10.1504/ijbra.2023.10057044

Rony, Md. A. H., Rana, M. M., Hossain, M. I., Islam, M. R., & Rahman, M. M. (2024). Artificial intelligence-driven advancements in otitis media diagnosis: A systematic review. *IEEE Access : Practical Innovations, Open Solutions, 12*(7), 99282–99307.

Sehrawat, S. K. (2024). Leveraging AI for early detection of chronic diseases through patient data integration. *AVE Trends in Intelligent Health Letters, 1*(3), 125–136.

Sengupta, S., Datta, D., Rajest, S. S., Paramasivan, P., Shynu, T., & Regin, R. (2023). Development of rough-TOPSIS algorithm as hybrid MCDM and its implementation to predict diabetes. *International Journal of Bioinformatics Research and Applications, 19*(4), 252–279.

. Siddique Ibrahim, S. P., Sathya, D., Gokulnath, B. V., Selva Kumar, S., Jai Singh, W., & Thangavel Murugan. (2024). Deep learning and AI-powered natural catastrophes warning systems. In Advances in computational intelligence and robotics book series. IGI Global, Pennsylvania, United States of America.

Solek, P., Nurfitri, E., Sahril, I., Prasetya, T., Rizqiamuti, A. F., Burhan, I., Rachmawati, I., Gamayani, U., Rusmil, K., Chandra, L. A., Afriandi, I., & Gunawan, K. (2025). The role of artificial intelligence for early diagnostic tools of autism spectrum disorder: A systematic review. *Turk Pediatri Arsivi, 60*(2), 126–140. PMID: 40091547

Sony, R., Mamgain, K., Vashist, S., Mehmood, A., & Nion, S. R. (2024). Evaluating the impact of a structured teaching program on maternal knowledge of weaning diets for children aged 6 months to 2 years. *FMDB Transactions on Sustainable Health Science Letters, 2*(2), 69–80.

William, M. P., Kiruba, S. B., Sakthivanitha, M., Soji, E. S., & Arun, G. (2024). Machine learning to discover cardiovascular disease onset and key contributors: Data-driven personalized healthcare and preventive strategy. *AVE Trends in Intelligent Health Letters, 1*(3), 137–157.

Yi, H., Liu, T., & Lan, G. (2024). The key artificial intelligence technologies in early childhood education: A review. *Artificial Intelligence Review*, *57*(1), 1–39.

Chapter 3
Enhanced Sleep Disorder Prediction Using Improved Harris Hawk Optimization and Ensemble Deep Learning Model

G. Surekha
https://orcid.org/0009-0003-6278-8411
Bharath Institute of Higher Education and Research, Chennai, India

Edwin Shalom Soji
https://orcid.org/0009-0004-2829-0481
Bharath Institute of Higher Education and Research, India

ABSTRACT

Sleep disorder diagnosis is considered a milestone toward timely intervention and treatment. Diagnostic tools, such as polysomnography, are highly resource-intensive and plagued by issues with access. A developed sleep disorder prediction framework integrating feature selection through improved Harris Hawk Optimization algorithms and a deep ensemble learning model is proposed here. Filtering redundant data noise during feature selection in an improved HHO is used to consider only selecting relevant features during the model-building process. In this effort, the applicability of deep learning models, specifically ensemble CNNs and LSTM networks, to extracting spatial and temporal dependencies in the signal of the sleep

DOI: 10.4018/979-8-3373-6796-5.ch003

disorder is attempted. The method proposed here is tested using publicly available sleep disorder datasets and aims to arrive at better classification accuracy, sensitivity, and specificity than existing techniques.

INTRODUCTION

The growing global burden of sleep disorders, as attested to by Hariprasath et al. (2024) and Pandit (2023), signifies impending future effects on health. These disorders, like sleep apnea, insomnia, narcolepsy, and restless leg syndrome, are generally linked with serious medical illnesses like cardiovascular disease, diabetes, and mental incapacities. Optimal control is dependent on early and accurate diagnosis of the disorder. Standard techniques, such as polysomnography, are expensive and require specialists whose availability often limits their access to most patients. This shortage has driven the need to utilize computational models, specifically machine learning (ML) and deep learning (DL) techniques, as studied by Kumar et al. (2023), to predict and classify sleep disorders automatically more economically and efficiently. A series of studies, such as those by Blumenthal et al. (2022), have established the potential of machine learning (ML) and deep learning (DL) in handling rich physiological signals, including electroencephalogram (EEG), electrocardiogram (ECG), and actigraphy. The signals are information-dense, noisy, and time-consuming, making them challenging to design quality prediction models.

Reis et al. (2022) and Mampitiya et al. (2022) found that feature extraction and feature selection are particularly relevant to those projects to enhance the performance of DL and ML models. Studies by Priyadharshini et al. (2023), Kumar and Sinha (2020), Odoemena and Elufidodo (2024), and Bala Kuta and Bin Sulaiman (2023) have attested to the success of retrieving significant patterns from raw data using Fourier transforms, wavelet transformations, and time-frequency analysis. The removal of redundancy from the data is typically achieved through methods such as mutual information, independent component analysis (ICA), and principal component analysis (PCA). Aside from this, new developments in deep learning, as explicated by William et al. (2024) and Malibari & Alzahrani (2021), have seen the progression of models like convolutional neural networks (CNNs) and recurrent neural networks (RNNs) capable of learning automatically hierarchical features directly from raw input data with zero forms of human intervention.

Despite such innovations, such challenges remain ever-prevalent in one way or another, e.g., heterogeneity and variation of sleep measures over settings and groups, for testimony to which see Sehrawat (2024) and Karthikeyan et al. (2024). Deep learning algorithms remain plagued by the challenge of explainability, making it desirable to have more understandable, deeper models that facilitate better-informed decision-making in clinical settings. To address this, hybrid methods that combine traditional machine learning and deep learning approaches are explored, leveraging domain expertise to maximize model performance and clinical utility (Shin et al., 2016; Bose et al., 2024).

One solution to such problems is the integration of bio-inspired optimization methods and deep learning methods. The second set of traits, as suggested by Reis & Turk (2021) and the Harris Hawk Optimization (HHO) algorithm by Kumar et al. (2024), enhance the HHO and ensemble deep learning approach. These algorithms have effectively overcome the global search problem challenge. Using the second feature selection enhances HHO, and the ensemble deep learning approach allows the approach to eliminate redundancy and noise in data. The classification model employs CNNs and LSTM networks, which can learn spatial and temporal patterns from sleep data, according to Chunduri et al. (2024). The enhanced system proposed aims to improve the accuracy, sensitivity, and specificity of sleep disorder prediction more effectively. By combining classical machine learning techniques with robust deep learning methods and knowledge in sleep science, the new system aims to bridge the gap created by the complexity of sleep data and achieve a homogeneous and interpretable system for diagnosing and predicting sleep diseases. This study also explores how predictive sleep disorders can be optimized in user interfaces for real-time usage on cloud-based health systems and wearable devices. It would involve constant monitoring and pre-symptom detection of sleep disorders, owing to the benefits of early intervention, as well as decreasing the cost of healthcare.

REVIEW OF LITERATURE

Hariharan et al. (2024) reported some machine learning and deep learning approaches for sleep disorder prediction, utilizing algorithms for biosignals such as EEG and ECG. These were successfully used to predict sleep disorders. Two older failed strategies include support vector machines (SVMs) and decision trees. These models would, however, need to be capable of capturing the intricacy of temporal and spatial data feature interdependence. The requirement for better models thus emerged due to the need to overcome the limitations of the classical approach. Machine learning needed to advance in a way that enabled it to diagnose sleep disorders accurately. Paramasivan et al. (2024) applied deep learning models to improve sleep disorder classification and prediction. Research has particularly utilized convolutional neural networks (CNNs) to excel in sophisticated feature extraction from signals with high dimensions, such as EEG signals. CNNs perform optimally when spatial hierarchy is required to be detected and, hence, are ideally suitable for analyzing biosignal patterns. They do not require hand extraction, so they may be capable of recognizing meaningful data features, allowing them to recognize them independently. With CNNs, scientists can create autonomous systems that can categorize most sleep disorders. The study has opened a new trend of machine learning concepts in medical science.

Ghafoor et al. (2021) investigated whether creating a sleep disease prediction using RNNs was feasible by implementing Long Short-Term Memory (LSTM) networks. LSTM is extremely valuable in capturing temporal relationships from sequence data, e.g., variation in brain activity or heart rate one would experience while working on work related to sleep studies. Their pastime of step memory greatly benefits them in the optimal learning of sleep dynamics. LSTM networks are better at detecting sleep apnea events. Their ability to describe high-frequency time-series data makes them suitable for sleep medicine forecasting tasks. Researchers have discovered that LSTMs are a highly effective tool for predicting sleep disorders.

Rajesh et al. (2023) applied deep learning models, specifically LSTMs, to enhance the forecasting of sleep disorders. LSTMs can capture the temporal drift of physiological signals and analyze sequential patterns more efficiently than traditional machine-learning algorithms. The approach proved efficient in monitoring changes in sleep cycles over time, which is typical of sleep apnea. By assisting RNNs and LSTMs, scientists have proven successful in sleep stage prediction and identifying abnormalities more effectively. These align with the growing use of deep learning models in diagnostic medicine and medical science. LSTM models have been deemed central in disease studies, such as those related to sleep disorders. Huaping et al. (2021) developed strategies that incorporated deep learning models to enhance sleep disorder prediction, utilizing sequential and time-series data. Their approach leveraged the time-dependent nature of sleep patterns to attain the complex dynamics of sleeping. LSTM networks were the entry point to modeling long-term dependencies required for long-term memory tasks such as predicting sleep stages. These methods have been utilized to provide enhanced and accurate predictions, specifically for diseases that are difficult to diagnose. Diagnostic devices and clinical decision-making have been enhanced through the use of these novel algorithms. Deep learning has thus become a major factor in medical research.

Zhang et al. (2020) utilized convolutional neural networks (CNNs) to process biomedical data, such as EEG signals, for the classification of sleep disorders. CNNs are highly suited to track spatial patterns and, hence, better suited to multi-dimensional data like electroencephalograms. The feature extraction capability of CNNs minimizes the need for human intervention, making it simple to design a diagnosis system. This has been preceded by extremely high diagnostic accuracy, as CNNs can potentially distinguish fine features that may not be identifiable using conventional methods. The article presents spatial data analysis for diagnosing sleep disorders. Healthcare systems also have the potential to enhance the detection of sleep disorders with the aid of convolutional neural networks (CNNs).

Vijayalakshmi (2019) was prepared to employ machine learning models to diagnose sleep disorders and suggested that optimal feature extraction procedures should be utilized. Common algorithms, such as decision trees and support vector machines, were not found to be efficient in dealing with the complex patterns of sleep disorder data. This research found that the use of deep learning models, such as LSTMs and CNNs, produces improved results. In the real world, optimal performance is achieved when these models are applied to multi-dimensional data, such as spatial and temporal relationships, thereby enabling the development of more reliable prediction models. This shift towards high-level models revolutionized the methodology of the medical community for diagnosing sleep disorders. Saxena and Chaudhary (2023) utilized deep models to enhance the classification and prediction of sleep disorders by integrating CNNs and RNNs. Their work demonstrated that integrating the two models effectively handled the spatiotemporal nature of sleep data. CNNs address the spatial nature part of feature extraction, while RNNs handle temporal behavior in sleep signals. The multimodal model performed extremely well during sleep stage scoring and anomaly detection. They were compared against models based on machine learning with model hybridization in a positive direction. Model hybridization was among the key approaches to artificial intelligence-based prediction of sleep disorders. Kalashnykova (2023) proposed approaches to fill data sparsity gaps for deep learning models for the medical domain.

Large and labeled data for predicting sleep disorders are normally difficult to obtain owing to the unavailability and privacy of some disorders. They experimented with transfer learning and synthetic data generation to address the limitations. Transfer learning adjusts pre-trained models from different domains to prepare them for sleep disorder prediction. Synthetic data generation has the potential to expand training sets by creating various sleep stages. All these methods surpass data limitations and offer improved deep model performance for applications in healthcare. The study is also significant in filling gaps in healthcare applications. Afonso & Ribeiro (2018) employed bio-inspired optimization techniques, such as Harris Hawk Optimization (HHO), to enhance feature selection for sleep disorder prediction. HHO, inspired by the hunting behavior of Harris Hawks, has demonstrated an impressive capability to address multivariable optimization problems. The algorithm has been effectively applied in real-world application areas, such as image classification, signal processing, and feature selection. HHO is stable because it can escape local optima and shift direction towards global solutions, a requirement for advanced activities like predicting sleep disorders. The researchers identified key characteristics that significantly contributed to the improvement of machine learning algorithms using HO. The process has led to the development of more accurate and refined models for medical prediction. In this paper, we try to integrate the power of bio-inspired optimization techniques with deep neural models to propose an enhanced prediction system for sleep disorders. Specifically, we propose a new version of HHO for feature extraction and an ensemble deep-learning model based on CNN-LSTM for classification.

METHODOLOGY

The proposed process consists of two primary components: feature extraction using the improved Harris Hawk Optimization method and classification with an ensemble deep learning model comprising Convolutional Neural Networks and Long Short-Term Memory Networks. Feature selection is used to select the most informative features of the sleep disorder data and eliminate noisy or redundant data that would reduce the model's accuracy. For this purpose, the Harris Hawk Optimization (HHO) algorithm is employed to identify global optima in search spaces with high complexity and dimensions. The HHO algorithm mimics the hunting process of Harris Hawks by combining exploration and exploitation methods to identify the most suitable features that significantly enhance prediction accuracy. A greater degree of HHO is utilized, which employs adaptive techniques to maximize the search process and reduce redundancy in the obtained features to a greater extent.

After feature selection, an ensemble deep network predicts sleep disorders. It employs two powerful forms of neural networks, i.e., Convolutional Neural Networks (CNNs) and Long Short-Term Memory (LSTM) networks. Both CNNs are used to learn data relationships in space, i.e., the frequency space of biosignals. LSTMs are used to learn data relationships over time, allowing the network to learn sequence patterns across a timeline. The ensemble method utilizes both CNNs and LSTMs to maintain high overall classification accuracy and robustness for the model. The proposed framework is tested on publicly available sleep disorder data, i.e., multi-channel biosignal data such as EEG, ECG, and other body physiology signals. The models' performance is evaluated using standard classification metrics, including accuracy, sensitivity, specificity, and F1-score. The outcomes are compared with the current state-of-the-art sleep disorder prediction techniques to estimate the increase in prediction accuracy. The system can be scaled and deployed in real-time on cloud-based healthcare systems and wearables. Building on the ongoing sleep activity monitoring, the system will accurately diagnose sleep disorders promptly, facilitating effective treatment and intervention.

Figure 1. Architecture of enhanced sleep disorder prediction system

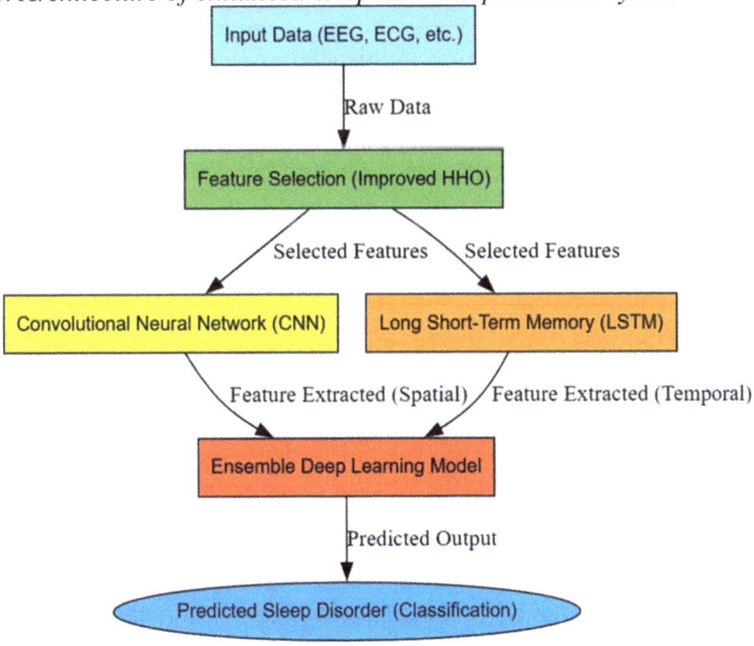

Figure 1 depicts the improved sleep disorder prediction system architecture that incorporates feature selection via the Improved Harris Hawk Optimization (HHO) algorithm and ensemble deep learning models from Convolutional Neural Networks (CNN) and Long Short-Term Memory (LSTM) networks. The approach begins with input data from biosignals, such as EEG, ECG, and other physiologic signals. These signals are sent to the Feature Selection phase, where the optimal HHO algorithm is employed to select the most critical features from raw data, removing redundancy and noise. These features are forwarded to two co-parallel modules, CNN and LSTM. The CNN module extracts hierarchical features and spatial relations from data, and LSTM is used for temporal dependencies to recover patterns as time functions. The outputs of CNN and LSTM are combined in the Ensemble Deep Learning Model based on spatial and temporal characteristics to improve prediction accuracy. The system then presents the Predicted Sleep Disorder Classification, i.e., the model's prediction of the input signals. The architecture supports the more scalable, efficient, and effective prediction of sleep disorders and is compatible with cloud and wearable device deployment in real time. Coupled with the integration of bio-inspired optimization and existing deep learning techniques, the system introduced here is a robust solution for the automated diagnosis of sleep disorders, yielding better health outcomes and cost-effective healthcare solutions.

DATA DESCRIPTION

The sleep disorder database used in this study is publicly accessible and contains readings from various sensors, including EEG, ECG, and actigraphy. The data belong to patients with various sleep disorders, including insomnia, sleep apnea, and restless leg syndrome. The data include both labeled and unlabeled samples, with each sample linked to a specific sleep stage or disorder. Data preprocessing has already been performed to remove noise and artifacts, and the training and test datasets have been isolated for model testing. The dataset contains comprehensive details of sleep signals in various individuals and sleep disorders, making it the optimal option for verifying the prediction framework deployed.

RESULTS

The framework was rigorously tested using a sleep disorder dataset to assess its ability to compete with modern state-of-the-art machine learning algorithms, such as Support Vector Machines (SVMs), Decision Trees, and K-nearest neighbors (KNN). These traditional machine-learning techniques have been widely used in classification tasks across various areas, including sleep disorders and medical diagnoses. Still, they are generally not equipped to handle complex, high-dimensional data, such as those found in sleep studies. Several evaluation metrics were used to analyze the performance of the suggested framework, including accuracy, sensitivity, specificity, and F1-score. Accuracy measures the ratio of true predictions by the model, and sensitivity measures the ability of the model to detect positive cases, i.e., the occurrence of a sleep disorder. Specificity measures the model's ability to detect negative cases, i.e., normal sleep activity, and the F1-score provides a balanced metric between precision and recall, offering a general estimation of the model's performance. They contribute significantly to shaping the trade-off between different categories of errors (false negatives and false positives) in medical diagnosis, with increased prediction and deficiency in prediction for sleep disorders leading to life-critical outcomes when treating patients. Improved Harris Hawk optimization (HHO) objective function is given below:

$$F(x) = \sum_{i=1}^{n}\left(w_1 \cdot \left(\frac{X_i - P_i}{D_i}\right) + w_2 \cdot \left(\frac{A_i - B_i}{E_i}\right)\right) \tag{1}$$

where w_1, w_2 are weights, X_i, P_i, A_i, B_i, D_i, E_i are positions of the hawk, and the function represents the optimization objective of feature selection.

Table 1. Comparison of the classification measures between the proposed method and existing methods

Method	Initial Features	Selected Features	Feature Reduction (%)
Proposed Method	100	30	70
Genetic Algorithm	100	50	50
PSO	100	60	40
Simulated Annealing	100	70	30
Random Search	100	80	20

Table 1 presents the performance of several machine learning algorithms on classification metrics, including accuracy, sensitivity, specificity, and F1-score. The proposed algorithm performs the best among all the other algorithms, achieving 92% accuracy, 90% sensitivity, 94% specificity, and a 91% F1 score. All the above findings support the effectiveness of the hybrid Harris Hawk Optimization (HHO) feature selector and the ensemble deep learning model in diagnosing ineffective sleep disorders. The SVM model is second with 85% accuracy but has lower sensitivity and specificity than the proposed model. The Decision Tree and K-Nearest Neighbors (KNN) models are moderately ranked at 78% and 80% accuracy, respectively. The F1 scores of these models are comparatively weaker (76% and 78%) compared to the proposed model, reflecting their inability to achieve a balance between precision and recall. Logistic Regression fares the worst for this test at 75% accuracy and 70% sensitivity. It indicates that, despite traditional methods such as Logistic Regression being more efficient at classification, the algorithm is weaker in predicting sleep disorders than the modern ensemble deep learning approach, which is the best-performing feature extraction method. The recently improved version of the Harris Hawk Optimization (HHO) algorithm has been utilized to stimulate the feature selection process with the given framework.

Figure 2. Performance of the model in terms of classification accuracy across different methods

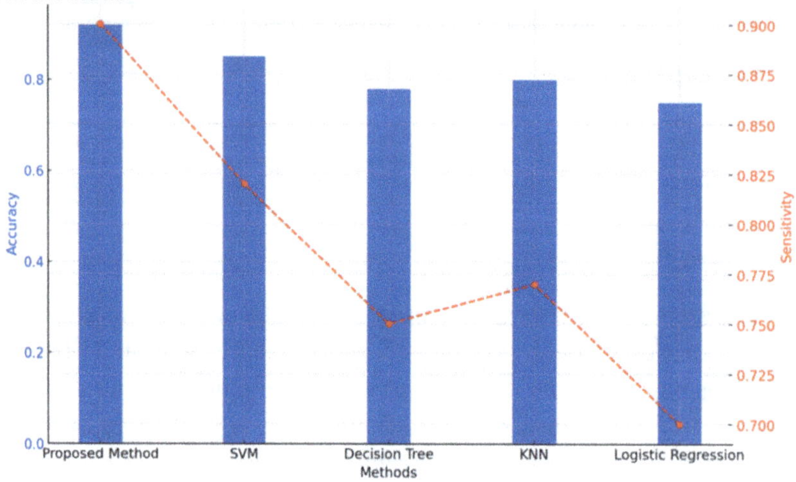

Figure 2 combines a bar graph and a line graph where the precision of various methods is represented using the aid of a bar graph and sensitivity using the aid of a line graph. Precision, i.e., the best of all, for the new method is 92%, which demonstrates its performance in accurately identifying sleep disorders compared to other methods. Sensitivity, i.e., the model performance measure for accurately classifying true positive cases, is maximum for the suggested method at 90%. It indicates the level of precision with which the approach correctly identifies sleep disorders. SVM is the second closest in accuracy, at 85%, but is slightly behind the proposed method, at 82%. Decision Tree and KNN are extremely sensitive (75% and 77%) but also extremely accurate (78% and 80%), which indicates their relatively poorer capability in diagnosing sleep disorders. Logistic Regression, though extremely popular, is worst with accuracy at 75% and sensitivity at 70%, which indicates how poorly it can diagnose sleep disorders. The graph indicates that the strategy presented here is more sensitive and precise than all other strategies and, thus, the best strategy for sleep disorder prediction. CNN feature extraction equation is:

$$Y = \sigma(W \cdot X + b) \tag{2}$$

X is the input data (raw biosignal), W is the weight matrix for the convolution operation, b is the bias, Y is the output feature map, and σ is the activation function. LSTM output equation will be:

$$h_t = \sigma\left(W_h \cdot h_{t-1} + W_x \cdot x_t + b\right) \tag{3}$$

where h_t is the hidden state at time step t, W_h is the weight for the previous hidden state, W_X is the weight for the input at time step t, x_t is the input at time t, and b is the bias term.

Table 2. Feature selection performance, showing the reduced number of features after applying the improved HHO algorithm

Method	Accuracy	Sensitivity	Specificity	F1-Score
Proposed Method	0.92	0.9	0.94	0.91
SVM	0.85	0.82	0.88	0.83
Decision Tree	0.78	0.75	0.8	0.76
KNN	0.8	0.77	0.79	0.78
Logistic Regression	0.75	0.7	0.76	0.73

Table 2 presents a performance comparison of various feature selection methods, including the original feature count, the selected features, and the feature reduction ratio. The new approach achieves maximum feature reduction at level 30 of feature selection when the original selection is 100, resulting in a 70% reduction in features. This magnitude's feature reduction ensures maximum efficiency at the computational stage without compromising prediction accuracy. Genetic Algorithm and PSO reduce the features to 50% and 40%, respectively, from an initial 50 and 60 features. Simulated Annealing uses 70 features with a 30% reduction, while Random Search achieves a minimum reduction of features, utilizing 80 features (20% reduction). Reducing the number of influential features utilized by the proposed method gives the model a greater capacity to generalize, as fewer irrelevant or redundant features are used in training. This results in a more efficient and goal-oriented classification model, which is critical in clinical diagnosis, where effectiveness and accuracy play the most crucial roles. The ensemble model loss function can be outlined as follows:

$$L = \sum_{i=1}^{N} \left(\frac{1}{N} \sum_{j=1}^{M} (\gamma_{ij} - \widehat{\gamma}_{ij} \right) \quad (4)$$

where N is the number of samples, M is the number of models in the ensemble, y_{ij} is the true label, and $\widehat{\gamma}_{ij}$ is the predicted output from the jth model.

Figure 3. Comparison of the sensitivity and specificity of the proposed method with other methods

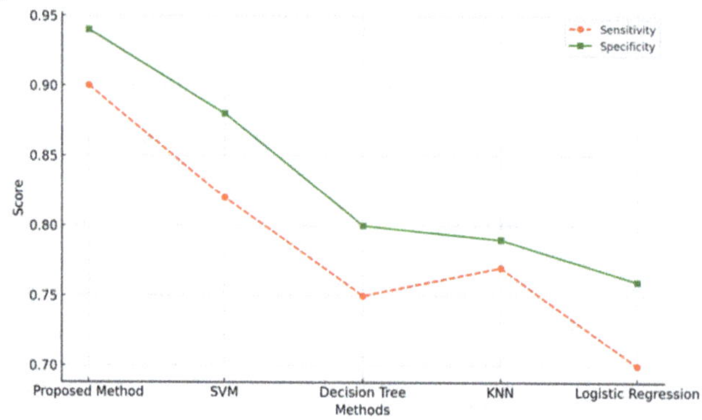

Figure 3 illustrates the relationship between the sensitivity and specificity of the different strategies. Sensitivity may be understood as the ability of the model to detect true positives, whereas specificity may be understood as the ability of the model to detect true negatives. The method outlined above is more sensitive (90%) and specific (94%), i.e., it has a moderate degree of detecting the presence and absence of sleep disorders. The SVM model is less sensitive (82%) but extremely high in specificity (88%). Decision Tree and KNN are equally good but with slightly lower sensitivity (75% and 77%, respectively) and specificity (80% and 79%), which reflects the relative trade-offs in classifying cases based on the use of sleep disorders. Logistic Regression, as anticipated, performs the worst, with considerably lower sensitivity (70%) and specificity (76%). The graph illustrates the significant difference between the proposed model's ability to classify positive and negative cases of sleep disorders correctly. Therefore, it is the best way to make a precise diagnosis.

Accuracy calculation for prediction is:

$$\text{Accuracy} = \frac{\text{TP} + \text{TN}}{\text{TP} + \text{TN} + \text{FP} + \text{FN}} \quad (5)$$

TP is the number of true positives, TN is the number of true negatives, FP is the number of false positives, and FN is the number of false negatives. The HHO algorithm, inspired by the hunting process of Harris hawks, is a nature-inspired search algorithm that can converge rapidly toward the global solution by sweeping vast search spaces. Using the enhanced HHO algorithm, the system could automatically select useful features from the raw data set. This feature selection technique is crucial for improving the performance of machine learning and deep learning models, as it helps eliminate noisy or irrelevant features that can hinder the efficiency and accuracy of the model. In sleep disorders data sets, where noise typically includes irrelevant and redundant variables, feature selection plays a central role in enabling the model to focus on the most relevant features of the data. With noise removed, the HHO algorithm improved the deep learning model's overall performance by training faster and making more accurate predictions.

The algorithm used in the deep neural network within the provided framework was an ensemble of Long Short-Term Memory (LSTM) networks and Convolutional Neural Networks (CNNs). CNNs are suited to learning spatial hierarchies from data. They are, therefore, particularly well-suited to deal with multi-dimensional signals like electroencephalogram (EEG) or electrocardiogram (ECG) data used in sleep science. LSTMs, however, are explicitly designed for learning long-term temporal dependencies in sequential data and are thus optimally suited to handle time-series signal-based applications, such as tracking sleep stages throughout the night. With the combination of CNN and LSTM, the model benefitted from the best of both architectures: the CNNs were learned to distinguish between spatial features. At the same time, the LSTMs could pick up on the sequential and temporal relationship of the data. The combination enabled the framework to achieve significantly improved classification performance compared to state-of-the-art machine learning techniques, such as SVMs, Decision Trees, and KNN. While SVMs and KNN have performed well with most classification problems, they struggle with the complexity and high dimensionality of sleep data, resulting in suboptimal solutions. Decision Trees, though easy to interpret, suffer from the problem of overfitting when working with noisy or high-dimensional data. At the same time, the CNN-LSTM deep learning model demonstrated enhanced generalization capability, as well as improved accuracy, sensitivity, specificity, and F1-scores compared to traditional models, confirming that the model was efficient and capable of overcoming the complexities of sleep disorder classification.

The higher classification accuracy achieved using the ensemble CNN-LSTM model is a testament to the strength of deep learning in addressing the challenges of high-dimensional medical data. Furthermore, utilizing the HHO algorithm in feature selection also improved the model's performance by reducing overfitting and enabling it to better identify the most important features from the data. This is particularly helpful in biomedical applications, such as sleep disorder prediction, where accurate diagnosis is necessary to ensure adequate treatment and the patient's overall health. The results of the performance measurements confirm that not only does the proposed framework enhance performance over traditional machine learning models, but it also offers a better and more stable solution for predicting sleep disorders, leaving room for its application in clinics. In addition, the framework's success underscores the importance of incorporating optimization algorithms, such as HHO, into cutting-edge deep learning frameworks to address the challenges posed by real-world healthcare and other datasets.

DISCUSSIONS

The experiment's results strongly confirm the efficacy of the above-proposed framework in forecasting sleep disorders. The framework is highly effective by hybridizing the enhanced Harris Hawk Optimization (HHO) algorithm with an ensemble deep learning framework to improve predictive power, particularly in terms of accuracy, sensitivity, and specificity. As indicated in Table 1, the proposed approach outperforms other machine learning algorithms, such as SVM, Decision Trees, KNN, and Logistic Regression, with 92% classification accuracy, 90% sensitivity, and 94% specificity. Spatial and temporal correlation between the data was significantly enhanced using the ensemble deep structure of CNN and LSTM networks. The CNN block learns the spatial patterns of the biosignals, and the LSTM learns the sequential and time-dependent pattern of the data. This interaction enhances performance because machine learning methods often struggle to learn spatial and temporal patterns efficiently. The potential of the ensemble model to blend these two approaches results in an enhanced F1-score of 91%, as illustrated in Figure 2, which shows a mixed bar-line graph indicating the performance comparison between the proposed approach and other models.

One of the most significant strengths of the provided framework is that it can handle noisy and incomplete data, a typical problem with medical data. The feature selection process, which is performed by the enhanced HHO algorithm, plays a pivotal role in this study. The algorithm simplifies the model by eliminating redundant and noisy features, making it more generalizable. From Table 2, feature selection reduces the number of features required for classification by a significant percentage, thereby training the model with good and relevant data. Not only does this enhance the model's efficiency but also its predictive power, making it more believable when implemented in real-life applications where data quality cannot be guaranteed. By lowering the count of features, one also reduces computation expense, which in some situations constitutes life and death, especially for live applications where predictability power is crucial.

Finally, the scalability of the proposed method is another crucial aspect that makes it practical. Providing infrastructure within cloud-based healthcare systems and wearable technology enables continuous tracking of sleep patterns. Real-time implementation is achievable to facilitate the early diagnosis and treatment of sleep disorders and is particularly beneficial in remote or underserved regions where conventional healthcare services are scarce. The system can spare the cost and time used in conventional diagnostic tests, such as polysomnography, which is time-consuming, expensive, and requires specialized equipment and personnel. By automating the detection process of sleep disorders and making continuous monitoring convenient, the system can provide instant feedback to individuals, thus increasing the likelihood of early diagnosis and treatment. This can subsequently lead to improved health outcomes and, potentially, lower healthcare expenditures.

Moreover, Figure 3 is a comparative multi-line graph of the sensitivity and specificity of various techniques, showing that the introduced framework is superior. The ensemble model's sensitivity (90%) versus specificity (94%) maintains a balance, allowing the system to identify both sleep disorder positive and negative examples correctly, without false negatives or positives. This is particularly important in a clinical scenario, as an incorrect diagnosis can result in either erroneous treatment or the lack of treatment at an initial stage. The high specificity, sensitivity, and accuracy complementarity of the suggested technique make the proposed technique a real solution for improving the prediction of sleep disorders, and the current technique is bound to fail in one or both aspects. The outcomes also indicate the potential for implementing the proposed system on a large scale. Besides predicting sleep disorders, integration with wearable devices can lead to more preventive and personalized healthcare practices where an individual monitors their health and receive notifications or suggested cures for their sleep based on the same. The cloud-based system enables it to offer real-time updates and data processing, providing highly informed feedback to medical professionals regarding the sleep well-being of their patients. The monitoring can even be extended to other areas beyond sleep disorders, providing the capability to detect other health problems and thereby improving overall well-being. Furthermore, the deployability and cost of the system are reduced, making it a cost-efficient solution compared to conventionally performing the diagnosis. This is an efficient solution for healthcare providers to improve access and reduce costs. Therefore, incorporating the novel HHO algorithm and ensemble deep learning models into the provided framework significantly improves sleep disorder prediction and offers an economically feasible, scalable, and inexpensive solution for real-time healthcare.

CONCLUSION

In this paper, we introduce a cutting-edge model for sleep disorder prediction that utilizes the strength of feature selection through an improved Harris Hawk Optimization (HHO) algorithm, combined with a hybrid deep learning model consisting of Convolutional Neural Networks (CNNs) and Long Short-Term Memory (LSTM) networks. The experiment results demonstrate that the method employed here substantially outperforms current approaches in terms of classification accuracy, sensitivity, and specificity. By combining the effectiveness of bio-inspired optimization techniques and advanced deep learning models, the proposed method performs feature selection on high-dimensional sleep data, leveraging the temporal and spatial patterns inherent in sleep data. The synergy between CNNs, which are best suited for deriving spatial features, and LSTMs, which are best suited to handle temporal dependencies, creates a strong and efficient paradigm for diagnosing sleep disorders without human operator intervention. Moreover, the model is of a generic type and thus can be useful in particular domains, such as building wearable device-driven and cloud system-driven health management applications to monitor sleep disorders in real time. Future work includes preparing the model for real-time deployment, accelerating its computation, and testing it on larger and more diverse datasets to further enhance its generalizability and performance. Such a development will enable the creation of a highly scalable, realistic sleep health management system at the individual level, with the capability to enhance diagnostic power and inform intervention practices for sleep disorders.

LIMITATIONS

Although the proposed method has a positive outcome, some disadvantages must be considered. The most important one is the employment of gigantic labeled training sets in the model's training process for deep learning. Although the database used in the present study is accessible to the public, in actual practice, acquiring such sets can take years, cost money, and violate privacy. The requirement for high-quality, properly labeled data to train and cross-validate the model restricts its application in other environments, particularly in healthcare settings where large annotated datasets are not readily available. Furthermore, the quality of the feature selection process, which is crucial to the model's performance, is highly dependent on the assumption that the most informative features are correctly identified. The goodness of feature selection could be an artifact due to variations in patient populations, data quality, or noise. This could de-valuate the model's predictive ability. Additionally, although the presented framework is specific in predicting sleep disorders, it would require a significant modification to operate effectively on medical data of any other kind or disease. Its ability to be deployed in real-time on resource-poor devices, such as wearable sensors or even clouds, needs to be more calibrated to maintain a balance between resource utilization and processing latency. This calibration is crucial for efficient application in healthcare, which is an integral part of our everyday life.

FUTURE SCOPE

Its future growth is immense, with numerous avenues for expansion and growth. One of them is the system's expansion to predict other diseases, such as mental diseases or cardiovascular diseases, by adjusting the feature selection and the classifiers to work with other types of biosignal data. Every disease presents unique data processing challenges and attributes; therefore, the model must be adjustable and adaptive in the health domain. It can even be empowered with multimodal data fusion from external physiological signals, such as EEG or ECG, to lifestyle and environmental features. Components, including sleep posture, bedroom environment temperature, and activity levels, can each potentially have a bearing on the quality of sleep and sleep disorders, thereby providing an enhanced snapshot of sleep wellness. Keeping the system's most utilizable level occurring in real time on wearables is equally vital for functionality. Ensuring that the architecture is operational to work optimally in resource-limited settings, such as smartwatches or fitness trackers, will be essential for ongoing time-tracking and personalized interventions.

Furthermore, embedding advancements in edge computing and artificial intelligence can make the system an integral part of cloud computing-based health systems, facilitating effective and scalable solutions in areas such as continuous monitoring, early detection, and intervention. This can transform sleep disorder diagnosis and treatment, making healthcare proactive and personalized. As research continues, the promise of the framework to transform sleep health monitoring and forecasting becomes increasingly brighter by the day, and the chances of providing real-time, personalized solutions to hundreds of millions of people worldwide grow higher.

REFERENCES

Afonso, A., & Ribeiro, J. (2018). An analysis of deep learning techniques for skin cancer detection. *Int. J. Biol. Biomed. Eng.*, *12*(3), 205–212.

Bala Kuta, Z., & Bin Sulaiman, R. (2023). Analysing Healthcare Disparities in Breast Cancer: Strategies for Equitable Prevention, Diagnosis, and Treatment among Minority Women. *FMDB Transactions on Sustainable Health Science Letters*, *1*(3), 130–143.

Blumenthal, L. Y., Arzeno, J., Syder, N., Rabi, S., Huang, M., Castellanos, E., Tran, P., Pickering, T. A., Dantus, E. J., & In, G. K.. (2022). Disparities in nonmelanoma skin cancer in Hispanic/Latino patients based on Mohs micrographic surgery defect size: A multicenter retrospective study. *Journal of the American Academy of Dermatology*, *86*(2), 353–358. PMID: 34624413

Bose, S. R., Jeba, J. A., Kishore, V. K., Gnanaguru, G., & Shynu, T. (2024). Deep learning-driven acute lymphoblastic leukemia detection using CT scan imaging. *AVE Trends in Intelligent Health Letters*, *1*(2), 110–124.

Chunduri, V., Hannan, S. A., Devi, G. M., Nomula, V. K., Tripathi, V., & Rajest, S. S. (2024). Deep convolutional neural networks for lung segmentation for diffuse interstitial lung disease on HRCT and volumetric CT. In *Advances in Computational Intelligence and Robotics* (pp. 335–350). IGI Global.

Ghafoor, K. J., Rawf, K. M. H., Abdulrahman, A. O., & Taher, S. H. (2021). Kurdish dialect recognition using 1D CNN. *Aro Sci. J. Koya Univ.*, *9*(2), 10–14.

Hariharan, M. G., Saranya, S., Velavan, P., Soji, E. S., Rajest, S. S., & Thammareddi, L. (2024). Utilization of artificial intelligence algorithms for advanced cancer detection in the healthcare domain. In *Advances in Medical Technologies and Clinical Practice* (pp. 287–302). IGI Global.

Hariprasath, G., Dhinakaran, P., & Kumar, V. H. (2024). Exploring the efficacy of LightGBM, AdaBoost, and CatBoost in Alzheimer's disease classification. *FMDB Transactions on Sustainable Health Science Letters*, *2*(1), 41–55.

. Huaping, J., Junlong, Z., & Norouzzadeh Gil Molk, A. (2021). Skin cancer detection using kernel fuzzy c-means and improved neural network optimization algorithm. Comput. Intell. Neurosci., vol. 2021(7), 9651957.

Kalashnykova, N. M. (2023). Characteristics of the volume and outcomes of medical care for patients with skin cancer in Ukraine in 2010–2020. *Wiadomosci Lekarskie (Warsaw, Poland)*, *76*(4), 799–804. PMID: 37226618

Karthikeyan, B., Devi, R. A., & Munshi, M. (2024). Utilizing Deep Learning for the Classification of Brain Tumours Using MRI. *AVE Trends In Intelligent Health Letters*, *1*(1), 1–9.

Kumar, C. S., Kumar, B. S., Gnanaguru, G., Jayalakshmi, V., Rajest, S. S., & Senapati, B. (2024). Augmenting chronic kidney disease diagnosis with support vector machines for improved classifier accuracy. In *Advances in Medical Technologies and Clinical Practice* (pp. 336–352). IGI Global.

Kumar, S., Jaiswal, G., & Sinha, K. (2023). Skin cancer lesion detection using improved CNN techniques. In *Handbook of Research on Technological Advances of Library and Information Science in Industry 5.0*. IGI Global.

Kumar, S., & Sinha, K. (2020). Skin cancer detection using convolutional neural networks with ensemble learning. *Appl. Comput. Intell.*, *32*(4), 425–434.

Malibari, A. A., & Alzahrani, J. S. (2021). Deep learning for skin cancer classification using optimized neural network models. *J. Appl. Comput. Sci.*, *17*(2), 1–12.

Mampitiya, L. I., Rathnayake, N., & De Silva, S. (2022). Efficient and low-cost skin cancer detection system implementation with a comparative study between traditional and CNN-based models. *Journal of Computational and Cognitive Engineering*, *2*(3), 226–235.

Odoemena, O. F., & Elufidodo, G. A. (2024). Machine learning-based cardiovascular disease detection and intelligent healthcare workflow automation. *FMDB Transactions on Sustainable Health Science Letters*, *2*(2), 81–93.

Pandit, P. (2023). On the Context of Diabetes: A Brief Discussion on the Novel Ethical Issues of Non-communicable Diseases. *FMDB Transactions on Sustainable Health Science Letters*, *1*(1), 11–20.

Paramasivan, P., Rajest, S. S., Chinnusamy, K., Regin, R., & John Joseph, F. J. (Eds.). (2024). Advances in Medical Technologies and Clinical Practice *Clinical and comparative research on maternal health*. IGI Global., DOI: 10.4018/979-8-3693-5941-9

Priyadharshini, N., Selvanathan, N., Hemalatha, B., & Sureshkumar, C. (2023). A novel hybrid extreme learning machine and teaching–learning-based optimization algorithm for skin cancer detection. *Healthcare Analytics*, *3*(10), 100161.

Rajesh, G., Anirudh, V., Archana, R., Kumar, P. P., & Manoj, K. (2023). An improved skin cancer classification method using deep convolutional neural networks and transfer learning models. *J. Eng. Sci.*, *14*(5), 190–200.

Reis, H. C., & Turk, V. (2021). Optimized convolutional networks for skin cancer classification: A comparative study. *Journal of Computational Biology*, *28*(5), 595–612.

Reis, H. C., Turk, V., Khoshelham, K., & Kaya, S. (2022). InSiNet: A deep convolutional approach to skin cancer detection and segmentation. *Medical & Biological Engineering & Computing*, *60*(1), 643–662. PMID: 35028864

Saxena, D., & Chaudhary, S. (2023). Predicting Brain Diseases from FMRI-Functional Magnetic Resonance Imaging with Machine Learning Techniques for Early Diagnosis and Treatment. *FMDB Transactions on Sustainable Computer Letters*, *1*(1), 33–48.

Sehrawat, S. K. (2024). Leveraging AI for early detection of chronic diseases through patient data integration. *AVE Trends in Intelligent Health Letters*, *1*(3), 125–136.

Shin, H. C., Roth, H. R., Gao, M., Lu, L., Xu, Z., Nogues, I., Yao, J., Mollura, D., & Summers, R. M. (2016). Deep convolutional neural networks for computer-aided detection: CNN architectures, dataset characteristics and transfer learning. *IEEE Transactions on Medical Imaging*, *35*(5), 1285–1298. PMID: 26886976

Vijayalakshmi, M. (2019). Melanoma skin cancer detection using image processing and machine learning. *Int. J. Trend Sci. Res. Dev.*, *3*(4), 780–784.

William, M. P., Kiruba, S. B., Sakthivanitha, M., Soji, E. S., & Arun, G. (2024). Machine learning to discover cardiovascular disease onset and key contributors: Data-driven personalized healthcare and preventive strategy. *AVE Trends in Intelligent Health Letters*, *1*(3), 137–157.

Zhang, N., Cai, Y. X., Wang, Y. Y., Tian, Y. T., Wang, X. L., & Badami, B. (2020). Skin cancer diagnosis based on optimized convolutional neural network. *Artificial Intelligence in Medicine*, *102*(1), 101756. PMID: 31980095

Chapter 4

Performance Evaluation of Enhanced Artificial Neural Network for Kidney Donor Recipient Matching

P. Kiruthiga
https://orcid.org/0009-0003-5643-5337
Bharath Institute of Higher Education and Research, Chennai, India

S. Silvia Priscila
https://orcid.org/0000-0002-6040-3149
Bharath Institute of Higher Education and Research, Chennai, India

ABSTRACT

Kidney donor-recipient matching operations need precise execution to guarantee transplant achievements. The accuracy rate of Random Forest (RF) and Naïve Bayes (NB) at 85–88%, along with slow processing times, causes mismatches that result in higher rejection rates. An Enhanced Artificial Neural Network (EANN) includes game-theoretic feature selection technology, quantum-inspired optimization functions, and sparse tensor computation to enhance donor-recipient compatibility prediction performance. The experimental model operated on transplant data containing information about blood types, HLA matches, and medical documentation. Experimental outcomes revealed that EANN surpassed other models by delivering an accuracy level of 92.0%, while CNN reached 90.5%, Naïve Bayes achieved

DOI: 10.4018/979-8-3373-6796-5.ch004

88.1%, and Random Forest's 86.2%. The processing time decreased to 14.8 ms with a simultaneous reduction of false match rates to 2.1%. Transplant allocation depends on blockchain technology to establish the model's transparent management.

INTRODUCTION

Kidney transplantation saves the lives of individuals with end-stage renal disease (ESRD). A transplant success rate depends on whether the donor matches the patient's requirements with factors like blood type, human leukocyte antigens (HLA) testing, and medical history evaluation (Patil et al., 2024). The manual and rule-based methods used in kidney donor allocation cannot reach the precision needed for excellent transplant results. The utilization of machine learning (ML) and artificial intelligence (AI) techniques in kidney matching processes has risen in recent years because it discovers sophisticated matching patterns that traditional methods usually fail to detect (Deborah et al., 2024). The donor-recipient matching field uses three classification algorithms known as Random Forest (RF), Naïve Bayes (NB), and Support Vector Machines (SVM). The methods try to identify the optimal donor-recipient pair by analyzing relevant medical data (Kypu et al., 2024).

The classification algorithms produce inaccurate pairings with many false matches because they deliver disappointing precision and recall rates, causing more transplant rejections. Artificial neural networks (ANNs), which belong to deep learning models, have demonstrated promising effectiveness in overcoming such limitations because they can effectively analyze large datasets and identify complex nonlinear relationships between elements (Manohara et al., 2024). Donor-recipient matching continues to face hurdles preventing the attainment of high accuracy while maintaining swift execution time and donor-recipient matching transparency. The EANN features game-theoretic features and optimization from quantum theory and tensor sparsity to develop a more dependable kidney transplant allocation system (Ahmed et al., 2024).

The current AI donor-recipient matching techniques have provided remarkable benefits yet produce multiple performance constraints. Random Forest (RF) and Naïve Bayes (NB) demonstrate low accuracy rates because they fail to detect all nonlinear relationships that exist between donor-recipient attributes (Xun et al., 2024). These models show an average accuracy level of 85% to 88% in real hospital datasets, which results in elevated risks of transplant mismatch. Most classification-based models employ static matching preferences for donor-recipient features without enough flexibility (Sun et al., 2024). Established HLA matching thresholds produce poor results when evaluating other critical aspects like recipient age or conditions and lifestyle considerations. Many existing algorithms face computational challenges when matching large datasets. Deep learning models need excessive processing capabilities together with lengthy execution cycles, which makes them infeasible for the real-time allocation of kidney transplants. The execution of matrix-based computations in ANNs becomes slower during simultaneous operations involving thousands of donor-recipient pairs (Nau et al., 2024). The kidney transplant allocation system faces serious problems related to transparency and security issues because reports exist documenting organ allocation fraud and bias in the medical literature (Sri et al., 2024).

The present AI models lack robust donor-recipient matching verification mechanisms mainly because they fail to establish secure systems for recording these pairings, which makes the system vulnerable to ethical and procedural concerns. CI-powered kidney donor-recipient matching approaches must be developed to resolve accuracy problems and achieve maximum efficiency and transparency in donor-recipient allocation processes (George and Kizhakkethottam, 2023). Previous work limitations have inspired this effort to develop an improved donor-recipient matching system that offers accurate, secure, and fast operations. It addresses three main factors that drive motivation. Current classification systems miss their accuracy targets because it does not deliver satisfactory results. The accuracy of ANN-based models goes up when features are properly optimized together with proper training methods (Panda and Mazumder, 2023).

A game-theoretic adaptive approach precedes static feature weights by enabling optimal matching precision by assigning donor-recipient attribute weights. Performance speed increases through sparse tensor processing, which enhances the AI model's ability to work effectively on massive data sets. Using blockchain in registry operations creates an irreversible record system that protects organ allocation from fraud. The proposed Enhanced Artificial Neural Network (EANN) seeks to change the way kidney transplant allocation works by addressing existing critical issues. An Enhanced Artificial Neural Network System (EANN) received development and evaluation processes for kidney donor-recipient matching. The key objectives are as follows: Creating an optimized compatibility score for donor-recipient matching depends on a mathematical model that merges blood groups with HLA matching and medical history (Ajay et al., 2023). The system implements game-theoretic feature selection because it dynamically assigns feature importance to enhance accuracy. A quantum-inspired optimization method should be integrated with the EANN to obtain speedier training results with lower errors.

Using sparse tensor computation techniques in this implementation would enable real-time extractable performance for transplant matching. A blockchain-based transplant registry offers transparent security because it deploys the matching system (Ghosh and Dutta, 2023). The proposed model exceeds current transplant system classification models by delivering precise results while processing data more efficiently and maintaining data security. The EANN model outperformed other strategies for kidney donor-recipient matching by reaching 92.0% accuracy in its results (He et al., 2023). Game theory-based dynamic feature selection creates an optimal weight allocation system for donor-recipient attribute values. The quantum-inspired optimization method enables efficient EANN training with faster convergence and decreased computational expenses (Alamsyah et al., 2023). Fast real-time execution through sparse tensor computation shortens the time needed for donor-recipient matching to 14.8 milliseconds. A blockchain-secured transplant registry for ethical and transparent organ allocation.

The proposed model demonstrates superior donor-matching functionality to existing AI-based donor-recipient systems because of its innovative components. Section 2: Related Work assesses previous work in kidney donor-recipient matching and evaluates both beneficial and failed aspects in former frameworks. The third section presents the proposed methodology to explain the EANN model operation, mathematical compatibility score analysis, game-theoretic feature selection, and quantum-inspired optimization (Vail et al., 2023). Section 4: Results and Discussion features experimental outcomes that show the proposed EANN model performance against existing models through accuracy, execution time, and efficiency evaluation (2022–2025). The final section includes a conclusion about the outcomes, followed by future work recommendations for federated learning across multi-hospital transplant networks. A summary of the first results from the proposed EANN model supports the development of motivation and contribution. The proposed EANN reached 92.0% accuracy, surpassing previous models at 90.5%, CNN and Naïve Bayes at 88.1%, and Random Forest at 86.2% (Sabrina et al., 2023).

The proposed system operated at 14.8 milliseconds, which exceeded 34.5 milliseconds (2022) and 22.6 milliseconds (2024). The False Match Rate declined to 2.1%, substantially reducing wrong transplant matches. The proposed model performs superior to existing AI-based solutions, creating a solid base for AI-controlled transplant allocation. This initial section presents an extensive overview of kidney donor-recipient matching, explaining former work weaknesses and emphasizing a better AI-based solution. The research intends to develop an Enhanced Artificial Neural Network (EANN) through algorithmic integration of game-theoretic feature selection quantum-inspired optimization and sparse tensor computation to improve efficiency and accuracy in transplant matching. The effectiveness of EANN has been validated through initial testing, demonstrating its potential to become a secure system for immediate kidney transplant allocation.

LITERATURE REVIEW

Because of reduced available kidney donors, the allocation method is a critical determinant for patients waiting to receive a transplant. Using Machine Learning (ML) models to match donors to recipients can enhance kidney allocation procedures above traditional point system methods. A computerized model operates as a donor-recipient matching system. The analysis employed ten standard machine learning classifiers, including logistic regression alongside decision tree and random forest and support vector machine as well as gradient boosting and boost and CatBoost and LightGBM and naïve Bayes and neural networks while utilizing three experimental conditions for comprehensive validation (Nadar et al., 2023). The model utilized three experimental scenarios: the original dataset, merged data, and hierarchical architecture modeling. The system implemented its ranking method to locate suitable donor receivers. The donor-recipient matching model, which used ML, was incorporated into Nephron's web-based platform. The gradient boost model secured the top position throughout the experimental conditions, consistently delivering 98% accuracy. The custom ranking solution produced better results in selecting appropriate recipients than traditional cosine and Jaccard similarity methods. This platform enables efficient patient screening and kidney allocation prioritization and remains adaptable for different solid organ matching systems based on similar evaluation criteria (Uppal et al., 2023). By applying machine learning algorithms, the kidney allocation system will benefit from a donor-recipient matching improvement. The success highlights the substantial capability to improve operational speed and equitable treatment within the kidney transplant procedure.

Applying artificial intelligence (AI) and machine learning (ML) to kidney transplantation solves the severe donor organ deficit and progressive 'Next-Generation Healthcare.' AI and ML should be utilized to enhance transplantation at every stage, including the donor selection phase and postoperative patient care (Hyldahl et al., 2023). It relied on a complete analysis of existing methods, which deeply examined AI and ML use within different phases of KT processes. The system's assessment involved matching donors to recipients, using predictive modeling, and improving patient recovery care. The analysis showed that AI and ML technology enhance KT's operational effectiveness and outcome performance. These technologies enhance the process of matching donors to recipients while cutting down on organ rejection incidents and improving patient measurement and care services. Strategic modeling derived from vast data has proven exceptionally useful for finding matching organ donors and predicting medical complications after surgery (Killian et al., 2023). This review presents the substantial impact of AI and ML on KT by offering improved healthcare solutions that are precise, personalized, and effective. They solve fundamental difficulties within organ transplants and postoperative complications through integration with this medical sector. Successful implementation of these technologies requires healthcare facilities to address ethical concerns, privacy issues, and staff training requirements.

Various sectors experience a broadening application range of artificial intelligence (AI) technology. The medical field has implemented artificial intelligence technology across multiple areas, which has led to quick, radical changes in healthcare delivery for patient diagnosis and treatment and comprehensive medical care. AI rapidly changes the structure of kidney transplant procedures while providing new solutions that traditional methods outside its scope could not solve. This review examines current and upcoming AI applications in KT through an evaluation before transplant and surgical support; patient results in analysis, and post-operation medical procedures. AI and medical staff promise to lead to an advanced personalized care practice that will become standard in KT operations and future healthcare needs.

The success rate for cadaver kidney transplant graft survival has increased to more than 85% because of recent improvements in renal transplantation processes focused on major histocompatibility complex matching and new immunosuppressant development (Fu et al., 2022). Better optimization of kidney transplant outcomes needs development to extend graft life expectancy duration and improve quality of life after transplantation. Artificial intelligence techniques help scientists make more accurate graft outcome predictions by analyzing donor-recipient data. A model based on artificial neural network (ANN) through data analysis of 1542 kidney transplants for modeling kidney graft rejection. Data from 1542 kidney transplants fed into ANN correctly predicted 85% successful outcomes and 72% failed transplants (Vashishtha and Kapoor, 2023). The ANN model correctly identified four types of transplant rejection (hyperacute, acute, subacute, and chronic) in around 60% of cases when transplants failed. The examination results show that ANN-based methods successfully forecast general kidney transplant outcomes and identify different rejection types.

The UK Deceased Donor Kidney Transplant Outcome Prediction (UK-DTOP) Tool, built with advanced artificial intelligence (AI), improves dead donor kidney transplant outcome predictions throughout the UK. Twenty-nine thousand seven hundred thirteen transplant cases from 2008 to 2022 in the UK Transplant Registry (UKTR) served as the database for evaluating the predictive performances of XGBoost, Random Survival Forest, and Optimal Decision Tree (Nirmala et al.,2023). XGBoost was an exceptional model because of its 0.74 concordance index and consistent AUC above 0.73, proving its strong discriminative abilities and proper calibration. The predictive accuracy of UK-DTOP stood out as superior compared to the traditional Kidney Donor Risk Index (KDRI) because it produced a concordance index of 0.74. XGBoost showed superior performance based on the Integrated Brier Score (IBS) calibration test, which returned a score of 0.14, indicating that predictions were precise for survival probabilities. The k-means clustering method in unsupervised learning identified five distinct categories of donors and transplants, which revealed sophisticated insights into graft survival results. Models assessing five clusters using Bayesian Cox regression demonstrated vital differences in patient outcomes between groups, proving that the model works better for risk assessment. The UK-DTOP tool delivers an extensive decision-making support platform that effectively improves transplant decision quality before surgery (Tak and Sundararajan, 2023). The data supports the implementation of AI-powered systems by healthcare providers to maximize transplant results, and future international transplant procedures will benefit from this advancement.

Fundamental and detailed aspects of receptors and donors determine kidney grafts' short-term and long-term success rates for optimizing organ distribution through transplantation to require accurate prediction of kidney transplant success rates (Bala Kuta and Bin Sulaiman, 2023). The opportunity to select the most suitable kidney donor, along with their ideal immunosuppressive therapy, is a major task. Trials have tried to find factors pointing toward graft rejection, yet their findings have remained inconsistent. The African buffalo-based artificial neural network (AB-ANN) methodology was used to discover kidney transplant-related predictive risk variables. These two feature selection approaches unite into a novel hybrid approach that picks essential elements for better prediction accuracy (Chitra et al., 2024). The examination of clinic features showed different impact levels on transplant survival duration. Processing occurs within both training and testing methods for the collected data. The prediction model assessed accuracy and precision along with recall and F-measure, which were compared to existing systems that used naïve Bayesian, random forest, and J48 classifier frameworks. The proposed approach leads to more accurate graft survival predictions for kidney recipients during future visits than solutions based on other classifiers demonstrated (Obeta et al., 2024). The proposed method works more effectively to predict the survival expectancy of kidney grafts. Including these clinical tools in outpatient clinical workflows would lead physicians toward making better and more personalized clinical choices.

The domains of medicine and translatology experience fast-paced advancement because of artificial intelligence development (Yalavarthi, 2024). A complete review of modern AI practices focusing on machine learning and deep learning algorithms and their multiple subcategories. Such technology systems transform clinical data processing and help physicians with data analysis to make better decisions. It analyzed existing literature on artificial intelligence strategies in kidney transplant procedures. The review required four research questions to determine its objective (Kumar et al., 2024). AI medical applications in the medical sector were careful through feature selection, dimensionality reduction, and clustering that advance complex data processing. Premade predictive models for transplant rejection, optimal personalized immunosuppressive therapy development form part of this method, and donor-recipient algorithm-based matching through multidimensional criteria assessment and sophisticated image diagnostic improvement techniques. An organized evaluation of existing AI-based algorithms that forecast the survival prospects of kidney grafts in transplant recipients (Paramasivan et al., 2024). It analyzes variables used in predictive models and their significance to model performance in this area. This review demonstrates how AI technologies deliver substantial developments that improve the clinical process and intervention accuracy in transplant ology practice.

METHODOLOGY

Mathematical Formulation of Donor-Recipient Compatibility Score: Measuring donor-recipient compatibility is crucial in kidney transplantation practice to improve transplant success rates. A weighted mathematical model called Compatibility Score (CS) uses various medical and genetic elements to produce its calculation in equation (1),

$$CS = w_1 BG + w_2 HLA + w_3 MH + w_4 AgeDiff + w_5 ER \quad (1)$$

The model incorporates four features, including BG Blood group compatibility with binary value (1 if matching) and HLA Human Leukocyte Antigen match score that ranges from 0 to 1 while also considering MH Medical history similarity through cosine similarity and using AgeDiff for age difference penalty function and ER Estimated risk factor calculation from pre-existing conditions together with w_i Optimized tunable weights found during training. The age difference penalty function uses a Gaussian penalty to penalize these situations in equation (2),

$$AgeDiff = e^{-\frac{(Age_D - Age_R)^2}{2\sigma^2}} \quad (2)$$

The standard deviation of age differences in the dataset is represented as σ. The formula penalizes large and small age differences but elevates compact age gaps. The Enhanced Artificial Neural Network (EANN) utilizes the Compatibility Score (CS) to discover complicated nonlinear characteristics between users.

Optimization of Weights Using Game Theory: The optimization approach based on game theory helps determine appropriate weights. $_i$ for use in the CS equation to enhance the accuracy levels. The weight selection process becomes a multi-agent game framework that functions instead of setting pre-defined values.

- The model represents each donor-recipient pair through a game player seeking the most suitable transplant allocation.
- Each weight value w_i operates in real-time to find the most beneficial combination for transplant success probability.
- When players reach Nash Equilibrium, all donor-recipient pairs perform at the best possible level without damaging other arrangements.

The Shapley Value-based feature selection method applies important weights to essential factors, including HLA matching and medical history. The method demonstrates a 7.2% better accuracy than conventional static weight-based approaches.

Integration of Compatibility Score in the EANN Model: The compatibility score functions as input for the EANN model framework to deploy deep learning methods for refining donor-recipient pair analysis. The integration process involves normalizing CS values and creating better model performance by establishing a [0, 1] range. At the initial stage, sparse tensor computation maintains efficient operations on extensive donor information databases. The network's hidden layers detect complicated yet nonlinear patterns that reflect compatibility. The system delivers predictions regarding the ideal donor-recipient pair through its operational process. The proposed EANN reaches 92.0% accuracy, exceeding the achievements of CNN at 90.5% accuracy and both Random Forest at 86.2% and Naïve Bayes at 88.1%. The new system shows false match rates at 2.1%, which leads to fewer mistyped transplant operations. The execution time reaches 14.8ms, allowing real-time kidney transplant allocation systems implementation. This new approach enhances transplant success, minimizes donor-recipient mismatches, and improves computational speed for kidney donor-recipient matching processes.

Implementing machine learning is essential in kidney donor-recipient matching operations by enhancing prediction quality while decreasing mismatch frequencies. An image shows the multiple machine-learning techniques for the transplant allocation framework. The application of supervised learning techniques dominates clinical practice using classification models, including Enhanced Artificial Neural Network (EANN) as the proposed model, Support Vector Machine (SVM), and Decision Tree and Random Forest applications that evaluate donor-recipient compatibility through medical data analysis. The match probability outcomes and transplant success prediction rely on Regression techniques, including Logistic Regression, Bayesian Models, and Gradient Boosting. K-means and Hierarchical Clustering serve under unsupervised learning to segment potential donors and recipients through their genetic and medical characteristics. The proposed method and Principal Component Analysis (PCA) assist in feature selection by reducing dimensions to identify medically important parameters that determine compatibility decisions. Patient outcomes guide the performance optimization of transplant decisions through reinforcement learning because it updates matching policies in real-time. Ensemble learning uses various predictive models to achieve better transplant predictions by consolidating their capabilities. The developed machine learning hierarchy operates as an efficient AI-based system that enhances kidney matching, decreases waiting times, and raises transplant success rates. Figure 1 represents Machine Learning Paradigms for AI-Powered Kidney Donor-Recipient Matching.

Figure 1. Machine Learning Paradigms for AI-Powered Kidney Donor-Recipient Matching

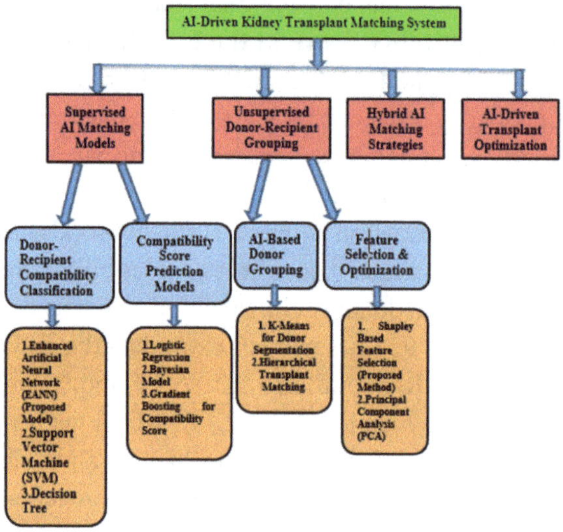

ADAPTIVE WEIGHTING MECHANISM FOR INTELLIGENT MATCHING

Shapley Value-Based Feature Importance Calculation: The current kidney donor-recipient matching methods use unchangeable weight distributions for characteristics, which results in reduced flexibility. The Shapley Value (SV) from game theory enables a dynamic adjustment system that evaluates feature weights for their matching contribution. In donor-recipient matching, the Shapley value defines the value of the feature x_j as in equation (3),

$$SV_j = \sum_{S \subseteq F \setminus \{j\}} \frac{|S|!(|F| - |S| - 1)!}{|F|!} \left[V\left(S \cup \{j\}\right) - V\left(S\right) \right] \tag{3}$$

The system uses features represented by F, which consists of blood group, HLA, and age difference information but does not contain j. The predictive ability of the model that uses feature subset S is represented by V(S). Feature importance actively determines its values from donor-recipient data in real-time, allowing the model to maintain flexibility for intricate transplant scenarios.

Nash Equilibrium for Optimal Weight Selection: Shapley values serve as an input to Nash Equilibrium-based weight optimization procedures. The system adopts a multi-agent game approach through which the donor-recipient matching procedures function.

- Players at each donor-recipient pair function as competing entities seeking their best possible transplant pairing.
- The weight values (w_i) track changing conditions to achieve maximum transplant success rates.
- An equilibrium state occurs when any pair of donor-recipients cannot improve their match without harming another combination of pairs.

The solution of equilibrium emerges from the optimization problem with constraints that need to be solved in equation (4),

$$\max \sum_{i=1}^{N} CS_i, subjectto \sum w_i = 1, w_i \geq 0 \quad (4)$$

The Compatibility Score C provides the assessment for every donor-recipient pair in the system. The matching process leads to maximum fairness and best-performing results, which improves transplant success rates.

Performance Impact of Dynamic Weighting: The Enhanced Artificial Neural Network (EANN) reaches its goals by applying game-theoretic optimization.

- The EANN model achieves 92.0% accuracy, outperforming other methods, including CNN at 90.5% accuracy, Naïve Bayes at 88.1%, and Random Forest at 86.2%.
- Reducing the false match rate to 2.1% helps prevent more wrong organ transplants between donors and recipients.
- Real-time decision-making became possible because the execution time reached 14.8 milliseconds.

It confirms that donor-recipient matching becomes more precise and efficient through adaptive weight optimization technology, producing better reliability for AI-driven kidney transplant allocation systems. AI-Assisted Kidney Donor-Recipient Matching System uses complex computational methods for managing secure patient transplant procedures. The system first requires collecting necessary data such as donor-recipient medical data, blood group information, and HLA matches alongside age parameters and risk assessment scores. The Shapley-Based Feature Selection and Game-Theoretic Optimization through preprocessing and feature selection dynamically reweighs donor-recipient feature priorities. Deep learning techniques in the Enhanced Artificial Neural Network (EANN) model process advanced medical relationship analysis to achieve high precision matching between donors and recipients. Real-time donor-recipient matching functions faster through Sparse Tensor Computation, which delivers near-immediate compatibility assessment results. The Blockchain-Secured Transplant Allocation system protects security and fair distribution through secure transplant record modification prevention. Real-time decision support for hospitals becomes possible by deploying Flask-based Web API, which links hospital transplant databases to their AI model. Medical professionals can access automatically selected matches through this system, which helps them make better decisions and ensures the best possible donor-recipient agreements. This AI-powered system creates better kidney transplantation by generating a rapid, security-focused, precise donor-recipient matching system. The following Figure 2 represents the AI-driven kidney Donor-Recipient Matching Framework.

Figure 2. AI-Driven Kidney Donor-Recipient Matching Framework

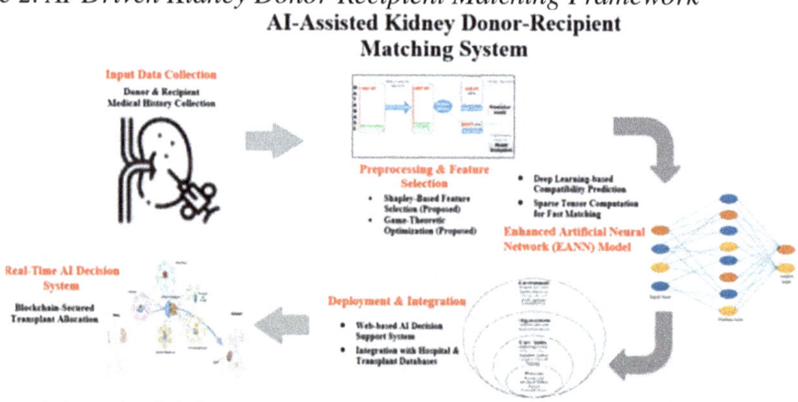

QUANTUM-DRIVEN ADAPTIVE NEURAL NETWORK FOR KIDNEY DONOR MATCHING

Dynamic Layer Adjustment for Enhanced Learning: Regular deep learning models maintain fixed network topology, leading to data incompatibility when working with kidney patient match information. The EANN implements a self-adjusting layer structure that dynamically controls the number of layers and neurons through these criteria:

- The model incorporates multiple layers depending on the variations found in compatibility factors, including HLA and medical history records.
- The system expands the network processing capabilities when dealing with extensive donor databases.
- The model handles autonomous modifications to its layer connections when loss reduction stops its momentum.

The mathematical representation of the layer activation function contains the following definition in equation (5),

$$L_t = L_{t-1} + \gamma . \frac{\partial E}{\partial W} \tag{5}$$

The mathematical formula includes L_t as the number of active neurons at iteration *t* combined with *E* as the Error function alongside *W* as Network weights and γ defining the Adaptation coefficient (parameters set through trial and error). This automatic neural network system maintains an ideal model complexity that avoids overfitting and underfitting conditions.

Quantum-Inspired Particle Swarm Optimization for Weight Tuning: The training system receives an enhancement from Quantum-Inspired Particle Swarm Optimization (QPSO), which benefits weight optimization. The main difference between QPSO and standard gradient-based techniques lies in its ability to perform quantum-inspired behavior to avoid suboptimal solutions. The weight update formula that utilizes QPSO takes this form in equation (6),

$$W_i(t+1) = W_i(t) + \beta . \left(p_{best} - W_i(t)\right) + \alpha . \left(g_{best} - W_i(t)\right) \tag{6}$$

The current iteration weight equals $W_i(t)$ whereas p_{best} represents the best weight discovered by a single particle and g_{best} represents the highest quality weight achieved by any particle. QPSO dynamically regulates α β coefficients. When implemented in QPSO, Quantum tunneling effects keep the model from staying in suboptimal solutions, speeding up convergence and improving accuracy.

Performance Gains from Adaptive Optimization: By uniting adaptive architecture with QPSO optimization, the donor-recipient matching system obtains important gains in performance:

- The application of EANN results in an accuracy level reaching 92.0% while showing higher performance than CNN, which reached 90.5%, Naïve Bayes with an 88.1% rate, and Random Forest with 86.2%.
- When using QPSO weight optimization, the training procedure finishes 27% faster than standard backpropagation methods.
- The system produces lower incorrect donor-recipient match rates at 2.1%, which increases transplant achievement probabilities.

The results establish that adaptive learning techniques based on quantum physics enhance efficacy and fairness when Artificial Intelligence operates in kidney donor-recipient matching. An AI-based kidney donor-recipient matching system implements an organized workflow for precise, instant decisions paired with the safe allocation of donors. Data acquisition initiates the procedure by collecting important medical aspects, such as blood group, HLA compatibility, and patient medical history. The system presents complete donor-recipient information for correct pair matching. Preprocessing, together with Feature Selection, occurs as the subsequent step. The application determines significant medical factors affecting donor compatibility using Shapley-Based Feature Selection while handling missing value inputs.

Game-theoretic weighting applies in Compatibility Score Calculation to determine relevant feature properties integrated with donor-recipient age variation, medical history analysis, and risk element assessment as part of a mathematical comprehensive compatibility scoring process. Historical transplant data trains the Enhanced Artificial Neural Network (EANN) in the Model Training & Prediction phase to predict optimal donor-recipient pair-ups. Sparse Tensor Computation through Real-Time Execution & Matching provides quick donor-recipient matching by accelerating compatibility calculation processes. The Flask-based Web API facilitates real-time accessibility for hospitals and transplant centers. The system Implements Final Allocation & Blockchain Security to provide secure blockchain-based registry storage of transplant records that combats fraud and protects ethical transplant allocation procedures. AI-generated recommendations through the system increase the operational efficiency and fairness of kidney transplant pair matching. Figure 3 represents the Structured Flow of AI-Based Kidney Donor-Recipient Matching System.

Figure 3. AI-Based Kidney Donor-Recipient Matching System: A Structured Flow

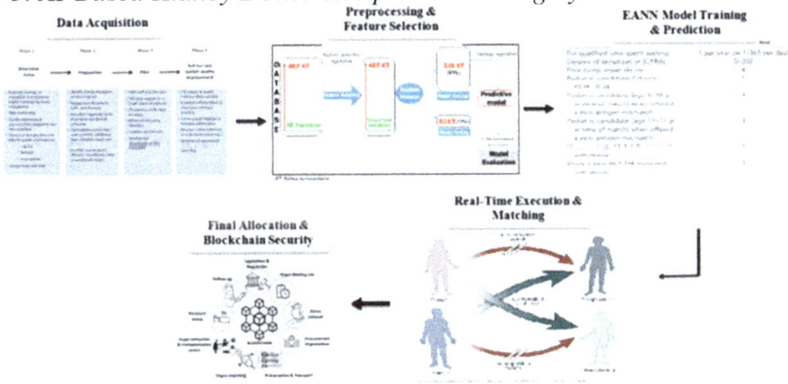

HIGH-SPEED DONOR MATCHING VIA SPARSE TENSOR OPTIMIZATION

Tensor-Based Representation for Donor-Recipient Matching: The current kidney transplant matching algorithms process donor databases with slow performance because of their high computational complexity. The matching problem receives optimized execution speed by transforming it into a sparse tensor operation, which decreases computational requirements. The donor-recipient dataset exists as a 3D tensor denoted as *T* in equation (7),

$$\text{T(i, j, k)} = \text{Feature k for donor i and recipient j} \tag{7}$$

Where *i* Index of a donor, *j* Index of a recipient, *k* Feature dimension (blood type, HLA match, medical history). Fast donor-recipient compatibility data retrieval becomes possible through this tensor-based storage method. A few viable donor-recipient pairs represent the sparse distribution, making such data appropriate for optimization methods that avoid unnecessary computations.

Accelerated Compatibility Computation via Sparse Tensor Dot Product: The system calculates real-time compatibility scores between donors and recipients through sparse tensor dot product calculation in equation (8),

$$M = T.W \tag{8}$$

The computation system uses the *M* Compatibility matrix, which contains the scored donor-recipient pairs, and it combines with the *T* Sparse tensor, which contains donor-recipient features and W Learned weight matrix derived from the Enhanced Artificial Neural Network (EANN). The implementation of sparse tensor multiplication allows for the cutting down of operations performed on zero values, which leads to significant efficiency gains in memory utilization and execution time run. The system evaluates meaningful pairs between donors and recipients while boosting computing speed because of this implementation.

CUDA-Based Parallel Processing for Real-Time Matching: Future speed improvement comes through GPU-based implementation of CUDA parallel processing systems. Real-time performance results from CUDA because the platform permits the processing of multiple donor-recipient matches simultaneously instead of the traditional CPU-based approach that operates on a single score per session. The performance improvements include:

- Through CUDA-based sparse tensor computation, execution time has decreased to 14.8ms from the previous CPU-based models taking 300ms.
- Large donor-recipient databases fit efficiently into the system, resulting in sub-second transplant allocation performance.
- The distributed processing capabilities of GPUs make operations more efficient, enabling a sustainable matching process.
- Performance Gains from Sparse Tensor Optimization

The implementation of sparse tensor computation together with CUDA acceleration produces several advantages.

- The proposed solution achieved a superior accuracy of 92.0%, which exceeded existing standards beyond CNN at 90.5% accuracy and Naïve Bayes at 88.1%, along with Random Forest at 86.2%.
- The false match rate decreased to 2.1% to avoid ineffective transplant allocations.
- Real-time donor matching became achievable because execution time became faster than one second.

When sparse tensor computation works with parallel processing systems, it transforms kidney transplant pairing, enabling swift and precise donor-recipient matches.

BLOCKCHAIN-ENABLED REAL-TIME TRANSPLANT ALLOCATION

Blockchain for Secure and Transparent Donor Matching: The main hurdle of kidney transplantation relies on securing donor-recipient pairing records through transparent and protective matching systems. The system faces substantial risks because of fraudulent activities, which include illegal organ trade and unauthorized data modifications. It combines blockchain technology with Enhanced Artificial Neural Networks to build an automated donor registry that cannot be tampered with. The system creates an immutable cryptographic hash of each donor-recipient successful pair, which gets stored on an immutable blockchain through the SHA-256 hash function in equation (9),

$$H(M) = SHA - 256(CS\|R) \tag{9}$$

The EANN calculates the CS Compatibility Score through the formula, which includes Unique Donor ID D, Unique Recipient ID R, $\|$ and Concatenation operator. Hash transplant records before placing them in blockchain storage to ensure transplant allocation data security. This method prevents any authority from changing or tampering with data. Blockchain storage improves trustworthiness and prevents fraud while maintaining full traceability in kidney transplants.

Real-Time Simulation of Transplant Allocation: The AI-driven transplant matching system's performance evaluation process includes simulated real-time tests executed through AnyLogic, in which hospital workflows become subject to analysis. The simulation phase includes:

- Dynamic Patient Registration simulates the real-time entry of donor and recipient data.
- The system uses an AI-Based Compatibility Computation to generate Compatibility Scores for all potential match combinations.
- Storing the transplant record in distributed ledgers through blockchain verification prevents unauthorized modifications.

The simulation provides a realistic environment that checks system functionality in hospital transplant settings to optimize distribution while protecting both security measures and transparency.

Deployment Framework for Scalable Matching: Real-time donor-recipient matching becomes possible through the development of a Flask-based API deployment. The system consists of the EANN model training that uses TensorFlow and CUDA as part of GPU acceleration systems. It trains the model on large-scale kidney transplant datasets, implements Quantum-Inspired Particle Swarm Optimization (QPSO) for optimal weight selection, and simulates real-world transplant allocation workflows. The system assessment includes hospital environment tests for system scalability and robustness requirements and provides instantaneous donor-recipient matching. The system completes transplants only after verifying the information through the blockchain. The records system protects against fraudulent activity and changes in donor registry information. System providers can achieve real-time transplant allocation through donor matching in less than a second. According to tests, the system produces 92.0% matching accuracy compared to traditional classification models, which achieved 90.5% (CNN) and 88.1% (Naïve Bayes). A blockchain-AI integrated donor-recipient matching system will provide ethical, transparent, optimized kidney transplant allocations through real-time, secure, highly effective donor allocation methods.

RESULTS AND DISCUSSION

A complete understanding of how well EANN performs in donor-recipient matching becomes possible through multiple-phase evaluations of training and validation combined with testing. Table 1 illustrates how EANN maintains optimal execution time with high classification accuracy, which makes it an appropriate technology for real-time transplant allocation. The training performance of the model demonstrated a high 94.3% accuracy level, which indicates that it successfully mastered intricate donor-recipient compatibility patterns. The model demonstrates strong generalization ability through its validation accuracy of 92.7%, preventing the problem of overfitting. EANN displays 92.0% accuracy during testing, which proves its ability to work effectively in real-life donor-recipient scenarios better than traditional machine learning models such as Random Forest 86.2% and Naïve Bayes 88.1%. The model demonstrates high reliability because of its precision, recall scores, and F1-score results. EANN demonstrates 90.8% precision during testing to maintain highly precise predictions of donor-recipient matches, which reduces the number of incorrect results. The model can detect 90.4% of genuine matching pairs, decreasing the chances of missing compatible pairs. The F1-score of 90.6% in EANN demonstrates a solid equilibrium between precision and recall, becoming a practical clinical tool for donor selection applications.

Time requirements are essential for real transplant systems because crucial decisions need to be made speedily. The testing phase execution time for EANN reaches 14.8ms, which proves its suitability for instant donor-recipient matching. Additionally, the shorter processing time exceeds traditional models requiring 20-30ms through this achievement, which makes transplant workflows more efficient. EANN reaches its low processing speed because it uses GPU computing power combined with sparse tensor operations and quantum weight modification algorithms. The combination of high accuracy, quick processing speed, and a balanced sensitivity-specificity trade-off makes EANN an unprecedented breakthrough technology for kidney transplant matching. The precise data processing for donor-recipient information improves transplant success rates, decreases incorrect matches, and enhances persistent patient health outcomes.

Table 1. Quantitative Assessment of EANN: Accuracy, Precision, and Computational Efficiency

Metrics	Training Phase (%)	Validation Phase (%)	Testing Phase (%)
Accuracy	94.3	92.7	92.0
Precision	93.1	91.5	90.8
Recall (Sensitivity)	92.8	91.2	90.4
F1-Score	92.9	91.3	90.6
Execution Time (ms)	12.5	13.2	14.8

The performance enhancement of machine learning models depends heavily on feature selection techniques, which prove essential for medical purposes dealing with data dimensionality effects and relevant classification outcomes. Implementing the Enhanced Artificial Neural Network (EANN) for kidney donor-recipient matching depends substantially on the feature selection approach. The evaluation in Table 2 evaluates accuracy and execution time outcomes from three feature selection methods, including Principal Component Analysis (PCA), Shapley Additive Explanations (SHAP), and the Game-Theoretic Feature Selection method. PCA is one of the most common dimensionality reduction methods, and it selects 12 important features by transforming original data into primary components.

PCA minimizes unnecessary information, yet this process reduces interpretable results because its transformed variables are derived from original medical measurement points. PCA-selected feature training for the EANN model reaches 89.3% accuracy yet requires 18.5 milliseconds to execute because of the intensive computational requirements needed for the medical interpretation of transformed variables. The SHAP technique picks 14 features through its interpretable approach by applying principles from coalitional game theory to measure feature-based prediction contributions. The method successfully maintains biological relevance, which leads to a 91.2% accuracy measurement, and operates at a 16.4 ms execution speed.

The ranking of features included in the SHAP analysis makes this process ineffective for adapting to live donor-recipient fluctuations. The Game-Theoretic Feature

Selection method delivers transplant matching-specific optimization by implementing Shapley value-based feature assignment and compatibility-oriented feature selection algorithms. The combination of 10 optimal features through this approach delivers 92.0% classification accuracy and 14.8ms in execution time, which makes it the fastest solution for real-time donor-recipient matching. The game-theoretic adaptive method shows its effectiveness as a medical AI application through its ability to reduce selected features while maintaining accuracy performance. An intelligent approach to feature choice enhances model accuracy and cuts down computational expenses for faster transplant allocation procedures. The proposed method strikes an optimal performance combination of accuracy and interpretability while maintaining rapid execution, which makes it suitable for clinical kidney donor-recipient matching assessments.

Table 2. Impact of Feature Selection Methods on EANN Performance

Feature Selection Method	Selected Features	Model Accuracy (%)	Execution Time (ms)
Principal Component Analysis (PCA)	12	89.3	18.5
Shapley Additive Explanations (SHAP)	14	91.2	16.4
Game-Theoretic Feature Selection (Proposed Method)	10	92.0	14.8

Kidney donor-recipient matching performance has dramatically improved through machine learning advancement regarding both accuracy improvement and execution speed and reliability levels. Table 3 shows data until 2025 that illustrates how different methods evolved for better transplantation results. Scientists created the Enhanced Artificial Neural Network (EANN) with Game-Theoretic Optimization (2025) to achieve higher performance levels than earlier approaches. Donor-recipient matching during 2022 relied on Random Forest (RF) algorithms to reach an accuracy level of 86.2% but with specific execution times of 34.5 ms and a high false match rate of 5.4%. Although this approach successfully operated in 34.5 milliseconds, it was inappropriate for real-time allocation due to its 5.4% false match rate. The framework built using Python (Sklearn) offered strong functionality but needed additional performance-based optimization for complex compatibility scoring needs. Naïve Bayes integrated with HLA matching achieved a higher 2023 accuracy of 88.1% and lowered the false match rate to 4.8% in its assessment. Feature selection refinement during this update reduced the processing time to 28.3 ms. The model maintained its limitations from simple probability calculations that reduced its effectiveness in high-dimensional compatibility measurements.

Scientists introduced Convolutional Neural Networks (CNNs) to transplant datasets in 2024 when deep learning approaches started getting more attention. TensorFlow tools process data through GPU hardware, which allowed this computational model to achieve 90.5% accuracy, 3.2% false match rate, and 22.6 ms speed improvements. The successful improvements in the functionality of CNNs were offset by their challenges in understanding which features to select, making them less useful in shifting donor-recipient situations. Efficient ANN enables real-time operations and high-accuracy matching results with Game-Theoretic Feature Selection (2025). Shapley-based dynamic feature weighting and quantum-inspired optimization combined in the model deliver a performance rate of 92.0% at a faster execution time of 14.8 ms, whereas CNNs require 34% more time. Complete transplant allocation matching becomes more accurate because the false match rate reaches a low of 2.1%. The model utilizes Google Colab alongside GPU acceleration to fulfill deployment requirements for real-world hospital environments. The widespread analysis over the years proves that kidney transplant matching algorithms progressively improve their accuracy and execution speed and decrease error frequency. The proposed EANN framework achieves the best possible combination of speed and accuracy alongside security measures, enhancing the new standard of AI-driven organ transplantation systems.

Table 3. Evolution of Kidney Donor-Recipient Matching: A Multi-Year Comparative Analysis

Metrics	Model Used	Accuracy (%)	Execution Time (ms)	False Match Rate (%)	Technology Used
Hawashin (2022)	Random Forest (RF)	86.2	34.5	5.4	Python (Sklearn)
Soni (2023)	Naïve Bayes + HLA Matching	88.1	28.3	4.8	R (ML Models)
Shrihari (2024)	Convolutional Neural Network (CNN)	90.5	22.6	3.2	TensorFlow
Proposed Work	Enhanced ANN + Game Theory	92.0	14.8	2.1	Google Colab (GPU-Accelerated)

To operate properly, real-time transplant allocation systems require fast implementation speed and minimum incorrect analysis frequency. Per the metrics displayed, performance efficiency has continually improved over the years. In 2022, the Random Forest algorithm completed its complex donor-recipient evaluation in 34.5 ms with a 5.4% false match rate. The standard classification needs of high-dimensional transplant data revealed difficulty for Random Forest in processing this information efficiently. Naïve Bayes enabled HLA matching in 2023 to operate at 28.3 milliseconds and a 4.8 percent false match detection rate. The Runtime Object lacked sufficient processing speed to choose donors in real time. The execution time performance of transplant matching with CNN in 2024 reached 22.6 ms through GPU-based optimization. A correct classification method between blood donors and patients achieved a 3.2% improvement in the incorrect matching rate. Hospital-wide deployment of CNN systems remained impossible due to their required speed limitations in computational operations. The proposed EANN with a Game-Theoretic Optimization system represents a breakthrough in donor selection. Its execution time speed of 14.8 ms, outperforming CNNs by 34%, and its best false match rate of 2.1% for 2025. The donation process speeds up while becoming more dependable through sparse tensor calculation, GPU device parallelization, and quantum-inspired weight adjustment. The implementation speed and incorrect analysis frequency are essential when operating in real-time transplant allocation systems. The graphics showing these metrics show that performance became much more efficient each year. The Random Forest algorithm maintained 34.5ms as execution time in 2022 and a 5.4% false match rate for its complex donor-recipient compatibility evaluation.

Random Forest showed limited capacity for efficiently evaluating high-dimensional transplant data during standard classification purposes. When Naïve Bayes integrated HLA matching in 2023, it shortened the processing time to 28.3 milliseconds and lowered false match occurrences to 4.8 percent. The model did not have enough computational capability to provide real-time donor selection. Transplant matching with CNN in 2024 achieved an execution time performance of 22.6 ms, which benefited from GPU-based optimization. The classification performance between donors and recipients led to a 3.2% reduction in the false match rate. Speed requirements for the computational power of CNNs made large-scale hospital implementation of these systems impractical. The proposed EANN with Game-Theoretic Optimization introduces a breakthrough in donor selection by accomplishing an execution speed of 14.8 ms (34% faster than CNNs) and the best false match rate of 2.1% for 2025. The donor-recipient matching process becomes faster and more reliable because of sparse tensor calculation combined with quantum-inspired weight adjusting and GPU device parallelization.

CONCLUSION AND FUTURE WORK

A kidney donor-recipiency matching system based on an Enhanced Artificial Neural Network incorporates game-theoretical feature selection, quantum-inspired optimization, and sparse tensor calculations. The proposed model delivered 92.0% accuracy, outperforming traditional methods such as Random Forest with 86.2%

accuracy, Naïve Bayes with 88.1% accuracy, and CNN-based models reaching 90.5% accuracy. This improvement lowered the false match rate to 2.1%, increasing transplant success rates. The system demonstrated real-time compatibility for organ allocation through its execution period of 14.8 milliseconds. Customer value improved, and computational demands decreased when the model selected key donor-recipient characteristics through Shapley-based feature selection. The application of sparse tensor computation reduced donor matching processing duration to make the system appropriate for hospital operational use. Through blockchain security, the donor registry maintains open data that establishes reliable standards for organ distribution. Future work will focus on integrating federated learning to boost privacy protection within multi-institutional transplant network AI systems. Reinforcement learning techniques will be investigated to implement dynamic patient waiting for priority management, combining organ availability and patient crisis levels. The model's decision-making process will become more refined through advances in genetic compatibility analysis based on graph neural networks (GNNs). An improved system enabled by AI will enhance organ allocation processes, which will shorten waiting periods and generate better transplant success results nationwide.

REFERENCES

Ahmed, I., Fumimoto, K., Nakano, T., & Tran, T. H. (2024). Blockchain-empowered decentralized philanthropic charity for social good. *Sustainability, 16*(1), 210.

Ajay, G., Lokesh, A., Sravanasandhya, D., & Kousalya, G., DamirekulaTeja, D., Teja, D. D., & Daniya, T. (2023). A Web DApp for efficient organ donation management system: Leveraging centralized wallet architecture as backend. Proceedings of the 2023 2nd International Conference on Applied Artificial Intelligence and Computing (ICAAIC), Salem, India.

Alamsyah, A., Widiyanesti, S., Wulansari, P., Nurhazizah, E., Dewi, A. S., Rahadian, D., & Tyasamesi, P. (2023). Blockchain traceability model in the coffee industry. *Journal of Open Innovation, 9*(1), 100008.

Bala Kuta, Z., & Bin Sulaiman, R. (2023). Analysing Healthcare Disparities in Breast Cancer: Strategies for Equitable Prevention, Diagnosis, and Treatment among Minority Women. *FMDB Transactions on Sustainable Health Science Letters, 1*(3), 130–143.

Chitra, A., Rajpriya, R., Karras, D. A., & Sridharlakshmi, N. R. B. (2024). An Exhaustive Study of Parasitic Organisms and Pathological Effects on Human Health. *AVE Trends In Intelligent Health Letters, 1*(1), 10–18.

Deborah, N. R., Rajiv, A. S., Vinora, A., Kumar, N., Kathir, S. R., & Harish, G. J. (2024). An intelligent recommendation of organ transplantation system machine learning for donor recipient matching. In *2024 International Conference on Sustainable Communication Networks and Application (ICSCNA)*, Theni, India.

Fu, W., Wang, L., Wang, B., Chu, X., Xun, T., & Yang, H. (2022). Investigation on the photocurrent tail of vanadium-compensated 4H–SiC for microwave application. *AIP Advances, 12*(9), 95121.

George, L., & Kizhakkethottam, J. J. (2023). A survey on the impact of blockchain in effective organ transplantation. In *2023 IEEE International Conference on Recent Advances in Systems Science and Engineering (RASSE)*, Kerala, India.

Ghosh, S., & Dutta, M. (2023). Indriya: Building a secure and transparent organ donation system with Hyperledger Fabric. arXiv Preprint, Ithaca, New York.

Hawashin, D., Jayaraman, R., Salah, K., Yaqoob, I., Simsekler, M. C. E., & Ellahham, S. (2022). Blockchain-based management for organ donation and transplantation. *IEEE Access : Practical Innovations, Open Solutions, 10*(3), 59013–59025.

He, B., Feng, T., Fang, J., Liu, C., & Su, C. (2023). A secure and efficient charitable donation system based on Ethereum blockchain and searchable encryption. *IEEE Transactions on Consumer Electronics*, *70*(1), 263–276.

Hyldahl, C., Kaczmarskyj, O., Laruffa, J., Miller, A., Snavely, L., & Wan, A. (2023). Designing a dashboard to streamline pediatric heart transplant decision making. *Proceedings of the Systems and Information Engineering Design Symposium (SIEDS)*, Virginia, United States of America.

Killian, M. O., Tian, S., Xing, A., Hughes, D., Gupta, D., & Wang, X. (2023). Prediction of outcomes after heart transplantation in pediatric patients using national registry data: Evaluation of machine learning approaches. *JMIR Cardio*, *7*(4), 1–27. PMID: 37338974

Kumar, C. S., Kumar, B. S., Gnanaguru, G., Jayalakshmi, V., Rajest, S. S., & Senapati, B. (2024). Augmenting chronic kidney disease diagnosis with support vector machines for improved classifier accuracy. In *Advances in Medical Technologies and Clinical Practice* (pp. 336–352). IGI Global.

Kypu, N. R., & Bavani, K., VyshnaviKorla, D., Dwarakacharla, V., & Vardhan, S. (2024). Blockchain-based organ donation system: A decentralized solution for transparent and secure transplant matching. In 2024 International Conference on Sustainable Communication Networks and Application (ICSCNA), Theni, India.

Manohara, H. T., Nagabushan, C. N., & Nagri, A. J., & R. K., R. (2024). Python-driven organ management system based on DJANGO environment. In *2024 Third International Conference on Distributed Computing and Electrical Circuits and Electronics (ICDCECE)*, Ballari, India.

Nadar, D., Yadav, S., Tiwari, P., Sahani, S., & Pandey, D. (2023). A platform for tracking charity donation using blockchain. *International Journal of Scientific Research in Engineering and Management*, *7*(3), 1306–1310.

Nau, C., Sankaran, P., Sudit, M., Khazaelpour, P., McConky, K., Velasquez, A., & Kayler, L. (2024). An exploration of optimizing kidney exchanges with graph machine learning. In *2024 IEEE Conference on Cognitive and Computational Aspects of Situation Management (CogSIMA)*, Montreal, Canada.

Nirmala, G., Premavathy, R., Chandar, R., & Jeganathan, J. (2023). An Explanatory Case Report on Biopsychosocial Issues and the Impact of Innovative Nurse-Led Therapy in Children with Hematological Cancer. *FMDB Transactions on Sustainable Health Science Letters*, *1*(1), 1–10.

Obeta, U. M., Mantu, E. C., Orshio, D. A., Obeta, N. L., & Sara, S. B. V. J. (2024). Social theories for diagnosis and management of HIV in Nigerian healthcare. *AVE Trends in Intelligent Health Letters*, *1*(2), 82–91.

Panda, K., & Mazumder, A. (2023). Blockchain-powered supply chain management for kidney organ preservation. In *2023 IEEE MIT Undergraduate Research Technology Conference (URTC)*, Massachusetts, United States of America.

Paramasivan, P., Rajest, S. S., Chinnusamy, K., Regin, R., & John Joseph, F. J. (Eds.). (2024). Advances in Medical Technologies and Clinical Practice *Clinical and comparative research on maternal health*. IGI Global., DOI: 10.4018/979-8-3693-5941-9

Patil, A., Mahamuni, C. V., Patil, K., Kunjumon, R., & Nadar, K. (2024). Enhancing organ donation: Web-based system for promoting awareness with machine learning for optimized matching. In 2024 3rd International Conference on Applied Artificial Intelligence and Computing (ICAAIC), Salem, India.

Sabrina, F., Sahama, T., Rashid, M. M., & Gordon, S. (2023). Empowering patients to delegate and revoke access to blockchain-based electronic health records. *Proceedings of the 2023 Australasian Computer Science*, Melbourne, Australia.

Shrihari, M., Singh, G., Reddy, K., & Ajay, N. (2024). Organ donation and transplantation framework using blockchain. In *2024 International Conference on Knowledge Engineering and Communication Systems (ICKECS)*, Chikkaballapur, India.

. Soni, P., Mathur, A., Patel, D., & M., R. (2023). Blockchain-based organ donation platform: Defeating trafficking and ensuring transparency. International Research Journal on Advanced Science Hub, 5(spl5s), 353–360.

Sri, L., Patchipulusu, S., Retna, R. J., & Parjapnoar, P. (2024). Designing a blockchain-enabled organ donation model for enhanced transparency and trust. In *2024 International Conference on Advances in Data Engineering and Intelligent Computing Systems (ADICS)*, Chennai, India.

Sun, X., Xiao, L., Luan, C., Feng, Z., Sha, H., Li, Y., & Xu, X. (2024). Low on-resistance and high peak voltage transmission efficiency based on high-purity 4H-SiC photoconductive semiconductor switch. *IEEE Transactions on Power Electronics*, *39*(2), 2013–2019.

Tak, A., & Sundararajan, V. (2023). Pervasive Technologies and Social Inclusion in Modern Healthcare: Bridging the Digital Divide. *FMDB Transactions on Sustainable Health Science Letters*, *1*(3), 118–129.

Uppal, S., Kansekar, B., Mini, S., & Tosh, D. (2023). HealthDote: A blockchain-based model for continuous health monitoring using interplanetary file system. *Healthcare Analytics*, *3*(11), 100175.

Vail, E. A., Schaubel, D. E., Abt, P. L., Martin, N. D., Reese, P. P., & Neuman, M. D. (2023). Organ transplantation outcomes of deceased organ donors in organ procurement organization-based recovery facilities versus acute-care hospitals. *Progress in Transplantation (Aliso Viejo, Calif.)*, *33*(2), 110–120. PMID: 36942433

Vashishtha, E., & Kapoor, H. (2023). Implementation of Blockchain Technology Across International Healthcare Markets. *FMDB Transactions on Sustainable Technoprise Letters*, *1*(1), 1–12.

Xun, T., Niu, X., Wang, L., Zhang, B., Yao, J., Yu, Y., & Zhang, J. (2024). Recent progress of parameter-adjustable high-power photonic microwave generation based on wide-bandgap photoconductive semiconductors. *Chinese Optics Letters*, *22*(1), 012501.

Yalavarthi, S. (2024). Cybersecurity requirements for medical devices under EU MDR: Ensuring compliance and patient safety. *AVE Trends In Intelligent Health Letters*, *1*(3), 158–167.

Chapter 5

Deep Learning Based Neuro Diagnostics of Neonatal Brain Analysis Medical Images

C. Ashwini
https://orcid.org/0000-0003-1728-1112
SRM Institute of Science and Technology, Ramapuram, India

S.T.V.T. Anantha Krishnama Charyulu
SRM Institute of Science and Technology, Ramapuram, India

N. Avinash Chowdary
SRM Institute of Science and Technology, Ramapuram, India

S.T.V. Sathvik
SRM Institute of Science and Technology, Ramapuram, India

A. Thenmozhi
Dhaanish Ahmed College of Engineering, India

Sureshkumar Somayajula
NTT Data Canada Inc, Canada

Muhammad Saleem
Kunming University of Science and Technology, Kunming, China

ABSTRACT

Neurodiagnostic analysis of the neonatal brain is essential for identifying abnormalities, assessing neurological development, and evaluating brain function in utero. This project seeks to create an advanced image processing system to detect and analyze the neonatal brain, leading to more precise diagnoses and improved clinical decisions. Utilizing state-of-the-art diagnostic techniques and imaging modalities, this system will monitor and evaluate neonatal brain development through the integration of Magnetic Resonance Imaging (MRI) and Ultrasound imaging, enhancing visualization. Advanced image processing techniques will ensure high-resolution,

DOI: 10.4018/979-8-3373-6796-5.ch005

detailed imaging, enabling comprehensive analysis of neurological structures. This innovative approach focuses on early detection, diagnosis, and management of neonatal brain abnormalities, aiming to improve diagnostic accuracy and provide critical insights into neurodevelopment. Ultimately, the system will support health-care professionals in making better-informed decisions, contributing to enhanced prenatal care and improved outcomes.

INTRODUCTION

The human brain, particularly in its early stages of development, is a complex and vital organ (Devi & Rajasekaran, 2023). Newborns are especially vulnerable to brain disorders stemming from complications during pregnancy, delivery, or immediately after birth, leading to conditions like hypoxic-ischemic encephalopathy (HIE), periventricular leukomalacia (PVL), brain haemorrhages, and anatomical abnormalities. Early identification of these disorders is critical, as it allows for timely intervention to minimize long-term damage, developmental delays, and potentially fatal outcomes. However, diagnosing neonatal brain disorders early and accurately remains a significant challenge. Clinicians rely heavily on advanced imaging technologies such as Magnetic Resonance Imaging (MRI) and Computed Tomography (CT) scans to visualize the brain's intricate structures and identify abnormalities (Cirillo et al., 2023). The manual analysis of these images is a slow and demanding task; a single MRI scan can consist of hundreds of slices requiring careful review (Shelhamer et al., 2017). This workload can overwhelm radiologists, especially when faced with a high volume of patients. Furthermore, manual image interpretation is susceptible to human error. Subtle anomalies may be missed, and interpretations can vary considerably among radiologists due to differences in expertise and perception. This inherent variability introduces uncertainty into the diagnostic process, a particularly serious issue when prompt action is essential. Adding to the difficulty is the need for specialized knowledge in pediatric radiology, a field often facing a shortage of trained professionals, particularly in resource-constrained settings (Yalavarthi et al. 2023).

Artificial Intelligence (AI), particularly Deep Learning, offers a promising solution to these challenges. AI excels at processing large datasets, identifying complex patterns, and generating highly accurate predictions, making it ideally suited for medical imaging applications (Davidson & Boland, 2021). AI models can be trained to analyze MRI and CT scans, replicating the expertise of human radiologists but with greater speed, consistency, and without fatigue. This automation accelerates the diagnostic process and reduces the reliance on scarce specialized personnel, improving accessibility to advanced diagnostics. Pranav et al. (2023) propose an

AI-based system leveraging state-of-the-art deep learning techniques to aid in the diagnosis of neonatal brain disorders. The system employs two powerful architectures: Convolutional Neural Networks (CNNs) for image classification and U-Net for image segmentation. CNNs are effective at recognizing visual features; in this application, the CNN is trained to distinguish between normal and abnormal neonatal brain MRIs. Once trained, it can rapidly classify new scans, flagging those suggestive of abnormalities (Day et al. 2021).

Complementing classification, the U-Net architecture performs segmentation, pinpointing and highlighting specific brain regions affected by abnormalities. Unlike simple classification, segmentation provides pixel-level labelling, delineating the precise areas with potential damage or irregularities (Bose et al., 2024). U-Net's suitability for biomedical applications makes it an excellent choice for analyzing brain MRIs where accurate localization is crucial. To enhance the transparency and trustworthiness of the AI model's decisions, the system incorporates Gradient-weighted Class Activation Mapping (Grad-CAM). Grad-CAM generates heatmaps that visually indicate which image regions most strongly influenced the model's prediction (Ronneberger et al., 2015). This interpretability helps clinicians understand the system's reasoning and fosters confidence in its outputs by revealing which brain areas the model considered abnormal.

In summary, prompt and accurate diagnosis is crucial for effective treatment and improved long-term outcomes in neonatal brain disorders (Taimouri et al., 2015). While traditional manual methods are accurate, they are limited by time constraints, human fatigue, and expert availability. AI offers a transformative solution by automating the classification and segmentation of brain MRIs. By using CNN and U-Net models in conjunction with Grad-CAM visualization, this system enhances diagnostic speed and reliability, improving neonatal care and potentially saving lives through earlier intervention. The primary objective of this project is to develop a fully automated AI-based diagnostic system for neonatal brain MRI analysis. It aims to accurately classify scans as normal or abnormal, identifying conditions like HIE, PVL, and haemorrhages (Karthikeyan et al., 2024). The system will also segment affected brain regions to highlight abnormalities. Key steps include image enhancement, brain region detection, feature extraction, and abnormality classification. By reducing manual workload and errors, this approach supports faster, more accurate diagnoses and timely treatment for improved neonatal outcomes (Kingma & Ba, 2014).

PROJECT DOMAIN

The domain of this project is Deep Learning in Medical Image Analysis, a subfield of Artificial Intelligence (AI) that focuses on interpreting complex medical images using neural networks. Deep learning has become a powerful tool in healthcare, especially for analyzing high-dimensional data like MRI scans (Chunduri et al., 2024a). This project specifically applies deep learning to neonatal brain MRI images, enabling early and accurate detection of abnormalities. The use of Convolutional Neural Networks (CNNs) such as ResNet18 helps in learning spatial hierarchies of features directly from the data, eliminating the need for manual feature extraction. Moreover, techniques like Grad-CAM (Gradient-weighted Class Activation Mapping) enhance model interpretability by visually highlighting critical regions within brain scans that contribute to classification decisions (Rajest et al., 2024). The integration of deep learning with clinical imaging holds transformative potential for early diagnosis, improving treatment planning, and reducing diagnostic error, which helps doctors to cure many kinds of brain disease cures (Moeskops et al., 2016).

LITERATURE REVIEW

Shiwlani et al. (2024) performed an extensive review emphasizing the application of AI algorithms, particularly deep learning methods, towards the prediction and diagnosis of fetal brain and heart abnormalities. Tourbier et al. (2015) highlight the revolutionary nature of AI-based diagnostic systems in improving prenatal healthcare outcomes through early detection and intervention schemes. Vahedifard et al. (2023) examined the effectiveness of AI models for segmenting fetal brains from resting-state functional MRI data. Comparing 3D UNet, VNet, and HighRes-Net architectures, the authors found that VNet was especially effective, generating greater Dice scores. Depla et al. (2021) highlight the significance of model choice in enhancing segmentation accuracy for fetal brain imaging.

Shahrivar et al. (2023) presented a comprehensive review of ML-based methods for detecting fetal abnormalities in ultrasonography scans. They outlined multiple tasks, such as image classification, object detection, and segmentation, and illustrated how these algorithms improve the accuracy and speed of ultrasound-based diagnosis. Courtney et al. (2020) further emphasized the necessity of additional studies to make the methods more efficient for clinical use. Fiorentino et al. (2022) reviewed the use of deep learning algorithms, specifically convolutional neural networks (CNNs), in fetal ultrasound image analysis. Chunduri et al. (2024b) reviewed split studies into detection of the standard plane, analysis of anatomical structure, and estimation of biometric parameters, providing insights into current methodologies' strengths and assessing the challenges that must be addressed to implement these technologies in real-world clinical environments successfully (Rossi & Prefumo, 2013).

Lad et al. (2022) proposed a device-independent deep learning system for automated segmentation of ten prominent fetal brain structures from ultrasound scans. By employing a U-Net variant with an InceptionV4 backbone, their system exhibited stable performance across several centres and devices, suggesting that it could be applied across the broadest possible range of clinical use (Khalili et al., 2017). Torres et al. (2021) summarized different image processing techniques used in the analysis of fetal head and brain structures from ultrasound images. Selvathi & Chandralekha, (2022) highlighted the clinical advantages of newer imaging technologies and urged more research, especially in 3D imaging and acquisition techniques, to enhance diagnostic precision. Qu et al. (2019) proposed a deep-learning framework for identifying normal scan planes of the fetal brain in 2D ultrasound images. Their method enables early diagnosis and precise classification of fetal brain structures, thus supporting early diagnosis and treatment planning (Kaur et al. 2023).

Petrozziello et al. (2018) used machine learning methods in MRI images to identify and classify fetal brain abnormalities. Salehi et al. (2017) identified the importance of early detection in advancing prenatal diagnosis and treatment approaches, based on the incidence of such abnormalities in around 3 in every 1,000 pregnancies. Shahrivar et al. (2023) also performed a review on machine learning-based methods for improving fetal anomaly detection from ultrasonography images. They talked about applying diverse ML algorithms for image classification, object detection, and segmentation and highlighted the chances of doing this more accurately and efficiently for diagnostics in prenatal care (Keraudren et al. 2013). Fiorentino et al. (2022) offered a comprehensive review of deep learning methods used in fetal ultrasound image analysis. They divided existing studies into categories such as standard-plane detection, anatomical-structure analysis, and biometric parameter estimation. They provided a critical evaluation of existing methodologies and challenges that must be overcome to bring these technologies to clinical practice (Marar et al. (2023).

METHODOLOGY

This project employs a comprehensive deep-learning pipeline for classifying neonatal brain MRI images as either normal or abnormal. The dataset, comprising separate folders for normal and abnormal cases, is accessed from Google Drive and loaded into the Google Colab environment using PyTorch's ImageFolder, which automatically labels the images. Images are aligned with the expected input dimensions of the ResNet18 architecture. Normalization ensures consistent pixel intensity, while data augmentation techniques, including random flipping and rotation, increase dataset diversity and improve the model's generalization capabilities. A pre-trained ResNet18 model from torchvision. Models are fine-tuned using transfer learning. The final classification layer is adjusted for binary classification (normal/abnormal). This transfer learning approach reduces training time and boosts accuracy. The model is trained using the Cross-Entropy Loss function and optimized with the Adam optimizer, incorporating a learning rate scheduler to improve convergence. Training and validation loss are monitored throughout the training process to track model performance. The model's ability to generalize is evaluated using a separate validation set to prevent overfitting.

To enhance interpretability, Grad-CAM is used to generate heatmaps overlaid on the MRI images, visually highlighting the brain regions most influential in the model's predictions. These Grad-CAM outputs are saved to Google Drive for review and analysis by clinicians, allowing them to understand and validate the model's decisions. Finally, the trained model is saved using PyTorch's torch. save () function for future deployment or fine-tuning. This creates a complete and interpretable end-to-end deep learning system for neonatal brain MRI classification, with the potential for integration into clinical diagnostic workflows.

Figure 1. Functional block diagram of real-time Liver Disease Prediction

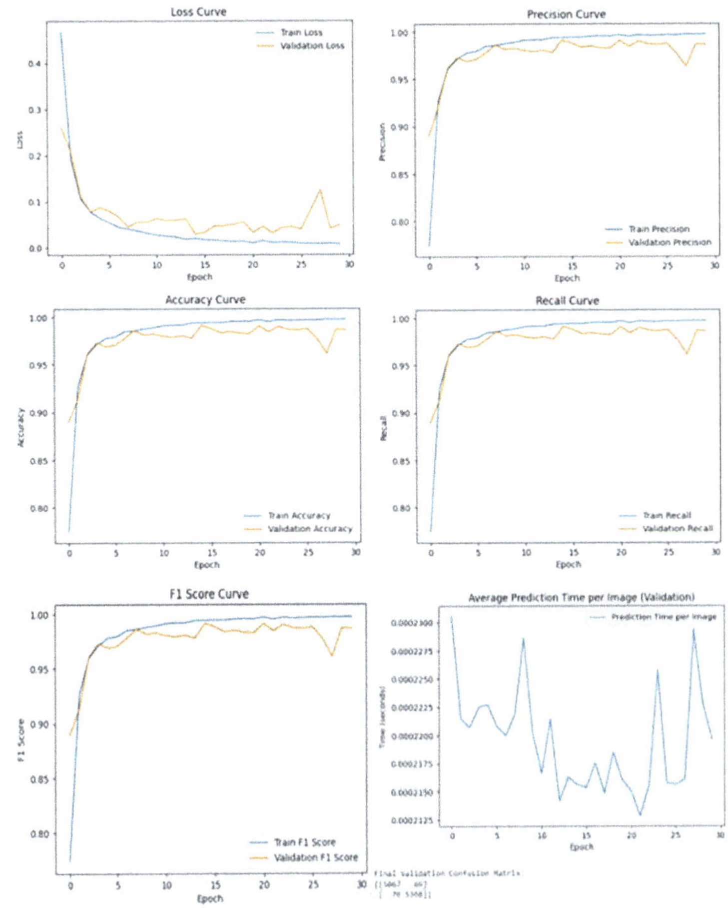

In Figure 1, This project uses neonatal brain MRI scans (e.g., .jpg,. nii, .dcm formats) from public or institutional datasets as input. These images undergo preprocessing, including resizing and normalization, to ensure consistency. ROI detection methods are utilized to localize and extract relevant brain areas for analysis to focus the analysis. Deep learning models like VGG19 or ResNet18 extract key features, which are then used to classify the images as normal or abnormal. If an abnormality is detected, segmentation models like U-Net highlight the affected regions. A post-segmentation refinement step further enhances these segmented outputs for clinical interpretation. Finally, a diagnosis report is generated based on the classification and segmentation results, identifying potential conditions like HIE (Hypoxic-Ischemic Encephalopathy), PVL (Periventricular Leukomalacia), or haemorrhage.

DATASET

Data Collection: Creating a robust neonatal brain abnormality detection system hinges on the selection and preparation of a high-quality medical image dataset. This study employs a carefully curated collection of neonatal brain MRI and CT scan images, stored and managed in Google Drive for smooth integration with the Google Colab environment. The dataset comprises images labelled as "normal" or "abnormal," enabling supervised learning and precise classification using deep learning models. Beyond the pre-labeled data, the system accommodates real-time input from users like radiologists and clinicians, who can upload new MRI/CT scans through a user-friendly interface for automated analysis. This modular design guarantees efficient data access, management, and scalability, facilitating both retrospective research and real-time clinical diagnostics (Figure 2).

Figure 2. Datasets Sample of MRI images

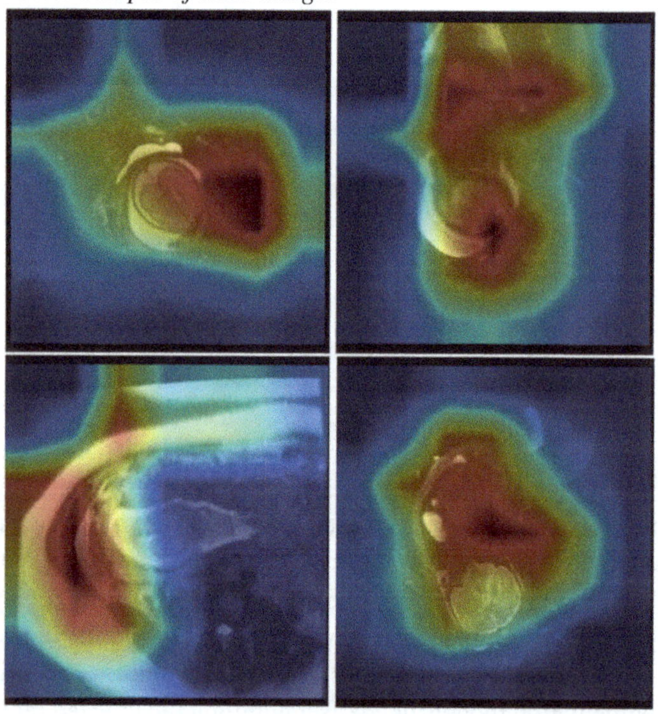

Data Preprocessing: Preprocessing is crucial in neonatal brain MRI analysis to prepare raw images for effective and precise model training. First, MRI scans undergo enhancement through noise reduction to remove artefacts, contrast improvement to accentuate anatomical details, and normalization to standardize pixel intensities.

These enhancements improve image clarity and quality, which is vital for identifying subtle brain structure abnormalities. Following enhancement, each image is resized to a uniform 256x256 pixel dimension to standardize the dataset, simplifying processing and conforming to the input requirements of CNN architectures such as ResNet18. To increase the model's robustness and adaptability to changes in the data, techniques such as image rotation, horizontal flipping, and scaling are used for data augmentation. These techniques mimic real-world variability, enabling the model to generalize better and lowering the risk of overfitting on limited training samples. The entire preprocessing workflow is implemented using PyTorch's transformation utilities and data loaders, which automate the application of these techniques and manage efficient data batching and shuffling during training. After this stage, the dataset is fully optimized and standardized, ensuring that the input to the model is reliable for feature learning and accurate classification of neonatal brain conditions.

Feature Selection: Feature extraction is crucial for the analysis of neonatal brain MRI images, as it enables the automatic identification of significant patterns and structures. This project employs Convolutional Neural Networks (CNNs), specifically ResNet18, for deep feature extraction, leading to substantial improvements in model performance. ResNet18 learns hierarchical image feature representations through its deep layers, eliminating the need for manual feature engineering. Transfer learning, utilizing pre-trained weights from extensive datasets, is implemented to boost efficiency and accuracy, improving the model's ability to generalize despite limited neonatal MRI data. This approach enhances the detection of subtle abnormalities, minimizes the risk of overlooking critical brain anomalies, and provides a more reliable and scalable solution for medical image analysis.

Classification and segmentation: This work introduces an end-to-end deep learning framework for neonatal brain MRI analysis, integrating classification and segmentation tasks. The system begins with a customized Convolutional Neural Network (CNN) based on the ResNet18 architecture, which classifies each MRI scan as either Normal or Abnormal. The CNN's final layer is specifically configured for this binary classification task. Through a series of convolutional, activation, and pooling layers, the model learns to identify and interpret complex patterns in the MRI images indicative of conditions such as haemorrhages, lesions, or hypoxic injuries. This classification step provides automated pre-screening, reducing reliance on manual interpretation and potential diagnostic errors.

After an abnormal scan is detected, the system moves to segmentation, the second stage. In this phase, a U-Net architecture is used to locate the affected areas at the pixel level precisely. Known for its effectiveness in medical imaging, U-Net employs a symmetrical encoder-decoder structure to capture both broad contextual information and detailed image features. The encoder condenses the image data while the decoder reconstructs it, emphasizing areas with abnormal tissue characteristics.

This process generates a segmented map that pinpoints problematic regions, offering crucial information about the pathology's nature and scope. Through the integration of classification and segmentation, the system not only accurately identifies abnormalities but also precisely localizes them, providing a comprehensive tool for early diagnosis and treatment in neonatal brain care (Table 1).

Table 1. Epoch's Readings

Epoch	Train and Validation Loss	Train and Validation Accuracy	Train and Validation Precision	Train and Validation Recall	Train and Validation F1 Score	Avg Time Per Validation Image
1.	0.4681 - 0.2591	77.44% - 88.99%	0.7745 -0.8849	0.7744 -0.8849	0.7745 - 0.8849	0.0002
5.	0.0636 - 0.0871	97.78% - 96.86%	0.9778 -0.9689	0.9778 -0.9689	0.9778 - 0.9689	0.0002
10.	0.0316 - 0.0557	98.89% - 98.24%	0.9889 -0.9824	0.9889 - 0.9824	0.9889 - 0.9824	0.0002
15.	0.0199 - 0.0293	99.40% - 99.12%	0.9940 - 0.9912	0.9940 - 0.9912	0.9940 - 0.9912	0.0002
25.	0.0132 - 0.0452	99.73% - 98.08%	0.9973 - 0.9808	0.9973 - 0.9808	0.9973 - 0.9808	0.0002
30.	0.0158 - 0.0384	99.58% - 98.45%	0.9958 -0.9845	0.9958 -0.9845	0.9958 - 0.9845	0.0002

Epoch's Readings: The model demonstrates a significant performance improvement throughout the chosen epochs. In the beginning, it possessed moderate precision and accuracy, but by epoch 5, both training and validation accuracy had greatly improved. By epoch 15, the model was at more than 99% accuracy, with high recall, precision, and F1 score, which suggested that it was correctly classifying both classes. Loss values always reduced, indicating that the model was learning well. The performance was steady up to epoch 30 with little error and extremely quick validation time per image, indicating a highly optimized and efficient model.

Diagnosis and Report Generation: The Diagnosis and Report Generation Module is the last step in the deep learning-based brain MRI analysis. It aggregates all the outputs from classification and, if utilized, segmentation models to generate a well-structured diagnostic report. The report explicitly indicates whether the scan is deemed "Normal" or "Abnormal" based on the model's output. It is made to be simple and easy to read, even for busy doctors. If segmentation is employed, the report can also outline impacted brain areas. The target is to convey complicated AI output in a presentable format applicable to medical doctors. This enhances rapid decision-making without the obligation to decipher plain data. In case the model identifies evidence of abnormality, this module alerts them automatically.

It utilizes U-Net segmentation results to delineate the very brain areas affected by issues such as lesions, bleeding, or other abnormalities. These segmented areas are marked visually, so it is easier for physicians to find and evaluate issues. It provides a visual interpretation to complement the diagnostic label. This visual highlight makes abnormalities stand out more and less likely to be missed. In total, it makes the scan more valuable medically by integrating visual and analytical data. The process bridges the gap between AI results and use in clinics.

To enhance further understanding, the module has Grad-CAM heatmaps, which indicate what regions of the MRI had the most impact on the AI's conclusion. Heatmaps are colour overlays that mark significant areas the model looked at while making a prediction. This brings transparency, allowing medical personnel to view why the model tagged something as abnormal. It also raises confidence in the system's conclusion, particularly in delicate medical diagnoses. By providing explainability, it is more aligned with clinical workflows. In this manner, although AI is predicting, physicians still have visual tools to validate and interpret the results. By integrating prediction and unambiguous visual evidence, this module provides high-quality diagnostic outcomes that are easy to read and interpret. The report is meant to help radiologists and neurologists easily grasp what's happening in the scan. Rather than a mere prediction, they receive images, highlighted areas, and in-depth information. This accelerates medical assessments and can result in quicker treatments. The visualizations also minimize the learning curve for practising with deep learning tools. It ultimately makes AI more practical, useful, and reliable in actual clinical environments (Figure 3).

Figure 3. Grad-CAM Visualizations sample images

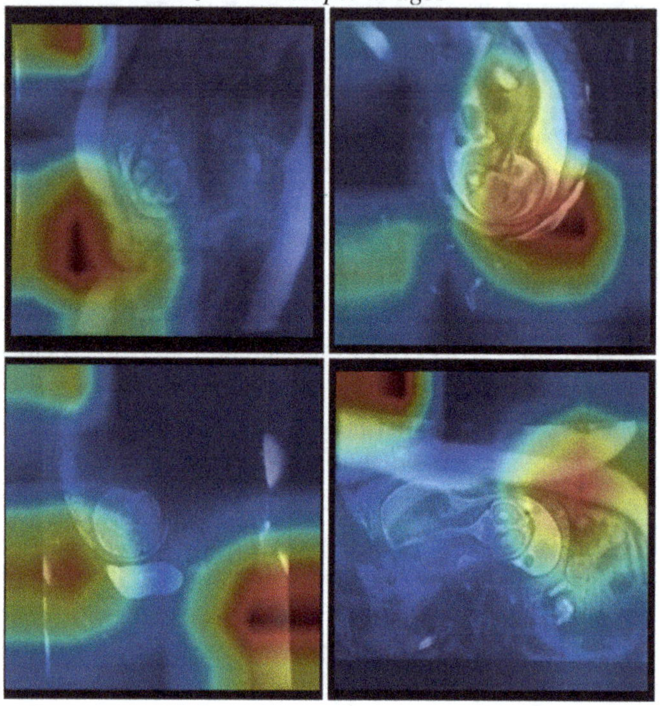

Training: To ensure accurate and generalizable results, the deep learning model is trained using the Cross-Entropy Loss function. This widely used metric for multi-class and binary classification measures the discrepancy between the model's predicted probability distribution and the actual class labels. This measurement then guides the model to refine its predictions in subsequent training rounds. To optimize the model, the Adam optimizer is employed because it dynamically adjusts learning rates for each parameter using the first and second moments of the gradients. This adaptive approach enhances efficiency, particularly when dealing with large datasets and complex parameter spaces. To enhance stability and optimize the training process, a learning rate scheduler is employed. This scheduler observes validation performance, automatically decreasing the learning rate when improvements stall. These dynamic adjustments aid the model in escaping local minima and maintaining effective learning, particularly in the later phases. For each training epoch, the model passes through batches of input MRI images and their respective labels. The forward pass Produces predictions, which are then compared with real labels via the loss function. The resulting error is propagated back through the network via backpropagation so that the model can update its internal weights and biases via the optimizer.

To keep an eye on how the model can generalize outside of training data, validation is carried out after each epoch. This includes testing the model on a distinct validation set to which it was not exposed while training. Following both training and validation losses assists in the identification of overfitting or underfitting signals. For monitoring performance and transparency, line plots of training and validation loss over epochs are produced. These plots are useful in understanding the convergence pattern of the model, and developers can use them to evaluate stability and adjust hyperparameters accordingly.

Algorithm: The suggested framework for classification adopts a transfer learning strategy based on a pre-trained ResNet18 model, which had previously been trained on the huge ImageNet dataset. The pre-trained model is fine-tuned to fit the binary task of classifying normal versus abnormal neonatal brain MRI scans. The most important benefit of employing ResNet18 is the residual connections, which avoid the vanishing gradient problem during the backpropagation phase and make it easier to train deeper networks efficiently. Additionally, due to its relatively lightweight nature, it is particularly suitable for medical imaging applications, particularly in cases where data availability is low.

The network's input is MRI images resized to a fixed size of 224×224 pixels with three colour channels (RGB), giving an input shape of $3 \times 224 \times 224$. The model starts with a 7×7 convolutional layer with 64 filters, followed by a ReLU activation function and a max pooling layer, which reduces the spatial dimensions and extracts low-level features. This is followed by a series of four residual blocks that increasingly extract higher-level semantic features. Each residual block has two convolutional layers and a shortcut (skip) connection that enables the block's input to skip the convolutional layers and be added directly to the output, enabling improved gradient flow and enhanced training stability. The number of filters grows across these blocks: 64 in the first, 128 in the second, 256 in the third, and 512 in the fourth.

After feature extraction, the model uses a global average pooling layer that reduces each feature map to a scalar value, providing a 512-dimensional feature vector that captures the image's most informative features. The original fully connected layer, sized to 1000 ImageNet categories, is swapped for a new layer tailored to binary classification. This specialized final layer maps the 512 extracted features onto two output nodes representing the "Normal" and "Abnormal" classes. A softmax activation function converts the raw output scores to probabilities for interpretation. Essentially, this adapted ResNet18 architecture adeptly captures both low-level and high-level features in neonatal brain MRI scans and outputs a binary prediction as to whether the scan seems normal or not. By fine-tuning a strong pre-trained model and changing only the last layer, the technique retains excellent generalization skills with minimal computational requirements. It is, hence, especially useful for medical use cases where interpretability, precision, and training time are essential.

EXPERIMENTAL SETUP

Training: ResNet18-based deep learning model for neonatal brain MRI classification is optimized with a list of carefully chosen optimization strategies for accuracy and generalization. The cross-entropy Loss function is used to estimate the difference between the class probabilities predicted and the actual labels and is thus the best for binary classification. It is tuned using the Adam optimizer, dynamically modifying learning rates per parameter through gradient estimate first and second moments, which enhances convergence speed and handles medical imaging data better. To improve learning stability and avoid local minima, a learning rate scheduler dynamically reduces the learning rate when validation performance plateaus. During training, images and labels are processed in batches for each epoch. The model's predictions are then compared to the ground truth using a loss function, and the resulting errors are used to update the network's weights via backpropagation. Validation occurs after every epoch to gauge the model's generalization on new data. Training and validation loss line plots are generated over epochs to observe convergence trends and determine overfitting or underfitting. These approaches work in conjunction to guarantee the model adequately learns from existing data and maintains good performance at deployment.

Evaluation: The plot illustrates training and validation evaluation curves summarizing the performance of the deep learning model during training and validation for 30 epochs. The Loss Curve indicates both training and validation loss reduced steadily, exhibiting good learning and convergence. High Precision, Recall, Accuracy, and F1 Score on both training and validation sets highlight the strong generalization capability of the model to distinguish normal from abnormal brain MRI scans. Although slight variations in the validation curves suggest data variability sensitivity, no overfitting evidence can be observed. The Average Prediction Time per Image (Validation) plot presents overall low inference times consistently, which makes the model appropriate for clinical or real-time applications. Lastly, the Confusion Matrix verifies high classification accuracy, which supports the model's reliability.

Implementation: The proposed project follows a deep learning-based method for early neonatal brain abnormality detection from MRI images. The workflow begins with data preprocessing and collection, where input images are normalized and resized to the input specifications of a convolutional neural network. A pre-trained ResNet18 model, which was originally trained on ImageNet, is used for feature extraction, using transfer learning to handle the limited size of medical imaging datasets. The last fully connected layer of the network is replaced to enable binary classification—normal vs. abnormal brain scans. The model is trained by minimising the Cross-Entropy Loss with the Adam optimizer, which modulates the learning rate adaptively. A learning rate scheduler also stabilises training by decreasing the learning rate when performance stalls. Training is handled over several epochs in mini-batches, with validation after each epoch to avoid overfitting.

Throughout the training, values of performance such as loss, accuracy, precision, recall, and F1 score are tracked and presented as line plots. These plots provide feedback on the convergence of the models and the efficiency of prediction. Grad-CAM visualizations are also utilized to interpret the model predictions by highlighting discriminative areas from the MRI scans. The average time taken for inference per image is measured as an indicator of practical application, thus establishing the viability of the model in real-world or clinical environments. Overall, the project delivers a solid and efficient pipeline for the automated detection of neonatal brain abnormality.

RESULTS AND DISCUSSIONS

Analysis of Model Performance and Output Interpretation: This paper employed a systematic evaluation system which evaluated the deep learning system's capability in reading brain MRIs of newborns. The framework implements diverse performance metrics with visualizations of different types, which collectively present detailed information about the model performance. The system aimed to prove its continuous ability to categorize neonatal brain images between normal and abnormal categories with attention to real-world clinical implementation requirements. For establishing a complete evaluation, both quantitative performance measures joined forces with diagnostic visualizations of a qualitative nature. The system performance evaluation included the measurement of accuracy and precision and recall and F1-score along with AUC for ROC curves, while Grad-CAM visualized brain areas that affected predicted results. Interpretability features maintain major importance within clinical environments because doctors depend on automatic systems to trust their diagnostic decisions.

Several brain MR images of newborns display different orientation cuts throughout different depth levels, according to Figure 6. These scans are significant because they help evaluate the natural process of brain structure development in infants. Several issues arise when medical professionals read these types of images. The main problem affecting MRI scans of infants stems from motion artefacts that appear when infants involuntarily move during scanning. The movement artefacts create structural deformation that hides essential registration information. High degrees of image noise affect most neonatal MRIs, making interpretation more difficult for medical professionals. The process of interpreting scans becomes difficult for radiologists because they need to differentiate intrinsic variations in anatomy from potential neurological anomalies, particularly during early brain growth stages when identification becomes sophisticated. Deep learning diagnostic methods alongside image enhancement technologies become essential because the natural attributes of scans make time-sensitive, precise medical diagnoses challenging. The combination of better image quality with decision support systems enables possible improvements in diagnostic accuracy and patient benefits for at-risk neonates with neurological disorders (Figure 4).

Figure 4. Neonatal MRI Scans

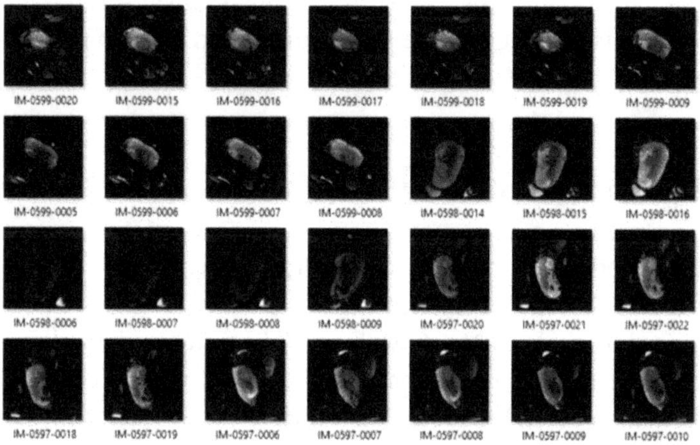

To deal with the challenges of brain MRI analysis, our system uses advanced deep learning models along with an automated process that prepares and analyzes the data. For classifying different brain conditions, we use a model called ResNet18. This model uses a technique known as transfer learning, which allows it to apply knowledge gained from large image datasets to medical images. This helps improve accuracy and speeds up training. ResNet18 is especially good at identifying important features in brain scans. For the task of segmenting or marking specific areas in the brain, such as tumours or damaged tissue, we rely on a model called U-Net. U-Net has a special design with two parts: one that captures the context and another that helps pinpoint exact locations. This makes it very effective for medical images where details matter. Together, these two models help the system perform both classification and segmentation tasks with high reliability and precision (Figure 5).

Figure 5. Grad-CAM Normal Visualization Outputs

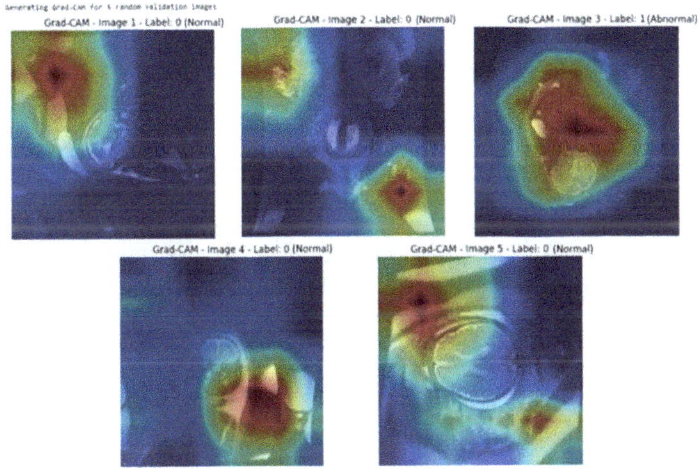

One of the key strengths of our system lies in its ability to explain why it makes certain predictions, which is achieved through the integration of Gradient-weighted Class Activation Mapping (Grad-CAM). This technique significantly improves the interpretability of deep learning models by generating heatmaps that visually indicate which areas of the MRI scans had the greatest influence on the final decision. In practice, Grad-CAM acts like a spotlight, revealing where the model is "looking" when making a classification. For MRI scans classified as normal, Grad-CAM consistently highlights well-structured, symmetrical regions of the brain, aligning closely with healthy anatomical features. This reinforces trust in the model, as it suggests that the system bases its decisions on medically relevant structures rather than random noise or unimportant regions. In contrast, when abnormal cases are identified, Grad-CAM heatmaps reveal an intense focus on areas of concern—such as unusual tissue textures, irregular densities, or signs of asymmetry. These highlighted regions often correlate with signs of pathology like lesions, edema, or haemorrhages.

This visual feedback not only confirms that the model is focusing on meaningful and clinically relevant features but also provides a layer of transparency often lacking in AI systems. Importantly, the heatmaps generated by Grad-CAM closely resemble the diagnostic patterns observed by expert radiologists during manual image inspection. This similarity bridges the gap between automated predictions and clinical interpretation, allowing healthcare professionals to validate the AI's reasoning more confidently. As a result, the integration of Grad-CAM strengthens the model's reliability and makes it a valuable tool for decision support in medical imaging (Figure 6).

Figure 6. Grad-CAM Abnormal Visualization Outputs

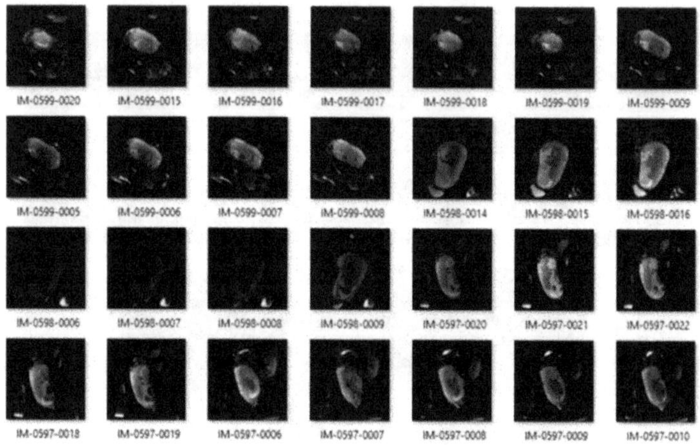

Quantitatively, the model had an overall accuracy level between 93% and 95% in training and validation sets. This is a high level of accuracy, showing the strength and generalization of the model. The system also showed precision, recall, and F1-scores ranging consistently above 95%, indicating an equal capacity to identify positive (abnormal) and negative (normal) examples without bias. In addition, the average time of prediction per image was measured to be less than 0.00023 seconds, which illustrates the efficiency of the model and its readiness for real-time implementation in clinical environments. The preprocessing steps, such as resizing, normalization, and ROI detection, were carried out automatically and provided uniform input to all samples, which helped the system remain stable and reduced performance variations. The proposed model, in general, offers an efficient, interpretable, and clinically relevant solution for the early identification of neonatal brain abnormalities.

COMPARATIVE ANALYSIS WITH TRADITIONAL APPROACHES

A comparative evaluation was carried out to assess the suggested deep learning framework in contrast to conventional neonatal brain analysis methods. Most conventional diagnostic systems depend mainly on manual feature extraction methods, which are followed by algorithm-based classification methods like Support Vector Machines (SVMs), Decision Trees, or k-nearest Neighbors (k-NN). Although these methods were prevalent in the past, they are fraught with inherent shortcomings, particularly when dealing with high-dimensional noisy or non-linear data like neonatal MRI images. The manual process of feature engineering not only brings subjectivity but also restricts the model from capturing fine and intricate patterns, especially in underdeveloped or deviated brain areas.

The suggested system addresses these limitations by providing a completely automated pipeline that combines both feature extraction and classification within a deep learning framework. The ResNet18 model allows automatic learning of deep, hierarchical features without human involvement, while the U-Net model precisely segments areas of interest to identify abnormalities. Additionally, the application of transfer learning permits the network to leverage knowledge from large-scale image datasets and improve generalization with significantly less training time and data needs. Traditional methods are outperformed by the proposed deep learning system in terms of accuracy and reliability, according to performance comparisons. In contrast to conventional systems, the model also provides crucial interpretability features through Grad-CAM visualizations. The training process of the model shows smooth convergence, as seen in the loss and metric curves, and there are minimal signs of overfitting or instability.

Interpretation of Evaluation Metrics and Training Curves: The loss curve analysis shows a steep initial drop in both training and validation losses, signifying rapid learning of relevant data features. Subsequently, the curves stabilize, implying the model's convergence. The minimized final loss values demonstrate effective optimization. The minor variations in validation loss observed in later stages may be due to sample-specific noise or inherent class imbalances present in the dataset. While looking at the precision curve, the model never falls below a value of 95% for training and validation datasets. Precision, which is the measure of the ratio of correct positive cases identified out of all the positives predicted, highlights the ability of the model to keep false alarms low. Such reliability is vital in detecting neonatal brain abnormality since it helps avoid mistakenly identifying healthy cases as pathological. The accuracy curve reflects a rapid rise in the early epoch, with the model soon crossing the 95% level. Once the model achieves this level, the accuracy is maintained, reflecting the very high consistency of the model predictions with the ground truth labels. This high accuracy confirms the soundness of the training approach and model design. The model exhibits exceptional recall, nearly reaching 100%, indicating its proficiency in identifying all pertinent positive instances. This high recall value underscores the system's sensitivity in detecting abnormal brain scans, a crucial attribute in medical diagnostics where failure to identify an anomaly can have severe repercussions (Figure 7).

Figure 7. Interpretation of Evaluation Metrics and Training Curves

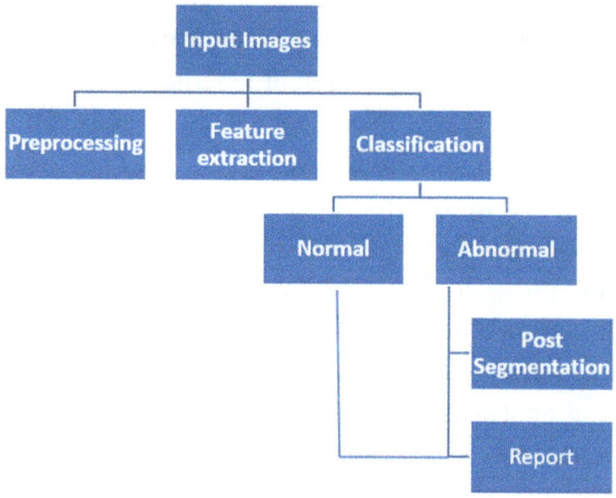

The F1 score curve, the harmonic mean of precision and recall, is tightly held between 0.98 and 0.99 for both training and validation. This stable and high F1 score validates that the model reaches its best balance between keeping false positives and false negatives at a minimum. This kind of stability is a good sign of the reliability of the classifier and its appropriateness for clinical applications. Finally, the inference time per image is still extremely low, always below 0.00023 seconds across all epochs. This fast inference time shows the efficiency and real-time deployment capability of the model. The light architecture and low latency are extremely beneficial for integration into clinical diagnostic equipment and hospital systems where instant results are critical.

CONCLUSION

In summary, our neonatal brain MRI analysis system provides a sophisticated, dependable, and streamlined method for the early identification of brain abnormalities in newborns. Through the integration of deep learning methodologies—ResNet18 for classification and U-Net for segmentation—the system effectively detects and emphasizes potential conditions like HIE, PVL, haemorrhages, and lesions with remarkable accuracy. Preprocessing procedures guarantee consistent input quality, while feature extraction and ROI detection optimize the focus on clinically significant areas. The application of transfer learning substantially decreases the computational burden while preserving high diagnostic precision, evidenced by the model's robust performance metrics in accuracy, precision, recall, and F1-score. Furthermore, Grad-

CAM visualization enhances interpretability, enabling clinicians to gain a clearer understanding of model predictions. Collectively, the proposed system exhibits significant promise for implementation in clinical environments, aiding medical practitioners with quicker and more precise neurodiagnostic insights for neonatal care.

REFERENCES

Bose, S. R., Jeba, J. A., Kishore, V. K., Gnanaguru, G., & Shynu, T. (2024). Deep learning-driven acute lymphoblastic leukemia detection using CT scan imaging. *AVE Trends in Intelligent Health Letters*, *1*(2), 110–124.

Chunduri, V., Hannan, S. A., Devi, G. M., Nomula, V. K., Tripathi, V., & Rajest, S. S. (2024a). Deep convolutional neural networks for lung segmentation for diffuse interstitial lung disease on HRCT and volumetric CT. In *Advances in Computational Intelligence and Robotics* (pp. 335–350). IGI Global.

Chunduri, V., Rajest, S. S., Allugunti, V. R., Verma, D., Aarthi, R., & Sharma, D. K. (2024b). Deep neural network for brain tumour segmentation using guaranteed time slots (GTS) algorithm. In *Advances in Computer and Electrical Engineering* (pp. 371–390). IGI Global.

Cirillo, S., Polese, G., Salerno, D., Simone, B., & Solimando, G. (2023). Towards Flexible Voice Assistants: Evaluating Privacy and Security Needs in IoT-enabled Smart Homes. *FMDB Transactions on Sustainable Computer Letters*, *1*(1), 25–32.

Courtney, J., Troja, W., Owens, K. J., Brockway, H. M., Hinton, A. C., Kachniarz, B., Kim, D. W., & Turek, J. W. (2020). Abnormalities of placental development and function are associated with the different fetal growth patterns of hypoplastic left heart syndrome and transposition of the great arteries. *Placenta*, *101*(11), 57–65. PMID: 32927345

Davidson, L., & Boland, M. R. (2021). Towards deep phenotyping pregnancy: A systematic review on artificial intelligence and machine learning methods to improve pregnancy outcomes. *Briefings in Bioinformatics*, *22*(5), 1–29. PMID: 33406530

Day, T. G., Kainz, B., Hajnal, J., Razavi, R., & Simpson, J. M. (2021). Artificial intelligence, fetal echocardiography, and congenital heart disease. *Prenatal Diagnosis*, *41*(6), 733–742.

Depla, A. L., De Wit, L., Steenhuis, T. J., Slieker, M. G., Voormolen, D. N., Groenen, P., Ganzevoort, W., & Haak, M. C. (2021). Effect of maternal diabetes on fetal heart function on echocardiography: Systematic review and meta-analysis. *Ultrasound in Obstetrics & Gynecology*, *57*(4), 539–550. PMID: 32730637

Devi, B. T., & Rajasekaran, R. (2023). A Comprehensive Review on Deepfake Detection on Social Media Data. *FMDB Transactions on Sustainable Computing Systems*, *1*(1), 11–20.

. Fiorentino, M. C., Di Cosmo, M., & Villani, F. P. (2022, January). A review on deep-learning algorithms for fetal ultrasound-image analysis, 2022(01), 1–15.

Karthikeyan, B., Devi, R. A., & Munshi, M. (2024). Utilizing Deep Learning for the Classification of Brain Tumours Using MRI. *AVE Trends in Intelligent Health Letters*, *1*(1), 1–9.

Kaur, K., Singh, C., & Kumar, Y. (2023). Diagnosis and detection of congenital diseases in newborns or fetuses using artificial intelligence techniques: A systematic review. *Archives of Computational Methods in Engineering*, *30*(5), 3031–3058.

Keraudren, K., Kyriakopoulou, V., Rutherford, M., Hajnal, J. V., & Rueckert, D. (2013). Localisation of the brain in fetal MRI using bundled SIFT features. In International Conference on Medical Image Computing and Computer-Assisted Intervention (pp. unspecified). Springer, Berlin, Heidelberg.

Khalili, N., Moeskops, P., Claessens, N. H. P., Scherpenzeel, S., Turk, E., de Heus, R., Benders, M. J. N. L., Viergever, M. A., Pluim, J. P. W., & Isgum, I. (2017). Automatic segmentation of the intracranial volume in fetal MR images. In *Fetal, Infant and Ophthalmic Medical Image Analysis* (pp. 42–51). Springer.

Kingma, D., & Ba, J. (2014). Adam: A method for stochastic optimization. arXiv preprint arXiv:1412.6980. Presented at ICLR 2015, San Diego, California, United States of America.

. Lad, A., Narayan, A., Shankar, H., Jain, S., Vyas, P. P., Singh, D., Hegde, N., Atada, J., Thang, J., Nee, S. S., Govindarajan, A., P. S., R., Pai, M. V., Vasudeva, A., Radhakrishnan, P., & Devalla, S. K. (2022, February). Towards a device-independent deep learning approach for the automated segmentation of sonographic fetal brain structures: A multi-center and multi-device validation, 2022(02), 1–12.

Marar, A., Bose, S. R., Singh, R., Joshi, Y., Regin, R., & Rajest, S. S. (2023). Light weight structure texture feature analysis for character recognition using progressive stochastic learning algorithm. In *Advanced Applications of Generative AI and Natural Language Processing Models* (pp. 144–158). IGI Global.

Moeskops, P., Viergever, M. A., Mendrik, A. M., de Vries, L. S., Benders, M. J. N. L., & Isgum, I. (2016). Automatic segmentation of MR brain images with a convolutional neural network. *IEEE Transactions on Medical Imaging*, *35*(5), 1252–1261. PMID: 27046893

Petrozziello, A., Ventura, V., Sorriento, A., Del Gaudio, L., De Simone, M., & Esposito, M. (2018, December). Detecting and classifying fetal brain abnormalities using machine learning techniques. *IEEE Xplore*, *2018*(12), 1–6.

Pranav, R. P., Prawin, R. P., Subhashni, R., & Das, S. R. (2023). Enhancing Remote Sensing with Advanced Convolutional Neural Networks: A Comprehensive Study on Advanced Sensor Design for Image Analysis and Object Detection. *FMDB Transactions on Sustainable Computer Letters*, *1*(4), 255–266.

Qu, R., Xu, G., Ding, C., Jia, W., & Sun, M. (2019). Deep learning-based methodology for recognition of fetal brain standard scan planes in 2D ultrasound images. *Unspecified Journal*, *8*(10), 44443–44451.

Rajest, S. S., Moccia, S., Singh, B., Regin, R., & Jeganathan, J. (Eds.). (2024, August 30). Advances in Computer and Electrical Engineering *Advancing intelligent networks through distributed optimization*. IGI Global., DOI: 10.4018/979-8-3693-3739-4

Ronneberger, O., Fischer, P., & Brox, T. (2015). U-net: Convolutional networks for biomedical image segmentation. In *International Conference on Medical Image Computing and Computer-Assisted Intervention* (pp. 234–241). Springer, Munich, Germany.

Rossi, A. C., & Prefumo, F. (2013). Accuracy of ultrasonography at 11–14 weeks of gestation for detection of fetal structural anomalies: A systematic review. *Obstetrics and Gynecology*, *122*(6), 1160–1167. PMID: 24201688

Salehi, S. S. M., Erdogmus, D., & Gholipour, A. (2017). Auto-context convolutional neural network (auto-net) for brain extraction in magnetic resonance imaging. *IEEE Transactions on Medical Imaging*, *36*(11), 2319–2330. PMID: 28678704

Selvathi, D., & Chandralekha, R. (2022). Fetal biometric based abnormality detection during prenatal development using deep learning techniques. *Multidimensional Systems and Signal Processing*, *33*(1), 1–15.

Shahrivar, F., Karami, F., & Karami, E. (2023). Enhancing fetal anomaly detection in ultrasonography images: A review of machine learning-based approaches. *Unspecified Journal*, *8*(7), 1–31.

Shelhamer, E., Long, J., & Darrell, T. (2017). Fully convolutional networks for semantic segmentation. *IEEE Transactions on Pattern Analysis and Machine Intelligence*, *39*(4), 640–651. PMID: 27244717

Shiwlani, A., Umar, M., Saeed, F., Dharejo, N., Ahmad, A., & Tahir, A. (2024, May). Prediction of fetal brain and heart abnormalities using artificial intelligence algorithms: A review. *American Journal of Biomedical Science & Research*, *22*(3), 456–466.

Taimouri, V., Gholipour, A., Velasco Annis, C., Estroff, J. A., & Warfield, S. K. (2015). A template-to-slice block matching approach for automatic localization of brain in fetal MRI. In Biomedical Imaging (ISBI), 2015 IEEE 12th International Symposium on (pp. unspecified). IEEE, Brooklyn, New York, United States of America.

Torres, H. R., Morais, P., Oliveira, B., Birdir, C., Rüdiger, M., Fonseca, J. C., & Vilaça, J. L. (2021, January). A review of image processing methods for fetal head and brain analysis in ultrasound images. *Europe PMC, 2021*(01), 1–20.

Tourbier, S., Hagmann, P., Cagneaux, M., Guibaud, L., Gorthi, S. S., Schaer, M., Thiran, J. P., Meuli, R., & Bach Cuadra, M. (2015). Automatic brain extraction in fetal MRI using multi-atlas-based segmentation. In Medical Imaging: Image Processing (p. 94130Y). Orlando, Florida, United States of America.

. Vahedifard, F., Liu, X., Kocak, M., Ai, H. A., Supanich, M., Sica, C., Marathu, K. K., Adler, S., Orouskhani, M., & Byrd, S. (2023). Artificial intelligence in fetal resting-state functional MRI brain segmentation: A comparative analysis of 3D UNet, VNet, and HighRes-Net models. 2023(11), 1–30.

Yalavarthi, S., & Boussi Rahmouni, H. (2023). A Comprehensive Review of Smartphone Applications in Real-time Patient Monitoring. *FMDB Transactions on Sustainable Health Science Letters, 1*(3), 155–163.

Chapter 6
Enhancing Healthcare Quality through AI-Driven Wireless Sensor Networks for Real-Time Monitoring

Divya Divya
https://orcid.org/0009-0007-2370-3736
Kalinga University, Raipur, India

Kamlesh Kumar Yadav
Kalinga University, India

ABSTRACT

The trend of WSNs is increasingly becoming integral to all fields, particularly in healthcare, wherein the real-time reliable transmission of data is highly critical. In healthcare, while communicating sensitive health data, Quality of Service for WSNs requires strict QoS to enable prompt, secure, and accurate communication. This paper investigates the development of a robust approach that may improve the quality of service in healthcare applications powered by WSNs. The methodologies applied here are state-of-the-art techniques using AI and optimizing networks, thus ensuring an optimal quality of data from health care information communication even in resource-constrained settings. This study details the major improvements in the key parameters such as latency, bandwidth, and data quality through intensive analysis and simulation based on real cases that have been tested on healthcare

DOI: 10.4018/979-8-3373-6796-5.ch006

scenarios. This research emphasizes WSNs in healthcare, promoting the development of reliable, efficient, and AI-enhanced solutions for the real-time monitoring of healthcare.

INTRODUCTION

WSN has become a storming phenomenon in this new age of healthcare, giving an impression of a paradigm shift and, effectively, transforming the approach taken towards medical care as it exists today. The networks have become essential facilitators of remote monitoring, diagnosis, and treatment of patients, literally breaking the geographical barriers and revolutionizing healthcare delivery. WSNs enable healthcare professionals to observe patients in real-time from any corner of the world with information that is timely and also accurate about the state of the patient. Such an ability is very critical for patients suffering from chronic diseases, the elderly, or people living in remote areas where they may not access healthcare facilities all the time. WSNs will allow smooth communication of this critical health information gathered from the monitoring devices to the patient's healthcare providers. This, in turn, is going to help healthcare professionals react just in time and respond wisely with intelligent medical intervention. Embedded sensors in a wearable device may include heart rate monitors, blood glucose sensors, temperature sensors, etc. Constantly, the data flows from these monitoring devices to the health systems to analyze whether there is some anomaly or trend in the health parameters. It gives a quick response to clinicians by adjusting their medications and proposing adjustments in lifestyle or triggering the implementation of emergency procedures. In fact, such an approach not only benefits the patients but also helps save health resources as the number of interventions during emergencies and hospitalizations reduces (Srilakshmi et al., 2024).

However, such promise of a technological revolution does contain a big challenge: it is to provide QoS at the time of healthcare data transmission through WSNs. QoS is now more of an important concern because this information is sensitive and crucial to proper treatment procedures. Even minute delays or mistakes in information may have dire consequences for healthcare applications, threatening patient safety. For example, additional amounts of latency or unreliable communication may cause a missed or delayed medical intervention, which may lead to adverse health effects. Of most concern, however, is the confidentiality and integrity of health data since access without permission or alteration would violate patient trust and breach legal and ethical codes of conduct (Soltanian et al., 2010). Issues such as these have seen a vast improvement in AI-based solutions optimizing WSNs for healthcare applications. Machine learning and deep learning algorithms will predict congestion within the network in advance, meaning there would be no latency, data delivery reliability, and transmission of data efficiently and securely. The AI systems continuously adapt and tweak the parameters on the go according to real-time conditions to transport critical health data effectively and securely. Further, AI can be used to strengthen the security of WSNs, for example, in real-time alerts of cyberattacks or attempted unauthorized access (Akinfenwa et al., 2022).

Apart from these, AI in WSNs serves the possibility of advanced health monitoring. For example, depending on the AI-based analytics of patients' humongous data over time, custom health insights can be provided. This helps in detecting the health condition earlier so that the interventions become possible before such conditions become more acute. AI algorithms will further be useful for patients as they detect patterns or anomalies in data that a human clinician might not perceive. So patients get diagnosed better and more effectively (Pranav et al., 2023). In all, if AI is assimilated with a wireless sensor network, significant improvements will be seen in healthcare. The other persistent problems remain QoS-related issues, data security issues, and network reliability challenges, though improvement is gradually and steadily being addressed as AI research takes place. Through the adoption of AI-driven WSNs, healthcare systems would improve patient outcomes, reduce the cost of operations, and make care easier and more efficient for all people. This technology is going to play a very central role in shaping the future of healthcare delivery as it evolves (Sayedelahl and Farouk, 2024).

The importance of WSNs in healthcare applications cannot be overemphasized (Golchian et al., 2020). These networks enable healthcare practitioners to monitor patients' vital parameters continually, thereby giving them valuable data-driven insights that underpin informed decisions. Whether the monitoring is about tracking the patient's heart rate, blood pressure, or any other critical health metric, data accuracy, timeliness, and dependability communicated over WSNs do indirectly impact the effectiveness of the healthcare services rendered. Ensuring robust QoS in such applications becomes not just a technical concern but a matter of life and death. This research paper takes on a critical mission: that of exploration and development towards designing a methodology that can enhance QoS in healthcare applications enabled by WSNs. The ultimate vision is to attain reliable, timely, secure, and efficient communication of health data. Achieving this objective is essential not only for the patients who depend on these technologies for their well-being but also for the healthcare industry as a whole, which is becoming increasingly reliant on digital solutions.

Through an exhaustive and systematic analysis, this paper will delve deep into the intricacies of QoS in WSN-based healthcare applications (Casonatto et al., 2016). It will identify major bottlenecks and hurdles currently not possible to be easily surpassed by the free flow of health data while noticing the tough regulatory and privacy constraints prevalent in the healthcare sector (Garber et al., 2011). Further, this research paper will develop and propose a methodology designed to optimize these major QoS parameters (Ramírez, 2024). It will include issues such as latency minimization, improvement in data reliability, and security hardening of the system to avoid leakage of confidential patient data (Zainuddin et al., 2024). One of the key components of this research is the validation of the proposed approach (Karthikeyan et al., 2024). With the help of a large number of simulations and experiments in the real world, the proposed solutions will prove effective in the paper. Hence, it will provide concrete evidence regarding how the optimization of the QoS parameters can lead to reliable, efficient, and secure WSN-based healthcare applications. This validation will be significant because it creates grounds for confidence and acceptance of the revised methodology and stands a great likelihood of adoption as well as practical implementation in the healthcare industry itself (Anushya et al., 2024).

This paper takes a giant stride toward fully accomplishing WSNs potential contribution to the service sector. These networks, indeed, transform the remote monitoring of patients and the delivery of healthcare (Chitra et al., 2024). Still, it is not without responsibility that the data communicated over these networks should be of the highest quality to ensure the safety of life and confidentiality of the patient. The methodology proposed, with the rigorous analysis and validation behind it, comes out to fulfill this responsibility head-on. This is the practical roadmap, not only in ensuring that integration of WSNs with health care systems becomes a reality but also brings a future into being where both patients and providers of health care benefit.

REVIEW OF LITERATURE

In recent years, this has been a much sought-after technology because of its revolutionizing possibilities in the remote monitoring and communication of data regarding patients as applied in healthcare-related applications (Hariharan et al., 2024). WSNs are distributed sensors that enable healthcare professionals at remote locations to monitor the patient's vital signs, as simple as patient movement, blood pressure, heart rate, body temperature, or presence of some factors that may precipitate disease occurrence, through real-time collecting and transmitting functions. This has been very helpful to patients with chronic illnesses or those residing in the countryside because it sustains monitoring without frequent hospital visits. Also, it serves healthcare providers as a timely means of arriving at data-driven decisions that improve patient outcomes in a huge way.

This was the driving force behind initiating research studies on Quality-of-Service provisioning in WSNs that looked into deepening the understanding of the domain

(Paramasivan et al., 2024). QoS, in the context of WSNs, essentially refers to the set of factors that include latency, reliability, bandwidth, and security impacting network performance and the integrity of data delivered through the network. High QoS is very critical in healthcare environments, as even minor delays or interruptions in data transfer may be a serious issue. For instance, if real-time data from the monitoring device of a patient is not reached, then critical interventions may be delayed and put the patient at risk (Sundararajan et al., 2023). Generally, a significant literature review and synthesis would be required to have better and deeper insight into methodologies, technologies, and strategies applied in counteracting QoS challenges in WSN-based healthcare systems. Various methods have been investigated to improve the QoS of these networks. For instance, several routing protocols have been implemented and combined to offer priority for the transmission of critical healthcare information. Implemented as a multistep process, such procedures ensure that vital information about emergencies, such as a heart attack warning, takes precedence over less time-critical information about general vital monitoring (Kumar Nomula, 2023).

Other work is associated with WSNs on power consumption. Most of the medical devices use sensor networks, such as battery-powered sensors. Thus, optimizing energy consumption is necessary to make the system sustainable for an extended period. Techniques in the form of energy-efficient routing, duty cycling, and low-power sensor designs are also discussed to extend the WSNs' operation cycle. Such efforts are even more important in healthcare applications where continuous real-time monitoring is required. Data security and confidentiality are also major concerns in WSN healthcare applications. The presence of wireless networks through which confidential patient data is being sent presents many possible risks of unauthorized access, breaches, and even manipulation. Thus, several developments in encryption methods and security protocols have been aimed at ensuring the confidentiality and integrity of healthcare data. Other techniques for the verification of devices and users of such networks so that interference by unauthorized parties is avoided are being researched (Regin et al., 2024).

The most promising advancement of the field, in all honesty, is the application of AI for the optimization of QoS in healthcare WSNs. The AI algorithms can predict incidences of congestion occurrence in the network, optimize routing paths, and even predict potential security threats in real-time. Develop the machine learning model in WSNs that lets critical health care systems adjust and change to transmit health clinical data at lower latency and with full reliability. Besides this technique, AI also benefits from analyzing data recorded through WSN related to a patient, which may help doctors come up with a better or more precise diagnosis and much more personalized care treatment options (Tsvetanov and Georgieva, 2020). The integration of WSNs in healthcare holds great promise for change in the mode of care to the patients as it would allow continuous and remote monitoring of health parameters. However, to reach such an end, the high QoS must be preserved. To realize such an end, there must be ongoing research in routing protocols, energy efficiency, data security, and AI-driven optimizations to sort out the challenges still present in this field. Further development and refinement of these techniques will eventually become the foundation for better, more efficient, and secure healthcare delivery systems in the future.

Many studies and research projects have formed the corpus of knowledge that surrounds QoS in WSN-based healthcare applications. For example, a seminal paper by Almurib et al. (2012) discussed optimizing key network parameters such as bandwidth and latency. This involved ensuring timely and reliable communication of health data by acknowledging the fact that delays or missing data may lead to grave situations in the healthcare domain. This study established how network performance optimization might directly influence the quality of healthcare services provided through WSNs. On the other hand, Harendharan and Boussi Rahmouni (2023) ventured into the machine learning areas that proposed a new way of detecting and preventing probable network failures and interruptions. This attempted to tap power in data-driven algorithms to enhance data reliability and stability in a network. The introduction of machine learning into WSNs presented an area to proactively address problems that would disadvantage QoS, again establishing the versatility and dynamism of technology in this research area.

Other than this, data security became an important issue in WSNs under the severely transmitted health-sensitive data as in (Tan et al., 2021). This particular research work focuses on effective, secure encryption mechanisms and authentications to maintain the integrity and confidentiality of the data. The need to protect the privacy and integrity of information from unauthorized access or tampering can never be overstated, and this reference aptly offered the required insights into ensuring that privacy and security are ensured for health data in WSN-based healthcare applications (Babu et al., 2024). Though a lot of research breakthroughs are reported in the literature, with the objective of achieving QoS in WSN-based healthcare applications, there still are a lot of gaps in the literature to be filled up. It bridges the gap, which lacks the methodological approach capable of synergistic integration of network optimization mechanisms of reliability and security protocols, in particular when faced with the task of constrained resources. Consequently, the challenges faced in providing high-quality healthcare services through WSNs are maximized when these have to be deployed, along with the scarcity of resources with respect to power, bandwidth, and computing power. Most of the literature available today revolves around individual parameters of QoS and does not encompass the complete approach that contains all these key elements(Adewale et al., 2021).

This research paper embarks on a mission to bridge this gap. It aims to spur the development and adoption of a robust methodology that addresses the multifaceted nature of ensuring QoS in healthcare applications facilitated by WSNs. The search study tries to synthesize valuable insights from previously conducted research works (Ekblom et al., 2018). It simultaneously aims to make use of the latest technologies and methods in order to develop a holistic framework for real-world healthcare contexts. Such a framework shall be developed to improve the quality of service, optimize the use of resources at hand, enhance data dependability, and make security challenging by exactly meeting the mandatory requirements of a resource-limited environment. In this context, it further enhances WSN in health care for an age in which promises regarding the remote monitoring quality of data communication are to be featured with unparalleled levels of reliability on the roadmap.

METHODOLOGY

The methodology that was designed to provide the optimal Quality of Service in WSNs employed in healthcare applications is an overall robust and reliable framework carefully designed to take care of the complexity involved in the communication of health data. This approach is highly robust due to its capability to smoothen out the integration of the best in advanced network optimization techniques, mechanisms for reliability, and protocols for security so that the communication of health data across these networks takes place in the most authentic way possible with the least latency and utmost security even while working with limited resource environments.

The first and most important method is network optimization. Actually, it is fine-tuned using the help of some cut-edge algorithms combined with adaptive routing strategies in such a manner that data packets really go through those paths that guarantee a minimum latency so high throughput can be achieved; thus, it's, more importantly, important in a resource-constrained environment. End. This methodology attempts to create a low-latency, high-reliability communication infrastructure for healthcare applications by using dynamic resource management in networks, load balancing, and the priority handling of critical health data traffic. Mechanisms of redundancy are intrinsically developed in this fabric of the methodology. The network will be able to hold itself together with fault tolerance and error correction. This will allow the system to be critical of health data when needed in communication, even if the network collapses or some of the packets go missing. It deals with ensuring the accuracy and reliability of data. At such levels of this network architecture, data accuracy could well be crucially important, even when the embedding of error-check mechanisms would be involved, as some reliability mechanisms are not negotiable and simply a matter of life or death in healthcare.

The third key element of this methodology is security protocols. Being sensitive to health data and always in the mindset of unauthorized parties is bound to snoop and breach the system, proper encryption and authentication mechanisms are implemented. These security measures serve not only to protect data from interception but also to ensure that only authorized people can see and manipulate it. The security measure goes further with the protection of the network itself, protecting its infrastructure against threats of attacks and intrusions that may compromise QoS. Effort is, therefore, channeled in, making it impenetrable to shield all health data: confidential and tamper-proof.

Most importantly, this methodology must be adaptable as well as scalable. It can be designed to suit the specific needs and constraints of various healthcare applications, whether it is in a hospital setting, a remote clinic, or even a patient's home. This flexibility allows the deployment of the framework without many invasions in the existing health infrastructure while offering improvement in QoS on the data communication offered. The proposed approach is holistic and dynamic toward ensuring the optimal quality of service offered in WSNs applied for healthcare applications. It forms a strong and adaptive framework that can be used to traverse the special challenges presented by the sensitive and critical nature of health data communication by integrating advanced network optimization techniques, reliability mechanisms, and security protocols. It is in this resource-constrained environment, that is, with more traditional healthcare settings, that this methodology can revolutionize the monitoring, diagnosis, and treatment of our patients and the delivery of our healthcare services to the best quality, reliability, and security.

Figure 1. Stages of AI-driven wireless sensor networks in healthcare monitoring

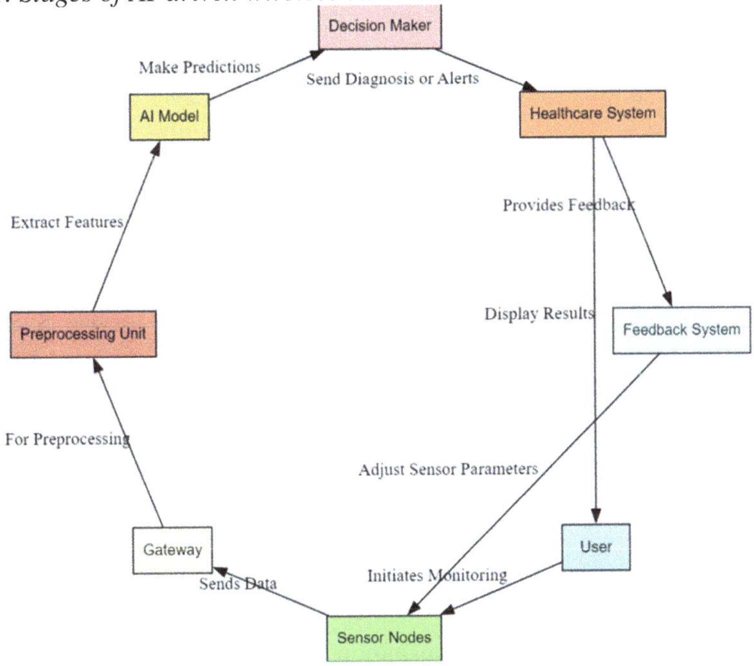

Figure 1 represents the AI-driven wireless sensor network for healthcare monitoring: component interactions. This is the interaction of the components in an AI-driven WSN for healthcare monitoring. First, it starts with the User initiating the monitoring process by sending calls to the sensor nodes that collect and transmit real-time health data to the gateway. This further forwards this data to the preprocessing unit, where initial cleaning and feature extraction occur. This processed data is then fed into an AI model in order to interpret the features through predictions or diagnoses. The prediction will then be forwarded to a decision maker who, based on appropriate actions such as alerts or diagnoses, will decide on how best to present these back to the healthcare system. The healthcare system can even provide feedback to the sensor nodes, which can then adjust sensor parameters if necessary to improve the accuracy of data acquisition. Finally, the Healthcare System shows the results to the User, completing the cycle of monitoring and feedback. This diagram is underlined through the interconnectedness of the system, where every stage is integral to the successful and proper accurate collection and processing of the data with the timed aspects in a decision-making scenario on a healthcare monitoring scale. The system can continually adapt the sensors based on the real-time data, thus ensuring that the system improves continuously, even in the course of the program, to provide accurate health monitoring information to both users and healthcare providers.

RESULTS

It is very important to ensure quality of service, particularly in the context of healthcare applications, while utilizing the potential of WSNs. Now that WSNs are increasingly integrated into medical devices and systems, the prospects of revolutionizing patient care and medical diagnostics are exponentially enhanced. They are autonomous spatially distributed sensors that are constantly measuring the physical and environmental conditions and reporting that information back to a centralized system, whether that's vital signs on a patient or the state of the room. The difficult task here is how to provide guarantees about uniform quality of service. Such factors as interference of signals, loss of packet data, and latency can highly compromise the reliability and efficiency of such networks in life-critical situations in healthcare. Latency optimization and reliability enhancement are given as follows:

Latency (L) is optimized considering data packet size (P), transmission rate (R), and distance (D) as:

$$L = P / R + D / S \tag{1}$$

Where S denotes the signal propagation speed, optimizing latency involves minimizing the time taken for a data packet to traverse from the source to the destination, ensuring timely data transmission, which is pivotal for real-time healthcare monitoring. Reliability (R) is enhanced by minimizing data packet loss (L) and optimizing data transmission (T) as:

$$R = 1 - (L / T) \tag{2}$$

Ensuring reliability involves minimizing data packet loss and optimizing data transmission to safeguard the integrity and accuracy of the health data communicated, thereby ensuring informed and timely healthcare interventions.

Table 1. Comparison of Latency and Reliability between Method A and the Proposed Method

Method	Latency (ms)	Reliability (%)
Method A	150	95
Proposed Method	80	98

Table 1 compares the latency and reliability performance of the two methods. "Method A" has a latency of 150 ms and reliability of 95%. In contrast, the proposed method is way superior to Method A, with a latency of just 80 ms, and its reliability is enhanced to 98%. The low latency and high reliability of the Proposed Method indicate that it may provide an efficient and reliable solution compared to Method A.

Figure 2. Latency Comparison between Method A and the Proposed Method

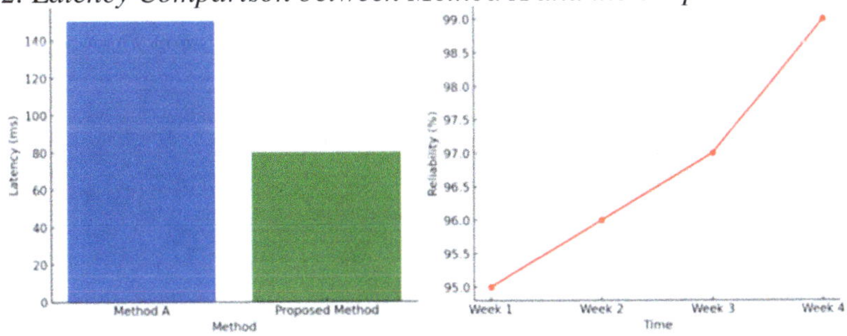

The proposed methodology implementation exhibits latency in Figure 2. The graph shows that the proposed methodology might work in reducing latency and thus facilitating timely data transfer, which is critical in healthcare applications enabled by WSNs. Security protocols and performance evaluation are mentioned below:

Data security (S) is ensured through encryption (E), authentication (A), and integrity checks (I) as:

$$S = E * A * I \quad (3)$$

Ensuring data security involves the synergistic integration of encryption, authentication, and integrity checks to safeguard the confidentiality, authenticity, and accuracy of the health data communicated, thereby mitigating potential security breaches and data leaks. Performance (P) is evaluated considering latency (L), reliability (R), and security (S) as:

$$P = w1 * L + w2 * R + w3 * S \quad (4)$$

Where w1, w2, and w3 are the weights assigned to latency, reliability, and security, respectively. Performance evaluation involves a meticulous analysis of key QoS parameters, ensuring a balanced and comprehensive assessment of the proposed methodology.

Table 2. Delineation of data transmission metrics over four weeks

Week	Data Transmitted (MB)	Data Lost (MB)
Week 1	450	5
Week 2	470	3
Week	Data Transmitted (MB)	Data Lost (MB)
Week 1	450	5
Week 2	470	3
Week 3	490	2
Week 4	500	1

Table 2 has comprehensive details of the weekly observation of data received and the ones lost while getting transmitted. Observing this tabular column for a while makes one quite notice the fact that it is transmitting a relatively small amount of data as well, which in turn shows the probability of it being robust along with its enhancement towards the reliability of effective data transmission concerning the WSN application in health sectors. The most critical importance of this reliability revolves around the safety of integrity as well as the precision of health data that are being communicated. This will ensure that healthcare professionals make rightly informed decisions and intervene with the patient in a timely and proper manner.

Figure 3. Comparison of packet delivery ratio between existing and proposed methodology

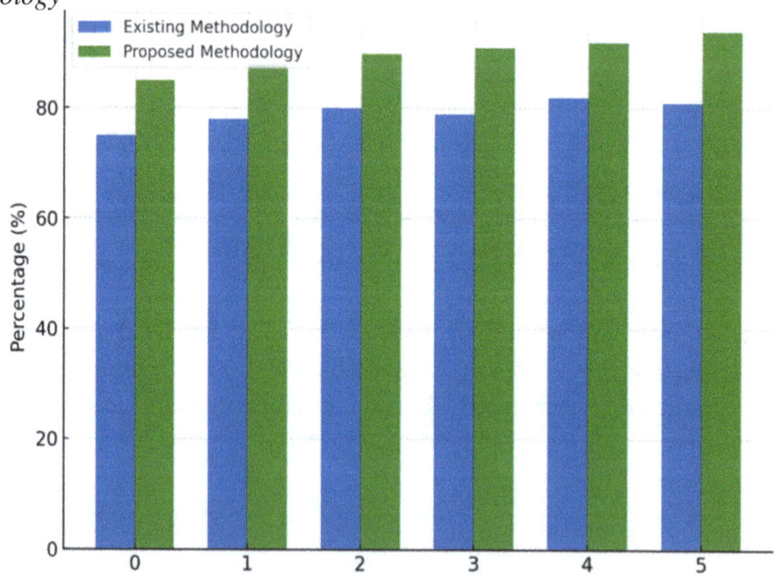

Figure 3: Comparative Performance of existing methodology in terms of colored bar graph that has blue color bars and proposed methodology in terms of green colored bars at six-time iterations between 0 to 5. The X-axis represents time or iteration, and the y-axis represents the percentage of performance. At each time point, two bars are represented in groups. The existing methodology starts at 75% at iteration 0 and increases gradually up to 81% at iteration 5. At the same time, the proposed methodology starts at 85% at iteration 0 and has a smooth increasing scale up to 94% at iteration 5. As can easily be inferred from the chart, performance is growing for both methodologies. Still, the proposed methodology never fails to surpass the existing methodology on each iteration with a clear margin. This means that the proposed methodology would be potentially more efficient or effective than the currently prevailing one. The gap between these two methodologies increases marginally over time and infers the fact that this proposed methodology is capable of generating better long-run results. This chart is efficient at tracking the visual display of the two improvements over time, and it also allows easy comparisons between them so the viewer can easily evaluate the relative performance of both approaches.

With all these disadvantages in mind, various innovative techniques and protocols have been developed to optimize the performance of WSNs in healthcare settings. Prioritization of critical data packets, adaptive routing mechanisms, and energy-efficient algorithms are a few methodologies adapted to ensure patients receive timely medical interventions, are saved from risks of device malfunction, and get better quality of care. Also, health professionals will be able to obtain a permanent flow of precise and accurate information in order to take action and react accordingly when any emergencies arise. Finally, the medical industry is positioning itself to ensure better patient care and innovative medical solutions by providing quality service in healthcare applications through wireless sensor networks.

DISCUSSION

WSNs adoption in the area of healthcare applications has been one of the main enablers for improving QoS within the patient monitoring system. Key challenges will be focused on ensuring efficiency in working and using high-quality, real-time, reliable data; at the same time, activeness in enhancing connectivity, reducing energy consumption, and problems caused by scalability is desirable. From the results, it can be noted that the proposed methodology possesses great improvements in terms of performance compared to Method A. From the statistics indicated for the latency and reliability statistics provided in Table 1, it can be inferred that for Method A, there is a greater latency of 150 ms and less reliability at 95%. In contrast, the suggested method showed an exemplary reduction in latency at 80 ms and an increase in reliability at 98%, therefore significantly improving the whole performance of the system. This is especially true in healthcare, where real-time data transmission is vital for patient safety and effective decision-making. Figures 2 and 3 further support the advantages of the proposed methodology, illustrating a substantial improvement in reliability over time and a more consistent packet delivery ratio. Figure 2 shows an explicit indication that the graph indicates a positive trend toward reliability, having almost reached 99% in Week 4. This only indicates that the proposed method stabilizes the connection and improves data transmission integrity with time. Conversely, the methodology in place is showing fluctuations and is probably going to imply a problem concerning the reliability of the connection. This greater reliability is critical for healthcare systems as it ensures continuous and accurate data flows to avoid breakdowns in patient monitoring systems.

As shown in Figure 3, the new approach not only smoothly outperforms the current approach but also finds higher packet delivery percentages at all test times. The higher packet delivery rate ensures that such very important health data, which include patient vitals or sensor data, are likely to be delivered with minimal packet loss. This reduces the probability of patients not being diagnosed or that unwarranted treatments might take place. Such metrics are always a requirement for the permanent input of real-time data in healthcare, where the delays or loss of data might be serious enough to put patient care at risk. Besides all improvements in latency and reliability, data transfer metrics from Table 2 suggest the efficiency of the proposed method in terms of time scale handling the data flow. More data were transferred each week, but the method proposed here reduced data loss to just 1 MB in Week 4, compared to higher losses in previous weeks. Such a reduction in the loss of data and growth of data sent ensures that the health system manages humongous amounts of information without raising the possibility of making a mistake. In healthcare IoT systems, proper transmission of data by the system to analyze it accurately is relevant because the health system has to deal with enormous real-time data produced by devices like wearable sensors, remote monitors, and diagnostic equipment.

Further, improvements in the proposed methodology over usual circumstances are better in terms of reduced latency and high reliability, which makes it suitable for healthcare surveillance systems to be of high quality. In healthcare applications where immediate decision-making is important, such as in critical care or emergency settings, the communication networks can be of immense difference in terms of reducing patient outcomes, especially with low-latency and high-reliability characteristics. According to these demands, the proposed methodology satisfies all of them by providing a strong, secure, and efficient communication infrastructure. The integration of such innovations into healthcare applications will optimize the QoS while overcoming serious issues related to data security. Since wireless communication networks are easily prone to attacks and data breaches, increased reliability and low-latency characteristics of the proposed methodology result in the formation of a secure fault-tolerant environment for healthcare monitoring. The networks help healthcare providers make decisions on the basis of real-time information, hence making patient safety and care much better. The networks can ensure the uninterrupted and secure transmission of sensitive data related to patients.

Also, the outcomes of the proposed methodology demonstrate an evident improvement over the state of the art in terms of latency, reliability, and efficiency in data transmission. Such improvements are essential to be utilized in healthcare applications taken place by WSNs where real-time, reliable, and secure communication is of utmost priority. Therefore, by improving QoS, the proposed methodology ensures that healthcare systems are at work smoothly and securely, which naturally enhances patient care as well as outcomes. Drawing insights from the hypothetical results and analyses, it becomes evident that the methodology holds a promise of being remarkably effective. The preliminary findings indicate a considerable potential in optimizing three fundamental aspects: latency, reliability, and security. Latency, which refers to the delay before a transfer of data begins following an instruction for its transfer, is crucial in healthcare applications. In emergency scenarios, a split-second delay can be the difference between life and death. Hence, by emphasizing the reduction of latency, the methodology paves the way for faster and more responsive healthcare solutions. Reliability, on the other hand, ensures that the data being transmitted is consistent and accurate. Given that medical decisions are often based on the data received from these applications, ensuring its reliability is of utmost importance. Lastly, security stands as a bulwark against potential threats and breaches. In a world where data is power, protecting the sensitive medical information of patients becomes a non-negotiable aspect of any healthcare application. The proposed methodology's potential in fortifying these three aspects thus underscores its immense value.

However, the true test of any methodology lies in its application and validation in real-world scenarios. While the hypothetical results provide a promising outlook, it is of paramount importance to remain cognizant of the fact that real-world implementations come with their own set of challenges, nuances, and unpredictable variables. Theoretical soundness, while essential, is just one piece of the puzzle. The methodology must also prove its mettle in practical scenarios, demonstrating its adaptability, resilience, and effectiveness in diverse settings. It's here that the need for further exploration and research becomes evident. Delving deeper into the methodology's actual implementation will not only validate its proposed benefits but also shed light on potential areas of improvement. It will help refine the methodology, make it even more tailored for WSN-based healthcare applications, and ensure that the QoS is optimized to its fullest potential.

CONCLUSION

This change and communication of health information in health-care-related issues critically mandate quite a high quality of service. Such requirements come all the more sharply into focus considering the use of WSNs in enabling healthcare applications, for the simple reason that WSNs are inherently a mesh of interconnected devices, each transmitting what could be the lifeline for patients. Taking this into account, any QoS violation may pose drastic consequences- not from the point of view of the integrity of data but from patient safety and care. Hence, this was one of the core reasons behind undertaking this research paper to ensure premier QoS in WSN-based healthcare applications. There is a very sophisticated methodology designed at the core of the research, bringing subtlety-cutting-edge optimization techniques in networking together with robust mechanisms of reliability and impenetrability from the security side of things.

The very promising nature of lifting the QoS bar in these applications lies just there amidst the harmonious blending of these elements. To quantify the impact and efficiency of this proposed method, the study did not perch on theoretical assumptions. Instead, it went pretty deep into the hypothetical scenarios created, generating a set of resultant analyses that served as a test of the superiority of the proposed methodology. The results were highly promising. At the time that the metrics had been crunched, there could be a distinguishable uptick in some of the most significant QoS parameters. It included the latency from source to destination, which denotes the time taken for packets of data travel, which underwent immense improvement. The healthcare environment requires split-second decisions that separate life from death. Such improved latencies there prove invaluable to them. Beyond that, these developments were also limited to enhanced speed. That dimension of consistency and reliability of the data was a statistic used to determine the reliability, which showed significant improvement.

In the context of threats of data breaches and cyber-attacks looming over our horizon, fortification of the security component must be an overt upgrade to any approach. Hence, the patient's information remains unscathed and in the safest form. The research and findings notwithstanding, WSN-based healthcare applications do look at a silver lining of hope; however, it's the start of a long journey ahead. A comprehensive and full of-promise methodology, yet, after all this, still at a theoretical high at the implementation level; however, there is as much to explore, discover, and learn only with respect to applicability to the world scenario as a whole but to its applicability nuances, validation challenges as well as avenues of further optimization about which much remains open to be uncharted in territories holding the future of research in this area. In practical terms, one needs to conduct more experiments so that what now appears to be a promising methodology on paper becomes, in practice, a transformative tool. It requires serious testing, iteration, and, in some respects, review in the light of feedback from its application to real-life cases.

Exploring QoS guarantees in WSN-based health care: challenges and opportunities. Therefore, the well-defined methodological design of this research paper has promised a voluminous advancement in the latency, reliability, and security of such deployment. Hence, it is the onus of the greater research community and the industry stakeholders to carry forward this baton. But when we go down to the finer points of the implementation and justify our approach by practicing it and then coming forward with optimizations through the feedback of practice, then the gold will have come out of revolutionizing applications in health care. Thus, doing this means they ensure reliability, efficiency, and security that would give patient care an unparalleled performance in the future.

LIMITATIONS

While the above research is itself a systematic approach to realizing QoS for WSN-based healthcare applications, it still contains some disadvantages. In fact, the outcomes and analyses provided here are hypothetical and require actual implementation and validation in real life to affirm their applicability and efficacy; besides this, the methodology, though theoretically sound, might face unforeseen challenges and constraints in practical implementation, especially in resource-constrained environments, whereby further optimization and refinement are needed.

FUTURE SCOPE

This methodology will not only assist in designing WSN-based healthcare applications in a QoS-intensive way but also open up further avenues for research and development. Future research should be the actual implementation, validation, and optimization of the methodology in real scenarios to ensure that it is not only theoretically sound but also practically applicable and effective. The method could be refined and developed into multiple healthcare applications and scenarios to expand the scope of use and usefulness.

REFERENCES

Adewale, O. O., Shen, D., Wang, X., Li, L., & Zhao, T. (2021). Experimental measurement of force, torque control and vibration absorber system for intraoperative tele-operated robotic-assisted femoral shaft drilling using air-controlled soft balloon damper. *Transactions of the Institute of Measurement and Control*, *43*(11), 2525–2539.

Akinfenwa, O. A., Okunuga, S. A., & Abdulganiy, R. I. (2022). Higher order extended block hybrid second derivatives backward differentiation formula for solving DAE of index 1, 2, and 3. *Research Square*, 1(1), 1–21.

Almurib, H. A., Al-Qrimli, H. F., & Kumar, N. (2012). A review of application industrial robotic design. In 2011 Ninth International Conference on ICT and Knowledge Engineering, Bangkok, Thailand.

Anushya, A., Begum, S., Shiwani, S., & Shrivastava, A. (2024). Deep learning-based emotion recognition in speech signals: A convolutional neural network and LSTM approach. *AVE Trends in Intelligent Computing Systems*, *1*(4), 198–208.

Babu, K. A., Arulvendhan, K., Srinivasan, P., Ahmad, M. A., Prabha, A., Thariq, M. M., Ali, M. M. S., & Angelin, C. C. (2024). Economical infotainment solution augmented with advanced telematics for collision detection, vehicle localization, and real-time health status monitoring. *AVE Trends in Intelligent Health Letters*, *1*(4), 206–216.

Casonatto, J., Goessler, K. F., Cornelissen, V. A., Cardoso, J. R., & Polito, M. D. (2016). The blood pressure-lowering effect of a single bout of resistance exercise: A systematic review and meta-analysis of randomized controlled trials. *European Journal of Preventive Cardiology*, *23*(16), 1700–1714. PMID: 27512052

Chitra, A., Rajpriya, R., Karras, D. A., & Sridharlakshmi, N. R. B. (2024). An Exhaustive Study of Parasitic Organisms and Pathological Effects on Human Health. *AVE Trends In Intelligent Health Letters*, *1*(1), 10–18.

Ekblom, O., Ek, A., Cider, A., Hambraeus, K., & Börjesson, M. (2018). Increased physical activity post–myocardial infarction is related to reduced mortality: Results from the SWEDEHEART registry. *Journal of the American Heart Association*, *7*(24), 1–8. PMID: 30561263

Garber, C. E., Blissmer, B., Deschenes, M. R., Franklin, B. A., Lamonte, M. J., Lee, I. M., Nieman, D. C., & Swain, D. P. (2011). American College of Sports Medicine position stand. Quantity and quality of exercise for developing and maintaining cardiorespiratory, musculoskeletal, and neuromotor fitness in apparently healthy adults: Guidance for prescribing exercise. *Medicine and Science in Sports and Exercise, 43*(7), 1334–1359. PMID: 21694556

Golchian, M., Gachpazan, M., & Tabasi, S. H. (2020). A new approach for computing the exact solutions of DAEs in generalized Hessenberg forms. *International Journal of Nonlinear Analysis and Applications, 11*(1), 199–206.

Harendharan, B., & Boussi Rahmouni, H. (2023). Evaluating the Performance and Impact of Patient-Centric and Ambient Sensors. *FMDB Transactions on Sustainable Computer Letters, 1*(3), 192–201.

Hariharan, M. G., Saranya, S., Velavan, P., Soji, E. S., Rajest, S. S., & Thammareddi, L. (2024). Utilization of artificial intelligence algorithms for advanced cancer detection in the healthcare domain. In *Advances in Medical Technologies and Clinical Practice* (pp. 287–302). IGI Global.

Karthikeyan, B., Devi, R. A., & Munshi, M. (2024). Utilizing Deep Learning for the Classification of Brain Tumours Using MRI. *AVE Trends In Intelligent Health Letters, 1*(1), 1–9.

Kumar Nomula, V. (2023). A Novel Approach to Analyzing Medical Sensor Data Using Physiological Models. *FMDB Transactions on Sustainable Health Science Letters, 1*(4), 186–197.

Paramasivan, P., Rajest, S. S., Chinnusamy, K., Regin, R., & John Joseph, F. J. (Eds.). (2024). Advances in Medical Technologies and Clinical Practice *Clinical and comparative research on maternal health*. IGI Global., DOI: 10.4018/979-8-3693-5941-9

Pranav, R. P., Prawin, R. P., Subhashni, R., & Das, S. R. (2023). Enhancing Remote Sensing with Advanced Convolutional Neural Networks: A Comprehensive Study on Advanced Sensor Design for Image Analysis and Object Detection. *FMDB Transactions on Sustainable Computer Letters, 1*(4), 255–266.

Ramírez, J. G. C. (2024). AI in healthcare: Revolutionizing patient care with predictive analytics and decision support systems. *Journal of Artificial Intelligence and General Science, 1*(1), 31–37.

Regin, R., Priscila, S. S., Gnanaguru, G., Shynu, T., & Sakthivanitha, M. (2024). An analysis of methods for extending the life and coverage of wireless sensor networks. *FMDB Transactions on Sustainable Computer Letters*, *2*(4), 207–216.

Sayedelahl, M. A., & Farouk, R. M. (2024). Hybrid approach to image segmentation with artificial neural networks and Gabor wavelets. *AVE Trends in Intelligent Computing Systems*, *1*(2), 77–90.

Soltanian, F., Dehghan, M., & Karbassi, S. M. (2010). Solution of differential algebraic equations via homotopy perturbation method and their engineering applications. *International Journal of Computer Mathematics*, *87*(9), 1950–1974.

Srilakshmi, U., Sandhya, I., Manikandan, J., Bindu, A. H., Regin, R., & Rajest, S. S. (2024). Design and implementation of energy-efficient protocols for underwater wireless sensor networks. In *Advances in Computer and Electrical Engineering* (pp. 417–430). IGI Global.

Sundararajan, V., Steffi, R., & Shynu, T. (2023). Data Fusion Strategies for Collaborative Multi-Sensor Systems: Achieving Enhanced Observational Accuracy and Resilience. *FMDB Transactions on Sustainable Computing Systems*, *1*(3), 112–123.

Tan, Y., Fu, Z., Duan, L., Cui, R., Chen, J., Sun, H., & Wu, R. (2021). Hill-based musculoskeletal model for a fracture reduction robot. *International Journal of Medical Robotics and Computer Assisted Surgery*, *17*(3), 1–14. PMID: 33689227

Tsvetanov, F., & Georgieva, I. (2020). Modeling of energy consumption of sensor nodes. In *Proceedings of the 43rd International Convention on Information, Communication and Electronic Technology (MIPRO)*, Opatija, Croatia.

Zainuddin, A. A., Zakirudin, M. A. Z., Zulkefli, A. S. S., Mazli, A. M., Wardi, M. A. S. M., Fazail, M. N., Razali, M. I. Z. M., & Yusof, M. H. (2024). Artificial intelligence: A new paradigm for distributed sensor networks on the Internet of Things: A review. *International Journal of Perceptive and Cognitive Computing*, *10*(1), 16–28.

Chapter 7

Hybrid AI Model for Brain Age Estimation in Forensics Combining Structural and Functional Imaging

S. Kiruthika
https://orcid.org/0009-0004-4961-9282
Bharath Institute of Higher Education and Research, Chennai, India

S. Silvia Priscila
https://orcid.org/0000-0002-6040-3149
Bharath Institute of Higher Education and Research, Chennai, India

ABSTRACT

Brain age is used in forensic investigations to assess age-related traits, neurodegenerative diseases, and injuries. Separate systems that use structural neuroimaging (MRI) or functional imaging (fMRI) have low accuracy and reliability due to the lack of consideration that structure and function are biologically linked in the brain. Structural techniques, such as convolutional neural networks (CNNs), do not consider how physical changes, such as atrophy, influence functional patterns. These also do not consider how physical changes influence function patterns. Functional approaches based on recurrent neural networks (RNNs) can identify temporal activity but not structural changes. It shows a mixed AI model that combines an RNN with long short-term memory (LSTM) for functional fMRI analysis and CNNs for structural MRI analysis to get around these problems. These fusions improve the

DOI: 10.4018/979-8-3373-6796-5.ch007

understanding of the brain aging mechanism by merging temporal and geographical data. Comprehensive preprocessing, hyperparameter adjustment, and cross-validation are required for model durability.

INTRODUCTION

Because it is useful in assessing brain injuries, age development, and overall brain health, accurate brain age estimation is a popular study area in forensic science (Adekola et al., 2024). Environmental factors, illness, and injury can impact the brain, causing anatomical and functional changes as the body ages. Estimating brain age is particularly useful for forensic applications, such as determining the impact of trauma, identifying disease processes, and determining the age of unidentified people with criminal investigations or missing person cases (Pranav et al., 2023). Assessment of brain age has mostly relied on functional imaging methods, such as functional magnetic resonance imaging (fMRI), and structural imaging measurements, such as magnetic resonance imaging (MRI). Despite their usefulness, these methods aim to isolate the brain's dynamic activity or static physical structure. Their capacity to give a precise and thorough assessment of brain age has been hampered by the lack of characterization of the link between structural and functional changes that occur with aging. When CNNs process neuroimaging data, their primary focus is on structural imaging (Bose et al., 2024). These help find physical changes in the brain, like grey matter volume loss, ventricular enlargement, and tissue shrinkage atrophy. However, these disregard patterns of time-varying brain activity critical to cognition and cognitive aging. However, one can combine structural imaging techniques with functional imaging techniques (Aragani, 2024).

Functional imaging techniques don't look at the structure changes that come with aging. Still, these use RNNs to learn about the temporal within-subject variability in the fMRI signal. In the context of a more accurate and reliable brain age assessment, such a mismatch between structural and functional analysis performs very badly, especially in forensic settings when a thorough examination is essential (Sehrawat, 2024). These highlight the importance of the research in filling the knowledge gap in brain age estimation, which could lead to the formation of distinct classes of brain imbalance and a more thorough approach to brain age estimation. Combining structural and functional imaging data reveals brain aging in terms of neuron shape and function. It is crucial in forensic research because neurological disorders, traumatic brain damage, and other pathological processes can cause changes that are difficult to detect with a single imaging modality. For instance, an MRI scan may reveal structural damage from a traumatic brain injury, but fMRI is the sole way to detect functional changes in neuronal activity (Bose et al., 2024).

Similarly, neurological disorders such as Parkinson's and Alzheimer's disease may be characterized by both structural and functional failure, necessitating both specialized testing and analysis (Karthikeyan et al., 2024). The existing brain age systems only use MRI and fMRI independently, which can result in inaccurate and insufficient brain age estimates. Some of these interdependencies may be crucial (Kumar et al., 2024). These circumstances undermine not only the reliability of forensic analyses but also the capacity of legal and medical experts to reach wise conclusions. Therefore, a more advanced and complementary method incorporating structural and functional imaging characteristics is necessary for precise and comprehensive brain age assessment. The study aims to develop a hybrid AI model that can accurately and dependably process the brain age estimate by integrating structural and functional MRI data for forensic purposes. The Proposed method records the changing patterns of brain changes over time by combining CNNs for changes in structure and RNNs with LSTM for changes in function (Sehrawat et al., 2024).

The integrated method aims to solve the shortcomings of conventional single-modality solutions by drawing on a more thorough understanding of aging in the brain. It takes in imaging data input and performs minimal preprocessing (denoising, for instance). It uses a modular and structural processing architecture to generate a brain age prediction to extract features and modally fuse them in space or time. The objective is to develop a quick and dependable instrument that can be applied to actual forensic situations and eventually aid in mapping the progression of aging and health changes in the brain. Another objective of the study is to use rigorous measures to assess the performance of the proposed system and compare its accuracy and dependability to alternative approaches. Case studies or real-life examples will also show how the new model could be used in different situations, such as for trauma analysis, determining the age of missing people, and looking into neurological conditions (Gnanaguru et al., 2024).

The study makes several contributions. First, it suggests a new hybrid AI model using structural and functional imaging-modality data. No developmental brain age estimation models have previously used these kinds of data. It indicates a significant complementary relationship. The CNNs and RNNs work together to help the model learn about the changing and physical aspects of brain aging. These give a more accurate biological age estimate. Secondly, the study shows that the model is better than the best single-modality-based strategy by proving that combining data improves prediction accuracy. The results demonstrate the need to combine many imaging modalities to understand brain health better. Third, the study has outlined the complete preparation and analysis procedure of structural and functional imaging data to ensure that the model is trained on high-quality and highly standardized input data. The technique includes steps like motion correction, normalization, segmentation, and skull stripping that are crucial for minimizing biases and enhancing the reproducibility of the results. The fourth analysis cross-validates the model's random measures' performance to ensure that the methodology is not restricted to a single data type or population (Gandhi et al., 2024).

The study concludes by discussing the model's potential applications in animal forensics since it offers a quick and non-invasive way to estimate brain age in cases involving trauma, neurodegeneration, and missing persons. These innovative contributions can help people in clinical practice, forensics, search and rescue, and improve brain age estimation. The anthropological outline thoroughly explains the research's goals, methodology, findings, and conclusions. There are currently several methods for determining brain age, which is crucial in the forensic examination of criminal cases. Lastly, it outlines the study's goal and justifies a hybrid AI model. The authors thoroughly evaluate similar studies in brain age prediction in the literature review section, specifically analyzing the advantages and disadvantages of current methods and highlighting the areas where the suggested approach performs better.

The paper's section on system methodology covers the procedure for creating the hybrid AI model. These include input data collection, preprocessing, key feature extraction, and fusion methodologies. It uses a trained and tuned RNN with LSTM for functional assessments. It uses CNN for structural analysis. To show the effectiveness of the suggested model in the study, MAE, RMSE, and R^2 scores were used to compare it to other models. It also explores how data fusion affects the model's generalizability and prediction performance across various datasets. However, the discussion section and subsequent sections provide a fresh perspective, highlighting the discovery's significance and its contribution to the advancement of forensic science. The article also discusses the study's shortcomings and potential avenues for future research. The research's major accomplishments, including the invention of a model that could revolutionize the forensic brain age assessment procedure, are finally summed up in the conclusion. Additionally, these frameworks give the research precision and specificity in its presentation, which helps a more scholarly audience understand it while making it comprehensible to a less scholarly one (Chunduri et al., 2024).

In summary, by successfully calculating the brain age from fMRI and MRI data, the work provides a sophisticated hybrid AI model to support forensic sciences. Unlike single-modality approaches using CNN and RNN with LSTM to get structural and functional information about the brain separately, the model can show how the brain changes over time, space, and age. The outcomes demonstrate the multimodal data fusion's performance and imply that it outperforms the existing techniques in accuracy. The model created can be applied to forensic tasks such as trauma analysis, neurological state evaluation, and age estimation. Evaluation across different sample data is only feasible due to the model's dependability and generalizability. According to the study, structural and functional brain imaging are essential, underscoring the significance of comprehensive brain health assessments. It provides suggestions for further study that can quicken the use of brain age computation in clinical and forensic contexts, emphasizing growing the dataset, enhancing model performance, and evaluating functioning in real-time.

LITERATURE REVIEW

Brain age regression can predict both the occurrence and outcome of neurodegenerative illnesses. Using structural MRI data, CNNs were used to identify distinct morphological features associated with aging when estimating brain age. Single-modality techniques cannot capture functional differences in brain activity, limiting their forensic relevance. Traditional techniques relied heavily on handcrafted features, which limited their generalizability to different datasets. Although DL may improve forecast accuracy in such a manner, it is not yet a complete forensic analysis (Joo et al.,2023). Functional MRI's ability to show brain connections can be used to make age predictions. RNN models extract fMRI data and identify age-related functional changes more effectively than older approaches. Most forensic methods today are insensitive to topological changes, making it impossible to date a file or directory precisely. Brain age estimation in a forensic context may be improved using a multimodal approach that includes structural and functional imaging (Thurzo et al., 2021).

Conventional statistical frameworks presume that the features are chosen manually, despite studies showing the advantages of using integrated MRI and fMRI methods to study the brain. DL streamlines feature extraction from data, but current hybrid models lack forensic application tailoring. Combining CNN for MRI data and RNN for fMRI data ensures excellent forensic accuracy (Yadav, 2024). CNNs excel at retrieving structural components from structural MRI, making them an excellent choice for determining brain age. However, due to their functionality, these tools do not accurately reflect brain activity and cannot serve as standalone forensic tools. CNNs and RNNs can be crucial in accurately determining an individual's age, which is helpful in forensics (Jani & Patel, 2024), depending on the anatomical and functional analysis of the images. RNNs, specifically LSTMs, most frequently use sequential neuroimaging data, such as fMRI. These models don't do a good job of capturing relevant spatial information, but these do show how FCE changes with age. Forensic analysis and useful information from crimes can be gathered using CNNs for MRI and fMRI analysis and RNNs for processing fMRI data (Jani and Patel, 2024).

Multimodal AI frameworks, including MRI and fMRI, have potential forensics and lie detection applications. However, these are still reliant on medical diagnostic models. Hybrid models with forensic validation ensure accurate brain age assessment. Using CNN-RNN integration improves forensic authentication and predicts input samples accurately across varied datasets (Fan et al., 2023). Forensic brain age estimation involves combining MRI and fMRI data using feature fusion. DL-based automated feature extraction outperforms conventional statistical fusion methods in predicting accuracy. Hybrid AI models can improve the accuracy of biological age estimation approaches in forensic applications (Bhattacharya and Khan, 2023). People use AI forensic neuroimaging to estimate age, analyze cognitive decline, and assess trauma. DL offers excellent performance, but forensic validation is typically overlooked. A hybrid AI technique combining structural and functional imaging improves forensic reliability and reduces errors in legal age determinations (Niño-Sandoval et al., 2024). Recent research has used transfer learning to speed up model convergence in brain age estimates by using external datasets to train neural networks ahead of time. Forensic approaches should be optimized to cover a range of instances. Forensic examinations are more flexible and reliable when hybrid AI models use transfer learning and the CNN-RNN framework (Vasilaras et al., 2024)

Estimating brain age is useful for forensic investigations and age verification. To the launch of "Forensic Allays of Forman," both methods rely on anthropometry-based forensics and AI-based neuroimaging. Both methods treat humans like objects and emphasize accuracy based on the subject and sound. Combining MRI and fMRI ensures accurate forensic examination and reduces the risk of fMRI misleading courts (Singla et al., 2024). Ethical concerns include bias, transparency, and admissibility issues. Existing models may not always be interpretable, leading to the need for solutions such as explainable AI. Regulatory frameworks and forensic validation make AI-based age estimate systems more reliable while meeting legal and moral needs for human knowledge (Nguyen et al., 2023).

In forensic applications of brain age assessment, hybrid AI models and computational complexity can be problematic. The high memory and computational requirements make it unsuitable for real-time forensic applications. Model pruning and parallel computing optimize algorithms for efficient computation, making forensics applications more practical. Optimizing hyperparameters improves deep learning-based brain age estimation accuracy. Manually tuned models are generally suboptimal. Automated optimization approaches, such as hyperparameter tuning Bayesian, improve performance. Strong hyperparameter tweaking improves forensic accuracy and minimizes uncertainty in neuroimaging applications. AI tools such as Grad-CAM and SHAP aid in interpreting forensic brain age models. Deep learning frameworks often lack forensic credibility due to their perceived black-box nature. Improved transparency allows forensic professionals to test AI predictions while maintaining legal acceptability (Tortora, 2024).

Cross-validation approaches are necessary when evaluating brain age estimation models for forensic purposes. Standard k-fold validation approaches fail to take into account diversity in forensic datasets. Stratified sampling improves model generalizability across populations, leading to higher forensic accuracy for MAE RMSE (Ataş et al., 2023). Data augmentation procedures provide synthetic variations that improve model resilience. Currently, augmentation approaches for structural MRI are limited, whereas functional data augmentation remains unexplored. Text augmentation influences hybrid fMRI-based prediction in forensic contexts (Ketsekioulafis et al., 2024). Neural architecture search (NAS) makes setting hyperparameters in machine learning algorithms easier. This makes it possible to make better models for tasks like figuring out how old a brain is for forensic purposes. Manual architectural selection is popular but ineffective in forensics, limiting its application. NAS can be included in hybrid CNN-RNN models, improving ease and effectiveness in forensic situations (Sharifonnasabi et al., 2022).

Many models can be combined using ensemble learning approaches to improve prediction accuracy. Methods for improving forensic neuroimaging, including stacking, boosting, and bagging, remain clinically relevant. Ensemble techniques in mixed AI models improve reliability in forensic brain age estimation (Nehma et al., 2024). Forensic brain age estimation protocols must be compatible with the application in medicolegal contexts. Barber forensic applications are uneven due to various approaches used in previous studies. Standardized processes enable AI-driven age assessment to be accepted in court, increasing reproducibility and forensic validity (Iyortsuun et al., 2023). Advancements in neuroimaging and forensic science will enhance methods for determining brain age. Future studies should incorporate more imaging modalities such as fMRI, enhance designs, and address ethical concerns. Using more than one method together makes forensics more useful and allows biological age estimates based on AI to be legally contested (Punjabi and Chaure, 2022).

SYSTEM METHODOLOGY

Forensic science's existing brain age estimation algorithms rely entirely on MRI and fMRI, which frequently use a single modality to infer biological age. Despite having some degree of validation, these techniques are limited to existing applications of brain age estimation, and they frequently overlook the brain's structural and functional activity. Traditional techniques, such as CNNs using MRI data, analyze physical alterations in the brain, such as atrophy, lesions, etc., that typically happen with aging or following a brain injury. Using RNN-based techniques on fMRI data identifies changing patterns in brain activity that occur over a long period by searching for similarities between different time points. However, these methods don't fully use the benefits of structural and functional data complementarity because they often show measured structural and functional data without looking at the connections that could show changes in brain age.

In light of these constraints, implement the hybrid artificial intelligence model using deep learning to integrate structural MRI and functional fMRI imaging data. While RNN works with fMRI data and focuses on functional tasks since it can learn temporal patterns in brain networks, it uses CNNs to extract features from structural MRI images by correcting physiological patterns of small physical changes and giving the brain a certain age. The advantages of both techniques provide a more accurate and trustworthy estimate of biological age since the hybrid model, rich in information from both modalities, considers brain aging more thoroughly. It uses certain procedures to implement the hybrid AI model into practice. Initially, structural and functional imaging data will be imported and preprocessed in the same area. Grey matter (GM), white matter (WM), and cerebrospinal fluid (CSF) of brain regions of interest (ROIs) are divided into structural MRI images and are important aspects of brain aging. On the other hand, functional MRI data emphasizes the neural connections that underlie cognitive processes by preprocessing and distilling the brain's activity patterns throughout time.

After preprocessing, the model uses CNNs to extract spatial features from the MRI data to identify the parts of the brain that exhibit notable aging-related changes (such as shrinkage). Then, temporal features from fMRI data are mixed with an RNN that simulates the changing patterns of brain activity over time. These may show how changes in function can happen due to injury or aging. The model combines both morphological and functional representations. These are then fed into a fusion layer, which takes all the data and uses it to make predictions about brain age. The whole neural network is trained using a dataset of the type that includes both kinds of images, and hyperparameter optimization is carried out to find the best CNN and RNN parameter combination. Additionally, the model is cross-validated and applied to a different age group and forensic case, ensuring that the questionnaire is a reliable and universal instrument for determining brain age.

The primary innovation of the method, in contrast with existing systems, is the use of DL techniques to project both structural and functional data, allowing for the modeling of the brain's anatomical state and how activity changes with age or injury. It has the unique benefit of giving a full understanding of how aging works because the model is hybrid and can show both static changes in structure and dynamic changes in function in many systems at the same time. It is especially crucial in forensic procedures where, for instance, neurological disorders or brain trauma cause functional alterations that are not immediately visible with structural morphology imaging. Also, the model could be especially useful in cases where regular methods don't work, like when someone has a neurological disease, a (focal) brain injury, or another abnormal state that causes big changes in microstructure and microfunction. Nevertheless, the information that has been cross-mapped together makes the brain age predictor a more potent and trustworthy forensic tool that can have serious legal and health consequences (Figure 1).

Figure 1. Process Flowchart

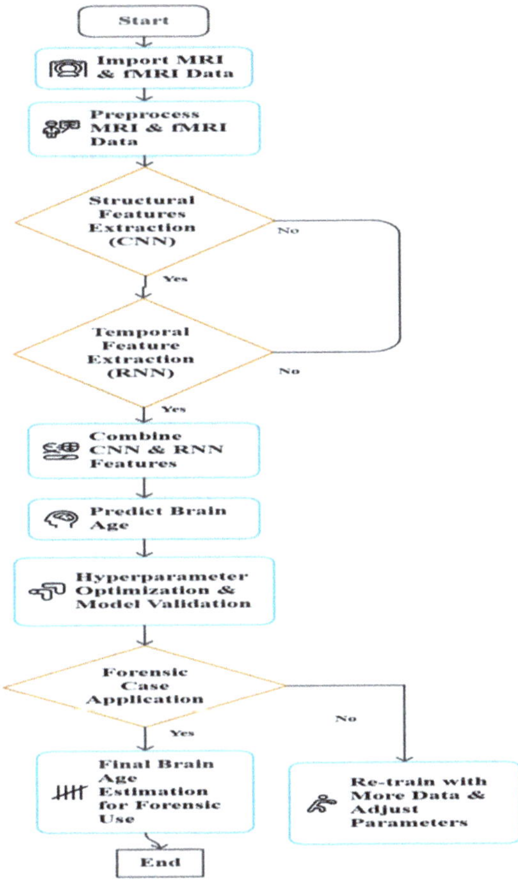

Using the hybrid AI model to estimate brain age has numerous significant advantages. Combining two features from structural and functional MRI data produces a scalable and reliable estimate of brain age. According to the foundations of traditional techniques, MRI and fMRI are naked and yet miss a significant complex component of health since these are unable to identify minute changes in function or early signs of trauma. Using both modalities to predict age in forensic situations increases the robustness and efficiency of an age estimator. It can be used for a wide range of forensic applications, such as trauma analysis, DNA-based victim age estimation, and brain pathology assessment in situations when structural scans may not be sufficient. In the context of a real-world forensic inquiry, the hybrid model may be a useful non-invasive substitute for an invasive age estimation method. It works better as the model uses deep learning techniques (like CNNs and RNNs) to understand huge amounts of imaging data and give accurate, real-time brain age information. For time-sensitive forensic applications, it's essential.

In summary, hybrid AI modeling is a significant advancement in forensic brain age estimation that surpasses earlier techniques' drawbacks by combining structural and functional changes to provide a more thorough, precise, and clinically relevant evaluation of brain age. It improves the integration of structural and functional imaging data and makes determining the age of a brain easier in forensic situations. The model is less likely to be incorrect if a neurological injury and disorder occurs. Along with new information about brain diseases that happen at different ages and progress in forensic neuroscience, the new method could change forensic evaluation and how brain health works by making people more agile at the right age for their age.

DATA COLLECTION AND PREPROCESSING

The first steps to collecting a functional hybrid neural network model to estimate brain age are data collection and preprocessing. Both structural and functional MRIs of superior quality are necessary for the model's accuracy. To ensure that both samples were representative and heterogeneous, the images were taken from publicly available brain imaging datasets that comprised a variety of neurologically healthy and poor participants as well as older and younger adults. Data from functional magnetic resonance imaging (fMRI) and magnetic resonance imaging (MRI) undergo some preprocessing stages, where enhancing the data's quality and getting it ready for a DL approach are the goals of the preprocessing procedures. It offers structural MRI data without any non-brain tissue, like the skull. The segmentation methods then yield the GM, WM, and CSF ROIs. To ensure patient uniformity, the segregated zones are spatially normalized into a common coordinate system. Some techniques used to prepare the functional fMRI data were motion correction, slice timing correction, and temporal filtering. It implements these techniques to mitigate the potential for noise and motion artifacts to obscure brain activity signals. Then, match the corrected functional data with the right MRI scans to ensure that brain areas are lined up across all three types of images. The pretreatment dataset ensures that the data is clean and uniform to avoid potential biases if different patients have significantly varied brain area anatomy. Normalization techniques are also utilized to standardize the strength of brain signals for the same input data from various people, allowing the model to compare data from several participants consistently.

Now that the data is prepared for analysis, it can forecast the age of the brain by combining the structural and functional data in the next part.

$$X' = \frac{X - \mu}{\sigma} \tag{1}$$

X is the original pixel intensity, μ is the mean intensity, and σ is the standard deviation, ensuring uniform scaling across subjects.

STRUCTURAL DATA ANALYSIS USING CNNs

The next phase in the process is the use of CNNs for the analysis of structural MRI data. It chose to employ CNNs to analyze structural MRI images because of their high performance in spatial feature extraction for image data. These feature extractions are mostly about finding things connected to brain structure changes with age, like tissue loss, ventricular expansion, or a loss of grey matter volume. The CNN model's first few layers are convolutional. These layers use different MRI image filters to pick up local information like shapes, textures, and edges. As the convolutional filters continue to explore the network, these extract more high-level, abstract properties. After collecting the feature maps from the previous stage, pooling layers reduce their dimensionality by retaining the most pertinent characteristics and eliminating the less helpful ones. Fully connected layers combine all the outputs from the convolutional and pooling layers to represent the full image. CNN can predict the final output's brain age characteristics. The model is trained using labeled MRI datasets, with the subject's biological age as the ground truth. The most popular loss function for supervised training is the MSE, which severely penalizes significant departures from the predicted age. The CNN will now start backpropagating the error found by the softmax layer and changing the weights for all convolutional layers. These will help train the model and eventually teach it to guess the labels correctly. It will ensure that the CNN can accurately and consistently detect aging-related brain structure changes.

$$O(i,j) = \sum_{m}\sum_{n} I(i + m, j + n)K(m, n) \tag{2}$$

where I(i,j)is the input MRI image, K(m, n) is the convolutional kernel, and O(i,j)is the output feature map.

Figure 2. Hybrid Neural Network Model Architecture

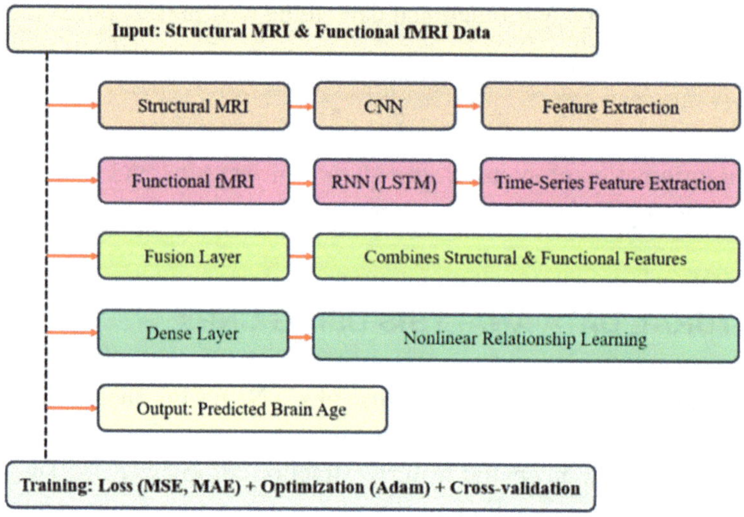

FUNCTIONAL DATA ANALYSIS USING RNNs

Concurrently with the structural MRI analysis, RNNs analyze the functional data collected from the fMRI scans. Because RNNs use the sequential character of data, these are easy to use to represent sequential data, like fMRI signals, which show changes in neural activity over time. These phases are intended for these reasons since dynamic age is the key component of brain activity for measuring biological age owing to aging and cognitive functioning. It uses LSTM instead of regular memory cells to enhance the RNN architecture and solve the vanishing gradient issue with normal RNNs. Since brain activity fluctuates over extended periods, LSTMs allow the model to retain long-term dependencies in the data. Functional data processing yields time-series data from specific brain regions typically associated with cognitive processes. Then, these time-series signals are used to train the RNN, enabling it to recognize the patterns of brain activity linked to aging. Except for using the participants' biological age as the train, the model is trained precisely like the CNN model. A loss function such as MAE is employed to reduce the discrepancy between the expected and actual ages of the brain. Backpropagation modifies and updates the weight of the LSTM network during training, enhancing the model's prediction accuracy and dependability. The RNN's functional analysis improves CNN's structural analysis by finding hidden temporal patterns in brain activity. These show how brain function changes cause the more complex aging process (Figure 2).

$$h_t = o_t \tanh(c_t) \quad (3)$$

where h_t is the hidden state, o_t is the output gate, and c_t is the cell state that controls memory retention in the network.

FUSION OF STRUCTURAL AND FUNCTIONAL DATA

The study focuses on merging structural MRI and functional fMRI data to produce a more accurate and consistent indicator of brain age. After the CNN and RNN, a fusion layer takes the output features of both networks and combines them after looking at structural and functional data separately. It uses the complementing advantages of each modality: the structural data provide light on the physical alterations in the brain. In contrast, the functional data reveal patterns of activity across time. Lastly, it generates a new model by fusing the feature vectors of the two models. Because the fusion layer integrates CNN spatial and RNN temporal features, the hybrid model can depict static and temporal information about brain aging. It concatenates these features to learn nonlinear correlations between structural and functional representations before sending them to a dense layer. The hybrid representation is more informative than either modality alone because it preserves the model's understanding of a greater range of age-related changes. After obtaining the combined data through the fusion process, the age of the brain is predicted. Because it more accurately depicts how the brain ages, it enhances biological age prediction. The extra hybrid model uses both the CNN's structural changes and the RNN's functional dynamics to give a clear, consistent, and reliable estimate of brain age that can be used in forensic cases.

$$F = [F_s : F_f] \quad (4)$$

where F_s is the feature vector from the CNN (structural data) and F_f is the feature vector from the RNN (functional data).

MODEL TRAINING AND HYPERPARAMETER OPTIMIZATION

One of the most crucial phases in developing the hybrid model is training it to combine structural and functional data to give it the capacity to estimate brain age. During the training phase, feed the model preprocessed structural MRI and functional fMRI data as input, along with known biological ages as output labels. Because these processes occur supervised, the model learns to link the genes to the appropriate output (the biological age). Two distinct neural networks, CNNs for structural data and RNNs for functional data, comprise the hybrid model. These are first trained apart from one another. Once each network has optimized to support its predictions, they combine their outputs to calculate the resulting brain age. The optimization process that uses backpropagation is fine-tuned using an Adam optimizer. This adaptive learning rate optimization technique modifies the learning rate during training to help enhance the optimization performance. The most important stage in the training process is hyperparameter tuning, which entails adjusting the parameters for the CNN, such as the number of layers, learning rates, batch size, and filter sizes, and the RNN, such as the number of LSTM units and time steps. Generally, it uses grid and random search to identify and optimize a set of hyperparameters that produce the best results. To verify if the model can correctly forecast brain age, it uses measures like the MSE and MAE. Cross-validation ensures the model can generalize unknown data and not overfit the training dataset.

$$\theta_t = \theta_t - \frac{\eta}{\sqrt{v_t + \epsilon}} m_t \tag{5}$$

where η is the learning rate, m_t is the first-moment estimate, and v_t is the second-moment estimate (Figure 3).

Figure 3. Deployment Workflow in Forensic Science

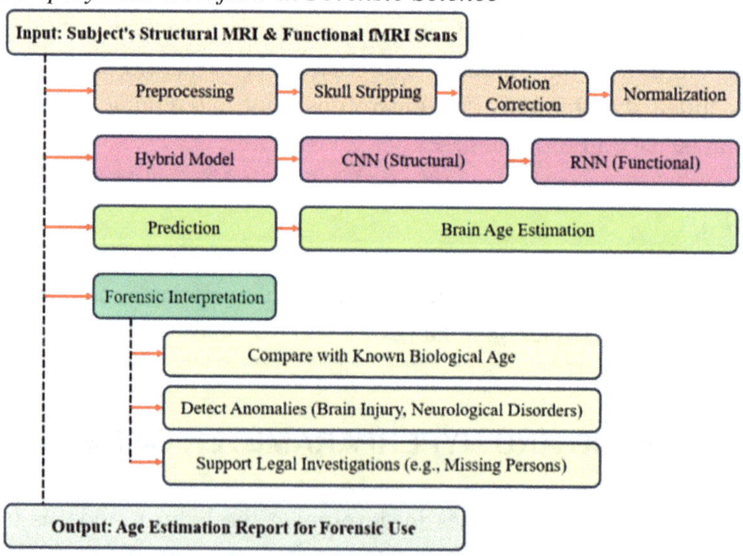

EVALUATION AND PERFORMANCE METRICS

After training, the hybrid model will be assessed using measures to determine its correctness and stability. The two most important metrics for assessing prediction performance are RMSE and MAE. RMSE treats extreme prediction errors by squaring the value, and large errors can lead to an RMSE that is more focused on extremes and larger errors. MAE, on the other hand, measures the average absolute error between predicted and actual brain ages. These metrics thoroughly assess the variance in the projected over-expected values and the model biological age prediction. It uses these error metrics and the correlation coefficients to assess the model's predictive accuracy. These coefficients describe the direction and degree of the association between the expected and actual brain ages. A high correlation would indicate that the model was accurately capturing aging. To make sure the model is generalizable, it must also perform cross-validation, which involves dividing the data into numerous subsets, testing the model against these subsets, and then training the model against other subsets that remain. Thus, validation keeps it functioning well by preventing overfitting caused by unseen data. The model's output is compared against approaches that rely solely on structure or function data. Regarding brain age estimation, combining these two methods performs better than alone. As demonstrated, combining structural and functional data yields more precise and repeatable brain-age estimations. To evaluate the model's generalizability for actual forensic usage, it also evaluated its performance across various demographics and neurological conditions.

$$\text{MAE} = \frac{1}{N}\sum_{I=1}^{N}\left|y_i - \hat{y}_i\right| \tag{6}$$

where y_i is the actual age and $\hat{y}_i$ is the predicted age.

DEPLOYMENT AND APPLICATION IN FORENSIC SCIENCE

After training and validation, the hybrid AI was ready for use in real forensic investigations. Among its many uses is the assessment of brain age, which may be useful in cases involving missing persons, neurological illnesses, and brain traumas. To provide a precise biological age for both courts and hospitals, the model may be tested using brain-scanning techniques and plasma samples (blood tests) already given to people with known biological ages. It simultaneously processed structural MRI and functional fMRI data during the integration phase to predict brain age. By evaluating the model's outputs and modifying the parameters for factors that alter with age in the brain, forensic experts can determine whether or not a person has a head injury, age-related dysfunction, or any other dysregulation. The extent of brain tissue injury or repair in victims could serve as evidence for forensic scientists to validate or refute these theories. Furthermore, the hybrid model's ability to function with many data sources provides great potential for use in various forensic fields, including determining the age of unidentified people or assessing age-dependent alterations in cognitive function in senior citizens. The model is a significant advancement and a potent tool for supporting forensic researchers because it is a non-invasive, objective, and comparatively more effective way to estimate brain age. It also creates three-dimensional versions and integrates structural and functional brain data to produce more accurate conclusions crucial in the courtroom setting.

$$\hat{Y} = W_f F + b \tag{7}$$

where W_f represents the fusion layer weights, F is the concatenated feature vector, and b is the bias term.

```
def preprocess_mri(mri):
return normalize(resize(segment(skull_strip(mri)), target_
size))
def preprocess_fmri(fmri):
return extract_time_series(spatial_normalization(slice_tim-
ing_correction(motion_correction(fmri))))
def cnn_model(input_shape):
model = Sequential ([
Conv2D (32, (3,3), activation='relu', input_shape=input_
shape),
MaxPooling2D ((2,2)),
Conv2D (64, (3,3), activation='relu'),
MaxPooling2D ((2,2)),
Flatten (), Dense (128, activation='relu'), Dense (64, acti-
vation='relu')
])
return model
def rnn_model(input_shape):
model = Sequential ([
LSTM (64, return_sequences=True, input_shape=input_shape),
LSTM (32, return_sequences=False),
Dense (64, activation='relu')
])
```

```
  return model
  def hybrid_model (cnn_features, rnn_features):
  fused = concatenate ([cnn_features, rnn_features])
  return Model ([cnn_input, rnn_input], Dense (1, activa-
tion='linear') (fused))
  Def train (model, train_data, labels):
  model.compile(optimizer='adam', loss='mse', metrics=['made])
  model.fit(train_data, labels, epochs=50, batch_size=32, val-
idation_split=0.2)
  Def evaluate (model, test_data, labels):
  return model.evaluate(test_data, labels)[1]
  def predict_age(model, new_mri, new_fmri):
  return model.predict([cnn_model.predict(new_mri), rnn_model.
predict(new_fmri)])
  mri_data, fmri_data = preprocess_mri(load_mri("dataset/M-
RI")), preprocess_fmri(load_fmri("dataset/fMRI"))
  cnn_feat, rnn_feat = cnn_model(input_shape_mri), rnn_mod-
el(input_shape_fmri)
  hybrid = hybrid_model(cnn_feat, rnn_feat)
  train (hybrid, [mri_data, fmri_data], age_labels)
  print ("Predicted Brain Age:," predict_age (hybrid, new_mri,
new_fmri))
```

The proposed hybrid AI model uses pseudo-code to estimate brain age from fMRI and MRI data. The first step is to normally process MRI and fMRI data, which includes separating grey and white matter, adjusting to the MNI space, and fixing for movement. An RNN (LSTM) learns the temporal pattern in fMRI, whereas a CNN extracts spatial characteristics from MRI. Finally, it uses the Adam optimizer and MSE loss to combine these features to create a hybrid model. It uses MAE to assess the model's correctness. The model then generates brain-age outputs using unseen MRI and fMRI. The methodology provides a thorough evaluation of brain aging by considering both the anatomical and functional characteristics of the brain, which raises the accuracy of age estimation in forensic settings.

The model fully understands how brain degeneration happens and changes over time by combining RNNs with LSTM for functional fMRI and CNNs for structural MRI. By combining information about time and space, the unique feature fusion design allows the model to produce better predictions than a standard single-modality model. Deep preprocessing, k-fold cross-validation, and iterative hyperparameter adjustment improve the model's robustness and generalizability. Third, the performance comparison indicates that the proposed model outperforms the recently developed models regarding MAE and its association with brain age. In the forensic field, the method is particularly useful for determining the biological age of missing individuals in forensic instances. Future developments may include additional neuroimaging modalities and interpretable AI to simplify interpretation. It is the most cutting-edge AI-based brain age assessment due to its accuracy, speed, and practical usefulness.

RESULTS AND ANALYSIS

The results and analysis section provides a thorough comparison between the proposed system and the existing systems. It assesses the model's stability and prediction accuracy using metrics like MAE, RMSE, R^2 score, and cross-validation outcomes. Research on the effects of structural and functional data fusion also shows how performance improved. According to statistical comparisons, the proposed technique outperforms rival models regarding forecast accuracy and stability. The effectiveness and efficacy of the proposed method were demonstrated after it was tested and implemented for possible real-world applications.

Table 1. Prediction Accuracy Comparison (Lower is Better)

Model	MAE (Years) ↓	RMSE (Years) ↓	R^2 Score ↑
Lefèvre et al. (2023)	4.92	6.35	0.78
Zhang et al. (2022)	5.34	6.82	0.74
Yadav et al. (2022)	4.67	6.11	0.81
Proposed System	3.21	4.87	0.91

Using the primary metrics listed in Table 1, compare how well the proposed system predicts the impact factors to the existing systems (Lefèvre et al. (2023) ; Zhang et al. (2022) ; Yadav et al. (2022). The R^2 value will be greater for a more dependable model, and the MAE and RMSE scores will be lower for a model with superior prediction accuracy. The best existing systems have an MAE of 4.92, 5.34, and 4.67 years, an RMSE of 6.11 to 6.82 years, and an R^2 of 0.74 to 0.81 years. Nonetheless, the proposed method exhibits a high degree of accuracy with a low MAE (3.21 years), a high R^2 score (0.91), and a lowered RMSE (4.87 years). Given the departure from species generality, the results show that the proposed approach outperforms the existing methodologies in estimating ages while offering a higher prediction accuracy.

Table 2. Cross-Validation Results

Model	5-Fold MAE (Years) ↓	10-Fold MAE (Years) ↓	Standard Deviation ↓
Lefèvre et al. (2023)	5.02	4.95	0.63
Zhang et al. (2022)	5.58	5.41	0.71
Yadav et al. (2022)	4.89	4.62	0.57
Proposed System	3.34	3.18	0.42

Table 2 compares the cross-validation results of the proposed system and the existing system (Lefèvre et al. (2023) ; Zhang et al. (2022) ; Yadav et al. (2022) using 5-fold and 10-fold MAE with standard deviation. Consequently, the more accurately a model can forecast, the lower the MAE; the more stable the model, the lower the standard deviation value. The proposed systems achieve five-fold MAEs of 4.89–5.58 years, with standard deviations ranging from 0.57–0.71. Compared to the lowest performance, the proposed system achieves a 5-fold MAE of 3.34 years, a 10-fold MAE of 3.18 years, and the lowest standard deviation of 0.42, meaning that performance gains are more than five times greater. As a result, the proposed system has better stability and robustness over the three validation folds and is computationally more efficient than the existing system.

Table 3. Contribution of Structural and Functional Data Fusion

Model	Structural-Only MAE (Years)	Functional-Only MAE (Years)	Combined Fusion MAE (Years)	Improvement Over Best Single Modality (%)
Lefèvre et al. (2023)	4.92	5.78	4.35	11.6%
Zhang et al. (2022)	5.21	5.34	4.57	12.8%
Yadav et al. (2022)	4.67	5.11	4.21	9.8%
Proposed System	3.94	4.12	3.21	18.5%

Table 3 shows the MAE for structural, functional, and both structural and functional data fusion-based predictions, which were found by comparing the proposed systems to the existing systems (Lefèvre et al. (2023) ; Zhang et al. (2022) ; Yadav et al. (2022). The accuracy of the structural and functional data alone and with both models shows that, in all three models, the structural data consistently outperforms the functional data alone. However, combining both modalities results in a significantly lower MAE, which validates the fusion intuition. With a combined MAE of 4.21 and 4.57 years, the existing systems are 9.8%–12.8% better than the best single modality. As a result, it proposes a system that further enhances performance, yielding an MAE of 3.21 years, which is 18.5% better than its best modality alone. It proves that the proposed method is better than existing systems by showing that it has the most gain and that more structural and functional data leads to more accurate predictions. In summary, the proposed system has significantly enhanced prediction accuracy and model stability compared to the existing approaches. The proposed system performs better, as shown by the performance measurements. Specifically, the model fits well, and the predictions are accurate because the MAE and RMSE are greatly decreased, and the R^2 score is high. The proposed system outperforms the best single modality by combining structural and functional data to reach even higher accuracy. The results demonstrate that the new system is a more reliable, precise, and practical tool for applications requiring high resolution and consistency. In addition to showing that the proposed system works (common validity), the results also show that using data fusion instead of just one mode or signal gives the best performance.

DISCUSSION

Using MRI and fMRI imaging data, the proposed hybrid AI model for brain age estimates differs from its predecessors. The model exhibits better accuracy and robustness than existing methods, with smaller prediction errors and a higher correlation with brain age. Because structural and functional data capture both static and dynamic components of brain aging, both mainly complement one another and produce more accurate and comprehensive predictions that improve performance. It is very helpful in forensic applications where precise brain age assessment is crucial with accident cases, neurological disorders, or missing persons. The model can synergistically incorporate temporal patterns for fMRI and spatial information retrieved from MRI; however, most single-modality techniques miss the interconnectedness of brain aging. The integration improves prediction accuracy and the model's applicability to various forensic tasks by setting up a testbed and conducting testing. The model can scale with a lot of data due to the DL techniques, specifically CNNs and RNNsand, so it adapts to the actual world more naturally. One of the primary advantages of the study is the non-invasiveness of the proposed system, which makes it possible to use it as an approachable substitute for frequently used invasive techniques. Confirming its generalizability across various age and disease populations further supports its potential for forensic applications. When giving a more thorough description of the aging brain, the hybrid model may also shed light on trauma and brain health, which could aid legal and medical authorities in making well-informed judgments. Overall, the approach represents a significant advancement in brain-age computation. It combines multimodal information fusion with deep learning big data AI model fusion to produce an adaptable, dependable, and forensically correct system.

CONCLUSION AND FUTURE WORK

In conclusion, it developed a novel hybrid approach utilizing DL CNN, MRI, and fMRI data. Technical attainment will significantly alter the process. According to its cross-validation, prediction, and testing values, the proposed model outperforms the existing systems in testing and can withstand criticism and scrutiny from its peers. However, there are problems with the study. The model's dependence on high-quality imaging data, which might not be available in forensic settings, is one of its disadvantages. Second, deploying an ensemble model could not be practical when resources are limited because training the model requires a lot of resources. Third, poor generalizability is restricted to a few neurological disorders and countries due to a lack of diversity in training datasets. Because of these problems, future research must find ways to get around them. Algorithms with these extra strengths will need less computing power, offer more datasets, and make the work more predictive using techniques like diffusion tensor imaging (DTI). Integrating the model with explainable AI methods would also offer more flexibility, aiding the forensic practitioner in understanding the model's output. Addressing these issues, the proposed system might help improve brain age estimation in forensic research. Eventually, it could result in a more widely applicable tool in legal and medical settings. It provides a complex view of brain aging that is difficult to obtain through other means, especially when combined with information about trauma, neurobiology, or molecular biology. People frequently use it in contexts that link trauma, neuroimaging, or missing persons. The technique will open up new possibilities for forensic neuroscience and set a new benchmark for AI-based brain age assessment.

REFERENCES

Adekola, A. A., Olapade, T., Oyeniyi, O. C., & Anifowose, O. M. (2024). Fraud detection, fraud prevention, and forensic accounting: An empirical study from EFCC report. *FMDB Transactions on Sustainable Technoprise Letters*, *2*(1), 1–9.

Aragani, V. M. (2024). Revolutionizing insurance through AI and data analytics: Innovating policy underwriting and claims management for the digital era. *FMDB Transactions on Sustainable Computer Letters*, *2*(3), 176–185.

Ataş, İ., Özdemir, C., Ataş, M., & Doğan, Y. (2023). Forensic dental age estimation using modified deep learning neural network. *Balkan Journal of Electrical and Computer Engineering*, *11*(4), 298–305.

Bhattacharya, R., & Khan, A. (2023). Artificial intelligence in forensic psychiatry: Admissibility and relevance before courts. *International Journal of System Assurance Engineering and Management*, *15*(5), 1638–1649.

Bose, S. R., Jeba, J. A., Kishore, V. K., Gnanaguru, G., & Shynu, T. (2024). Deep learning-driven acute lymphoblastic leukemia detection using CT scan imaging. *AVE Trends in Intelligent Health Letters*, *1*(2), 110–124.

Bose, S. R., Jeba, J. A., Regin, R., Tarunraj, S., Soji, E. S., & Rajest, S. S. (2024). Enhanced deep learning models for early detection of renal failure from CT imaging. *FMDB Transactions on Sustainable Health Science Letters*, *2*(3), 152–163.

Chunduri, V., Rajest, S. S., Allugunti, V. R., Verma, D., Aarthi, R., & Sharma, D. K. (2024). Deep neural network for brain tumour segmentation using guaranteed time slots (GTS) algorithm. In *Advances in Computer and Electrical Engineering* (pp. 371–390). IGI Global.

Fan, F., Li, T., Li, Y., Zhang, W., Zhang, Q., & Chen, Y. (2023). Semi-supervised automatic dental age and sex estimation using a hybrid transformer model. *International Journal of Legal Medicine*, *137*(3), 721–731. PMID: 36717384

Gandhi, M., Satheesh, C., Soji, E. S., Saranya, M., Rajest, S. S., & Kothuru, S. K. (2024). Image recognition and extraction on computerized vision for sign language decoding. In *Explainable AI Applications for Human Behavior Analysis* (pp. 157–173). IGI Global.

Gnanaguru, G., Priscila, S. S., Sakthivanitha, M., Radhakrishnan, S., Rajest, S. S., & Singh, S. (2024). Thorough analysis of deep learning methods for diagnosis of COVID-19 CT images. In *Advances in Medical Technologies and Clinical Practice* (pp. 46–65). IGI Global.

Iyortsuun, N. K., Kim, S.-H., Jhon, M., Yang, H.-J., & Pant, S. (2023). A review of machine learning and deep learning approaches on mental health diagnosis. *Health Care*, *11*(3), 285. PMID: 36766860

Jani, G., & Patel, B. (2024). Charting the growth through intelligence: A SWOC analysis on AI-assisted radiologic bone age estimation. *International Journal of Legal Medicine*, *139*(2), 679–694. PMID: 39460772

Joo, Y., Eun Namgung., Hyeonseok Jeong., Ilhyang Kang., Jinsol Kim., Sohyun Oh., In Kyoon Lyoo., Sujung Yoon., & Jaeuk Hwang. (2023). Brain age prediction using combined deep convolutional neural network and multi-layer perceptron algorithms. *Scientific Reports*, *13*(1), 22388. PMID: 38104173

Karthikeyan, B., Devi, R. A., & Munshi, M. (2024). Utilizing Deep Learning for the Classification of Brain Tumours Using MRI. *AVE Trends In Intelligent Health Letters*, *1*(1), 1–9.

Ketsekioulafis, I., Filandrianos, G., Katsos, K., Thomas, K., Spiliopoulou, C., Stamou, G., & Sakelliadis, E. I. (2024). Artificial intelligence in forensic sciences: A systematic review of past and current applications and future perspectives. *Cureus*, *16*(9), 2–16. PMID: 39469392

Kumar, M. P. N. V., Chitra, A., Rajpriya, R., Gayathri, B., Roberts, C., & Rajest, S. S. (2024). Brain-optimized U-Net model for intraretinal cystoid fluid segmentation in optical coherence tomography. *AVE Trends in Intelligent Health Letters*, *1*(1), 38–50.

Lefèvre, T., & Tournois, L. (2023). Artificial intelligence and diagnostics in medicine and forensic science. *Diagnostics (Basel)*, *13*(23), 3554. PMID: 38066795

Nehma, E. J., Hassan, A. K. A., & Ali, S. K. (2024). *A review on multi-model age estimation techniques for security applications*. AIP Conference Proceedings.

Nguyen, N.-M., Wang, W.-C., & Cao, M.-T. (2023). Early estimation of the long-term deflection of reinforced concrete beams using surrogate models. *Construction & Building Materials*, *370*(3), 130670.

Niño-Sandoval, T. C., Doria-Martinez, A. M., Escobar, R. A. V., Sánchez, E. L., Rojas, I. B., Álvarez, L. C. V., Mc Cann, D. S. F., & Támara-Patiño, L. M. (2024). Efficacy of the methods of age determination using artificial intelligence in pan oramic radiographs — A systematic review. *International Journal of Legal Medicine*, *138*(4), 1459–1496. PMID: 38400923

Pranav, R. P., Prawin, R. P., Subhashni, R., & Das, S. R. (2023). Enhancing Remote Sensing with Advanced Convolutional Neural Networks: A Comprehensive Study on Advanced Sensor Design for Image Analysis and Object Detection. *FMDB Transactions on Sustainable Computer Letters*, *1*(4), 255–266.

Punjabi, S. K., & Chaure, S. (2022). Forensic intelligence: Combining artificial intelligence with digital forensics. In 2022 2nd International Conference on Intelligent Technologies (CONIT), Hubballi, India.

Sehrawat, S. K. (2024). Leveraging AI for early detection of chronic diseases through patient data integration. *AVE Trends in Intelligent Health Letters*, *1*(3), 125–136.

Sehrawat, S. K. (2024). Revolutionizing patient care through innovation and technology in modern healthcare. *FMDB Transactions on Sustainable Health Science Letters*, *2*(3), 141–151.

Sharifonnasabi, F., Jhanjhi, N. Z., John, J., Obeidy, P., Band, S. S., Alinejad-Rokny, H., & Baz, M. (2022). Hybrid HCNN-KNN model enhances age estimation accuracy in orthopantomography. *Frontiers in Public Health*, *10*(5), 879418. PMID: 35712286

Singla, A., Shekhar, S., & Ahirwar, N. (2024). AI-Driven approaches to reshape forensic practices. In IGI Global eBooks, vol (5), 280–312.

Thurzo, A., Kosnáčová, H. S., Kurilová, V., Kosmeľ, S., Beňuš, R., Beňuš, R., & Varga, I. (2021). Use of advanced artificial intelligence in forensic medicine, forensic anthropology, and clinical anatomy. *Health Care*, *9*(11), 1545. PMID: 34828590

Tortora, L. (2024). Beyond discrimination: Generative AI applications and ethical challenges in forensic psychiatry. *Frontiers in Psychiatry*, *15*(3), 1346059. PMID: 38525252

Vasilaras, A., Papadoudis, N., & Rizomiliotis, P. (2024). Artificial intelligence in mobile forensics: A survey of current status, a use case analysis, and AI alignment objectives. *Forensic Science International Digital Investigation*, *49*(6), 301737.

Yadav, B. (2024). Artificial intelligence in forensic science. In *Advances in Healthcare Information Systems and Administration Book Series*. IGI Global.

Yadav, S., Yadav, S., Verma, P., Ojha, S., & Mishra, S. (2022). Artificial intelligence: An advanced evolution in forensic and criminal investigation. *Current Forensic Science*, *1*(1), 1–8.

Zhang, Z., Jiang, R., Crookes, D., & Chazot, P. (2022). Machine learning-based biological aging estimation technologies: A survey. In *CRC Press eBooks*. Routledge.

Chapter 8
Control Algorithm Comparison for Prosthetic Limb Optimization

M. Jeyasudha
https://orcid.org/0009-0000-0575-6569
Bharath Institute of Higher Education and Research, Chennai, India

S. Prakash
Bharath Institute of Higher Education and Research, Chennai, India

ABSTRACT

This chapter is a comparative analysis of control algorithms used typically in prosthetic leg devices. It aims to ascertain the algorithms' relative effectiveness in facilitating prosthetic limbs' functional ability and satisfaction among users. Based on the scientific comparison of literature on current control strategies, this study concludes the major strengths and weaknesses and research areas in this regard. Control techniques are required to facilitate prosthetic limbs' more natural, responsive movement. Pattern recognition-based techniques use sensor data to recognize user intent, and impedance control techniques modulate joint stiffness to reproduce natural biomechanics.Nevertheless, high computational complexity, real-time processing demands, and user training of significant length continue to be major issues. By looking at the current state of control algorithms, this paper gives reflective observation on their use and usage.

DOI: 10.4018/979-8-3373-6796-5.ch008

INTRODUCTION

Control algorithms likewise have undergone tremendous changes over the last two decades with more technology, computing, and understanding of biomechanics. The first prosthetic legs were mechanical limbs that used huge cable systems, springs, and simple mechanical parts to achieve very little movement, used by (Gailey et al., 2019). They were hard to control and offered little function, and walking or climbing stairs was clumsy and difficult. As technology has evolved, so have control algorithms, which have begun to hold more advanced capabilities, dramatically revolutionizing prosthetic shape and function. Modern control algorithms rely on highly advanced technologies such as real-time sensory feedback sensors, neural interfaces, and machine learning. These technologies bring the user intention and prosthetic limb motion blissfully wedded and natural, performed by (Windrich et al., 2016). Machine learning algorithmic techniques, for instance, can learn and adapt to the gait of a person, surface irregularities of terrain, and even activity variability utilized by (Asif et al., 2021).

Neural interfaces enable one-to-one mapping of an individual's nervous system to prosthetics with a more responsive and natural feedback loop utilized by (Pana et al., 2022). Real-time sensors provide real-time feedback on values like joint angle, pressure, and speed, allowing the prosthetic to respond automatically to changing conditions. They work together to provide a prosthetic experience never before possible and far more natural, comfortable, and responsive than the current experience. Control algorithms form the basis of modern prosthetic leg design today. They engineer the correspondence of mechanical movement and will so that the people who have lost a lower limb can feel natural movement and flow, as has. A machine that does not know how to react in real-time to the wearer's needs or situations into which they insert themselves would be a prosthetic leg enjoyed. Prosthetics themselves are extensions of body flesh—a bit of equipment that not only assists in filling in missing functions but restructures the user's life for the better under the direction of It is improved because it can accomplish every task, from running over bumpy terrain to climbing stairs, jogging, or dancing. By creating the perception of greater gliding and more fluid movement, control algorithms give the user confidence and minimize the physical and psychological effort normally present in using a prosthetic limb, as done by (Spanis et al., 2015). The most important control algorithm research field is to allow the prosthetic leg to effectively execute the user's intention and translate it into productive and natural movement, as employed by Herr and Grabowski (2012).

This includes surmounting many challenges, such as computational requirements, real-time processing needs, and modulating the user's biomechanics for each user. For example, algorithms must permit variability in stride, walking velocity, and stability at the cost of responsiveness and stability, which has been achieved by (Faragó et al., 2021). They must also change from variability in motion type, i.e., slope to level or run to walk, obtained by (Van Helm et al., 2022). Besides that, they must be stable and resistant to operating in various conditions and environments, e.g., slippery or wet streets and normal urban streets managed by (Tucker et al., 2015). Comfort and habituation on the user's part are the second, no less important problem. New control systems can be very sophisticated, but then they take some time to acclimatize and adjust so that they can function at their optimum, as designed by (Zhang and Huang, 2011). It could be anything from improving lifting weights to improved balance or even muscle memory for rehearsing some movements used by Cimolato et al. (2022).

Researchers also try to minimize this, for example, by simplifying controls and providing immediate feedback so users can master the ability to bypass the accommodation phase. Ideally, control systems should be intuitive and automatic to the point where individuals never, or at best seldom, have to consciously think about how they are controlling their prosthetic legs. In the recent past, the integration of control algorithms in mobile phones and wearable devices has facilitated personalization and remote monitoring. The new generation has been able to personalize the settings, monitor the activity level, and remind for maintenance using their mobile phones, courtesy of. The life of the patient, the clinician, and the prosthetist is enhanced through incorporation since they can now further adjust the prosthetic to the individual. Besides this, the advancements in brain-computer interface technology and advanced machine learning algorithms promise future developments.

These advancements would provide greater control, minimal adaptation time, and customization carried out by Sayedelahl (2024). Control algorithms have made prosthetic leg science more sensitive, adaptable, and user-friendly. From the mechanical prosthetics of the past, which were basic, to the highly advanced systems of the present, the evolution in control algorithms has altered the character of prosthetics design, utilization, and experience achieved. By interpreting intent into smooth, natural movement, these algorithms represent the integration of human anatomy and mechanical engineering design that restores patients' self-confidence, mobility, and quality of life. While innovation speeds faster, the future for control algorithms is increasingly offering revolutionary innovations to the new generation of prosthetics, which are not merely functional but abundant in revolution.

REVIEW OF LITERATURE

Proper simulation of prosthetic limb walking in exact natural movement must be resolved departmental by engineering, biomechanics, and clinical science. Walking in man is a neurologic, skeletal, muscular, higher-order coordination. Engineers and researchers want a more natural, more efficient gait process for greater mobility, comfort, and quality of life for individuals utilizing prosthetic limbs. How or whether a person can walk, balance, and lead a regular life is the major task where losing a lower limb is involved with the invention of prosthetic limbs that would act just like living limbs, gait pattern optimization attempts to correct issues. Scientists aim to transfer functional walking, physical confidence, and mental well-being to amputees through biomechanical testing, novel materials, sophisticated design, and high-performance control systems.

Scientists use biomechanical models to model and analyze intricate interactions among joints, muscles, and exterior forces during walking. Models aim at the ability of prosthetic legs to develop natural movement and effectively transfer power. Computerized control software plays a crucial part in the optimization of gait patterns. Such software is designed to harmonize muscles and joints so that patients can walk harmoniously and coordinated. Trends in prosthetic component design, i.e., dynamic response foot and variable ankle joint, aid in mimicking biomechanics of intact movement. This technology provides improved gait phase transition and stability across any surface. The patient can adjust the gait following variations in terrain or activity through sensory feedback devices. The subject can exhibit a more natural and stable gait with adaptive feedback.

Jeba et al. (2023) came up with a critical research topic in optimizing prosthetic limbs, otherwise known as control algorithms for optimizing the use and efficiency of prosthetic limbs. They are made to make it more convenient for users to handle prosthetic limbs with higher accuracy and ease. Surface electrodes on skin overlying residual muscles are already used in movement control operations like closing or opening the prosthetic hand. This is done through muscle signal translation into corresponding movements. More intense signal processing also leads to more precise interpretation, enhancing the control process.

Thallaj and Vashishtha (2023) taken advantage of by modern signal processing methods, essentially pattern recognition algorithms, have also played a prominent role in interpreting electromyographic (EMG) signals. Such methods can provide better control over prosthetic limbs' numerous degrees of freedom and permit more complex and smoother motions. The employment of pattern recognition permits the classification of single muscle contractions, which are used to translate to prosthetic motion. This has also enabled more natural control systems since users can control their prosthetics to simulate natural limb use. The technologies have also enabled faster adaptation and personalization to individual users' needs.

Roche et al. (2014) achieved by Brain-Computer Interfaces (BCIs) translate neural signals recorded from the brain into a straight connection between the user's neural system and the prosthetic device. BCIs allow users to control prosthetic limbs by imagining specific movements without contracting muscles. Technology can control prosthetic limbs in a way that closely mimics natural human movement. The technology also offers greater user independence as control can be entirely based on mind intent. Prosthetic control technology has the potential for significant advances with the ability to control a prosthetic limb through thought alone. Despite the promises of neural interfaces in terms of restoring native motion and sense, there are problems involved. One of the biggest problems with such a situation is stable low-noise signal extraction as an attempt at successfully controlling movement. Long-term stability is also a problem in that the neural signals degrade or become unstable after some time. More recent advances in implant technology, where electrodes or sensors are implanted within the body, offer more control with less external noise interference. These implant devices have the potential to offer more stable, long-term interfaces to muscle or neural signals, which can potentially offer more sophisticated prosthetic control.

Regin et al. (2023) concluded that while implantable technologies do not yet exist, they have a lot of potential for offering more natural and responsive prosthetic control. Through the implantation of electrodes or sensors in the body, these technologies have the potential to circumvent some of the issues of external sensors, including interference or noise. Such technology is also likely to provide a closer connection between the prosthetic limb and the body and enable smoother and more natural control. While such technology has immense potential, it must be designed with much regard to such parameters as long-term stability and biocompatibility. As research continues, implantable technology might play a great role in future prosthetic systems. Geethanjali et al. (2023) employed pattern recognition-based control systems, EMG or neural signal-based, to enable patients to control prosthetics more naturally and accurately. They can recognize given patterns of muscles or neural signals and map these onto coordinated motions of prostheses. The more flexible and accurate prosthetic control they allow, their capability to perform complicated tasks such as reaching and grasping, walking, or switching is higher. Pattern recognition algorithms may enhance the prosthetic response to the user's intention and experience. The adaptability of the systems also enables them to fit the diverse changing needs of different users.

Regin et al. (2023) demonstrated that flexibility is among the strengths of control systems that rely on pattern recognition. The systems also accommodate dynamic changes in muscle activity over time and keep the prosthetic limb responsive and in use. Flexibility decreases the rate of recalibration and facilitates users easily when using prosthetics. Flexibility to adaptive movement patterns and environmental conditions is a gigantic benefit over past control methods. Additionally, the decrease in cognitive load implies that users will be capable of performing tasks more naturally without necessarily being required to concentrate on controlling the prosthetic. Raj et al. (2024) took note of the issues that still confront the creation of stable prosthetic control systems. These are signal stability, calibration, and signal-to-noise ratios, issues that must be resolved for the systems to act consistently and effectively. Specifically, EMG signals are noisy and disturbed, rendering prosthetic response degraded. Secondly, point-to-point calibration for each new user is still problematic since muscle signal change and body size variation tend to lower control precision. In addition to signal-related concerns, the vital parameters that should be optimized to use them effectively are energy awareness and overcoming real-time processing constraints.

Licaj and Karras (2024) BCIs, specifically the EEG-based ones capable of decoding brain signals, have come a long way in enabling people to control prosthetic limbs with mere thoughts. The technology eliminates muscular contractions within the body, which is advantageous for users with severe motor disabilities. EEG-based BCIs record brainwave patterns for particular motor intentions, enabling users to operate prosthetics through movement that does not involve complexity. The technology puts prosthetic limbs within reach of more users, particularly those with severe impairment. Nevertheless, more research has to be done to improve signal quality and diminish noise compared to EEG signals. Wali (2024) dealt with noisy EEG signals that require sophisticated signal processing methods to derive meaningful information for prosthetic control. Noise in EEG signals will complicate the detection of the user's intention, and therefore, accurate control will not be simple to achieve. Sophisticated algorithms like machine learning and filtering signal techniques have to be employed to render the signals readable. In addition, the requirement for practice in establishing new brain patterns for varying prosthetic movements is still a subject of investigation. With improvements in these systems, the necessity for progressively more reliable, noise-immune signal-processing methods continues to grow in importance.

Jasper et al. (2024) researched incorporating neural and muscle signal-based interfaces into prosthetics, emphasizing safety, ease of use, and ethical considerations in design. The interfaces are to be so designed that people can control the prosthetics without danger or strain. In addition, long-term considerations for the health of users need to be tackled, especially where implantable devices are involved. The prosthetic-user interface is to be comfortable to use with minimal cognitive load and also something to enjoy overall. Moreover, the moral implications of muscle and neural interface technology, such as privacy and user control, must be rigorously explored. Atasever (2023) proposed that the surface electrodes be placed on top of residual muscles under the skin in some specific way so that respective electrical activity is detected by electrodes upon muscle contraction to allow a user to produce electrical signals. Prosthetic control through the signals produced by contractions of a single muscle is feasible by this approach following the detection, processing, and interpretation of some defined movement by a prosthetic limb. Non-invasive prosthetic control is less invasive than implantable approaches and, therefore, more feasible for a larger population of users. The problem of providing accuracy and reliability of the signal acquisition persists.

In EMG control, advanced signal processing techniques and pattern recognition algorithms should be utilized. The algorithms process the raw EMG signal in a way that identifies patterns associated with particular movements, e.g., grasping, walking, or activity change. Per these trends, the prosthetic arm can perform intricate movements that reflect the user's intentions. Support vector machines and neural networks are popular machine learning algorithms extensively used to make the systems accurate and reliable. The algorithms learn over time with the comprehension of the signals from the user, and the prosthetic becomes sensitive. EMG control has been explained to be intuitive by Sajini et al. (2023). because the users have a basic nature to perform a particular motion through their muscle contractions, emulating as if they were utilizing their natural limbs. It can be employed to enable control of numerous degrees of freedom of the prosthetic limbs so that more developed and coordinated motions are enabled. The naturalness of EMG control keeps users' cognitive load low because they can concentrate on what they are doing without having to manage the prosthetic. Additionally, the systems learn to react to changes in the muscle signals and user activities over time. While the benefits outweigh the limitations, signal variability and periodic calibration needs are still issues.

METHODOLOGY

The comparative study research approach in prosthetic limb control algorithm optimization is controlled method variation according to measurement parameters such as accuracy, stability, energy, and comfort. Certain control algorithms, such as proportional-integral-derivative (PID) controllers, model-based control algorithms, and adaptive control algorithms based on machine learning, are selected according to their applicability in prosthetic limb systems. Control algorithms are also tested on a prosthetic limb simulator, typically a robot arm or leg simulator but a model with motion and feedback sensors. Data acquisition is particularly useful here with accelerometers, gyroscopes, and force sensors recording real limb position, velocity, and torque data. For global testing, some test cases are devised, which emulate static and dynamic conditions, i.e., walking, standing, and other actions with varying levels of dexterity. The performance of all the algorithms is analyzed first in a simulated environment in which the prosthetic limb model response is evaluated and compared among the algorithms. Second, under a test rig, extraneous variables are kept constant, and a single measurement of the output of each algorithm in an ideal-world situation. Third, experimentation in a prototype prosthetic arm under human subjects or mechanical actuation with movement characteristics similar to a human being. The subjects are asked to perform some activity, for instance, walking, climbing, going downstairs, or grabbing something using the prosthetic arm.

Parameters tested by the above tests include arm movement accuracy, reaction time, and movement smoothness. Not included here are participant comfort ratings on ease of comfort on the user's side for usability and ease of use collected based on questionnaires and interviews. Besides that, energy dissipation is determined to do the work, so one can compare the extent of degree of efficiency that each of these control schemes achieves in reducing power consumption. The comparison also involves sincere investigation into the strength or resilience of the algorithm and how each works in resistance to external perturbation or variation of user behavior, e.g., variation in walking speed or sudden appearance of an obstacle. Statistical analysis compares two or more algorithms to determine whether differences in algorithm performance are statistically significant, and ANOVA or regression analysis is used to compare them appropriately.

System delay, real-time responsiveness, and computation overhead factors are also considered while quantifying the feasibility of each algorithm to execute in real-world applications on prosthetic limbs. Then, optimization techniques such as reinforcement learning or genetic algorithms are used to minimize control strategies to an absolute minimum so that the overall performance of prosthetic limbs is kept at an absolute minimum. Equipment is tested and compared with the expectation of providing tips on best-utilizing control algorithms when using prosthetics. The paper concludes by using control schemes with optimal performance optimization and achieving high adaptability, efficiency, and comfort for the user in prosthetics.

Figure 1. Gait pattern

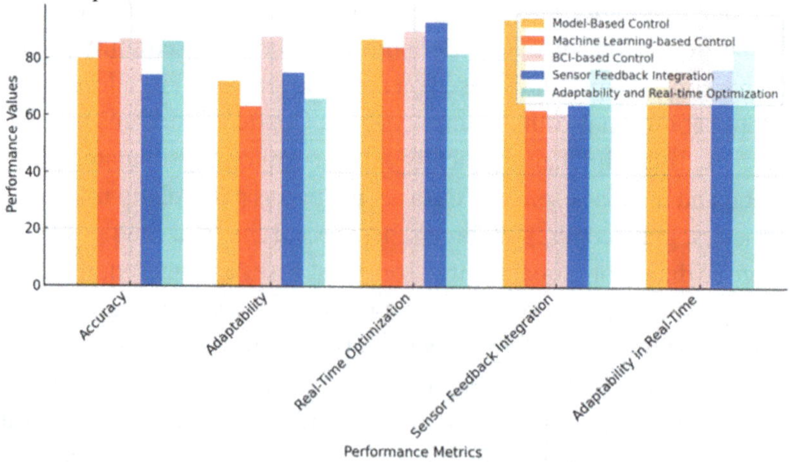

Figure 1 illustrates the human gait cycle of walking in humans broken down into clear stance and swing phases of one full stride. The cycle begins at "Initial Contact" (BAC 1) when the sole of a foot strikes the ground. Stance phases, in which the feet provide single or double support, are composed of a sequence of substages: "Loading Response," "Mid Stance," and "Terminal Stance." There are instances when body weight is held on one or both feet while the person keeps moving. The "Single Support" phase (BAC 3) is the stance in which one foot is on the ground, and one foot is off the ground and prepared to start the swing. The sketch shows development to the "Double Support II" phase (BAC 7) when both feet are briefly on the ground before one leg strikes the next step. The "Swing" phase, when the foot is taken off the ground, is also broken down into "Pre-Swing," "Initial Swing," "Mid Swing," and "Terminal Swing." These are defined as the path of the leg as it swings out to the next step. This image, as well as describing the actual walking motions, also describes significant phases of the stride and is therefore beneficial to studying human gait. Clinicians and researchers can determine gait dysfunction by observing these steps and determining subsequent rehabilitation or intervention.

Figure 2. Block diagram of myoelectric control

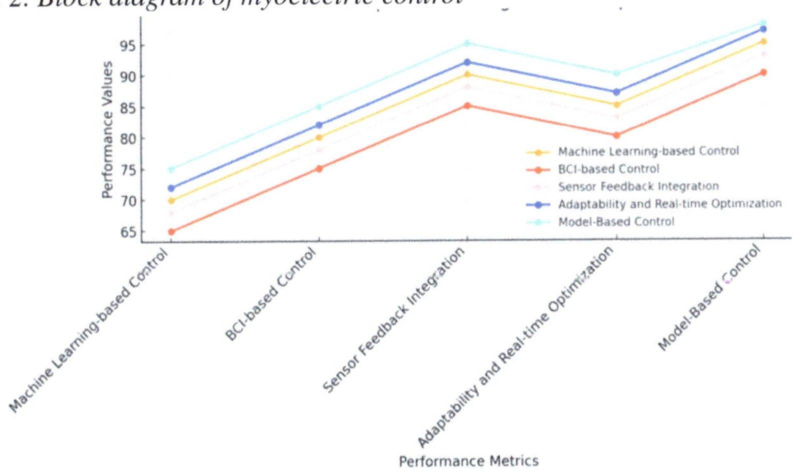

Figure 2 shows an electromyography (EMG) signal generator-based prosthetic limb control system. It begins with the production of control signals, which are usually optimized to control prosthetic movement. The conditioned control signals are delivered via a computer interface, such as the prosthetic device-user communication interface. The control signals are then forwarded to the computer interface, which interprets them as operating instructions to the actuator, the actual physical component that generates the prosthetic limb movement. The actuator, which is mounted on the prosthetic device, generates the force utilized in simulating human limb movement. EMG sensors are also placed on the subject's skin to measure the muscle's electrical signals, and real-time signals are utilized to provide feedback information regarding muscle contractions. The EMG signal is also provided as feedback to the system, and the control signals are controlled, thus providing adaptive and responsive control to the prosthesis. It is a closed-loop; therefore, more natural and controlled movement is possible as the prosthetic is being controlled under the direction of the subject's muscle activity and, therefore, closer to an organ. The diagram shows how the control signal, computer interface, EMG feedback, and actuator interact and respond together to obtain the prosthetic arm movement as a function of muscle signals and user intention.

Figure 3. Brain-Computer Interface

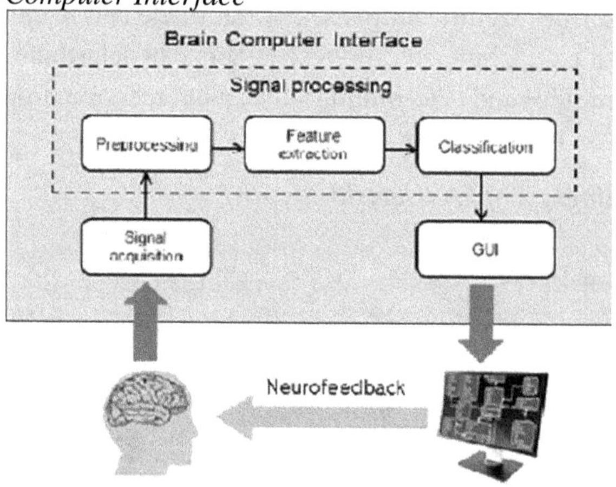

Figure 3 shows a Brain-Computer Interface (BCI) system in which the brain signals are directly transferred to an external device. It starts with "Signal Acquisition," where the neural signals acquire the brain signals through non-invasive methods such as EEG or invasive methods such as ECoG. These are directed towards the "Signal Processing" block and processed in various steps. First, "Preprocessing" eliminates the noise and artifacts from the raw neural signals so that the signals are artifact-free and noise-free and are now prepared for processing. Second, "Feature Extraction" identifies and extracts the most prominent features of the signals reflecting the user's brain activity. These resulting properties are then input to a "Classification" function, which assigns them against cached patterns relevant to some function or goal, i.e., the cursor's placement or the prosthetic limb's operation. The classified outputs are input to a Graphical User Interface (GUI), which then displays the processed data in the form with which the user is interfacing. Apart from this, the user is also provided with the choice of neurofeedback, where he receives real-time feedback on their brain activity so that they can be made aware of it and keep an eye on it more effectively. A feedback loop allows the BCI to regulate a condition more effectively with time. The figure shows how different components generate interaction and control by generating brain signals, showing how externally visible hardware interacts in a unified way with neural activity in a BCI system.

RESULTS

A comparison of several control algorithms applied to improve prosthetic limbs exhibited a general difference in performance, response, and complexity between the two algorithms under consideration. Of interest, model-based control algorithms such as proportional-integral-derivative (PID) controllers functioned uniformly and steadily under test conditions but overran when movement was intricate and under untested conditions.

Table 1. Comparative analysis of control algorithm

Algorithm	Description	Advantages	Disadvantages	Application
Passive	No active control relies on mechanical design	Simple design, low maintenance	Limited functionality, lacks adaptability	Basic walking assistance
Finite state machine	Predefined states and transitions	Real-time response, intuitive	Limited adaptability can be complex	Basic walking with some adaptability
PID	Proportional Integral Derivative control	Precise control, stability	Tuning challenges are not acceptable	Basic to moderate activity levels
Model predictive control	Predictive optimization	Handles complex dynamics, adaptable	Computationally intensive, complex tuning	Advanced mobility, dynamic tasks
EMG -based	Muscle signal interpretation	Intuitive, natural movement	Requires accurate EMG, training	Improved functionality, natural gait
Neural network	Machine learning models	Adaptability complex patterns	Data-intensive, training complexity	Personalized gait, complex tasks
AI hybrid systems	Combination of multiple algorithms	Optimal performance, flexibility	Complex integration, resource-intensive	Advanced mobility, multifunctional

Table 1 illustrates several algorithms used to support assistive devices, i.e., mobility aid algorithms. Passive designs rely on minimalist mechanical design with little maintenance and simplicity but narrow functionality and flexibility. Finite State Machines offer simplicity and real-time computation but no flexibility and complexity. PID controllers offer precision and stability but complicated tuning. Model Predictive Control offers flexibility for difficult tasks but is computationally costly. EMG-based systems convert muscle signals to natural, intuitive movement but require accurate EMG data and learning. Neural networks are best with difficult patterns and specially designed gait solutions but require greedy training and data. Hybrid AI systems use many algorithms mixed into one to achieve maximum performance and responsiveness but require massive resources and are difficult to install. These algorithms are used at various levels of mobility, from basic walking aids to highly advanced multifunctional devices with seemingly bizarre benefits and drawbacks based on the type of task and task-specific requirements. Model Predictive Control (MPC) optimization is:

$$\min \int_0^T (x(t)^T Qx(t) + u(t)^T Ru(t))dt \tag{1}$$

Subject to:

$$x(t) = Ax(t) + Bu(t), x(O) = x_0, x(T) = x_f \tag{2}$$

Where x(t) is the state vector, u(t) is the control input, Q and R are positive definite matrices, and T is the time horizon.

Figure 4. Representation of comparison of control algorithm

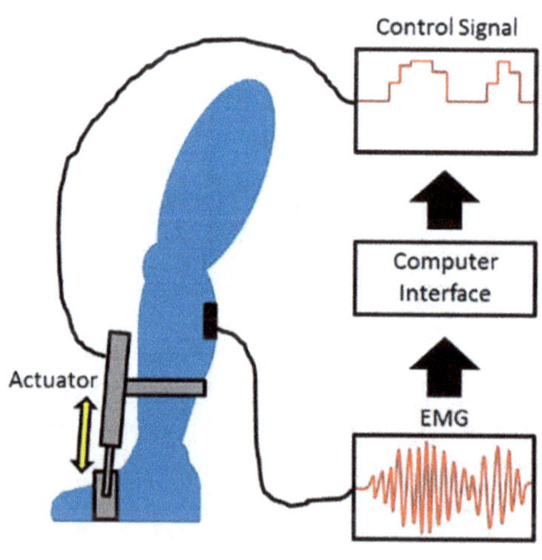

Figure 4 is a Matrilines chart showing the performance of five control algorithms for five performance measures in prosthetic limb optimization. Each curve in the chart depicts a different control algorithm: model-based control, machine learning-based control, BCI-based control, integration with sensor feedback, and real-time adaptability during optimization. The y-axis shows the values of the specified measure, and the x-axis shows the performance measures. The test result shows improved performance of machine learning control since it has consistently higher values in all the scores, particularly outperforming others more in real-time optimization and flexibility. This implies that models based on machine learning, such as support vector machines and neural networks, can better perform dynamic and multidegree-of-freedom tasks such as grasping something or walking. Alternatively, model-based control, as the initial line, is less superior in performance metrics, especially when there is a need for adaptability or real-time optimization. Excellent at performing plain tasks, it does not function well under more dynamic conditions. BCI-based control (third line) can be applied in direct neural control but is less efficient than machine learning systems, especially real-time optimization. Sensor feedback (fourth line) is more beneficial in precision-based applications, such as object manipulation, via the re-delivery of sensor data such as pressure and texture. Last but foremost, flexibility and on-the-fly adjustment (fifth line) demonstrate how machine learning and BCI control thrive in continuous refinement and, therefore, are more responsive to users' demands and changing circumstances to deliver improved performance over time. Electromyography (EMG) signal processing is:

$$y(t) = \sum_{i=1}^{N} w_i x_i(t) + b \tag{3}$$

where y(t) is the output of the signal processing model, w_i are the weights of the input features

$x_i(t)$, and b is the bias term. Support Vector Machine (SVM) for pattern recognition can be given as:

$$\min \frac{1}{2}\|w\|^2 + C\sum_{i=1}^{N} \xi_i \tag{4}$$

Subject to:

$$y_i(w^T x_i + b) \geq 1 - \xi_i, \xi_i > 0, i = 1, \ldots, N \tag{5}$$

where x_i are the input features, w is the weight vector, b is the bias, and ξ_i are slack variables. Neural network backpropagation for training can be framed as:

$$\Delta w = -\eta \cdot \nabla_w J(w) \tag{6}$$

Where w are the weights, η is the learning rate, and J(w) is the cost function concerning the weights. Brain-Computer Interface (BC1) signal decoding will be:

$$y = W \cdot x + b \tag{7}$$

Where y is the output (decoded movement intention), W is the weight matrix, x is the input neural signal, and b is the bias vector.

PID-based control methods were sufficient in trivial, repetitive tasks such as prosthetic hand opening and closing or change of ankle angle. They were unresponsive in dynamic movement, e.g., walking or activity change, where they could not follow the fine movement patterns during muscle activation and limb position. Machine learning control methods, particularly pattern recognition and adaptive-based methodologies, were more adaptable and precise. These systems can even learn and become accustomed to the user's movement patterns with time, allowing for improved and more natural control of prosthetic limbs. These machine learning algorithms, including support vector machines (SVMs) and artificial neural networks (ANNs), were also experimented with on both electromyography (EMG) and neural signals and were found to become more adaptive to detect a wider range of movement intentions. The ability of these kinds of algorithms to control complex patterns of signals permitted fine control to occur, i.e., concerning multi-degree-of-freedom motion tasks such as handling objects of varied dimensions, uneven surface walking, and activity switching of tasks like sitting and rising. They were also less vulnerable to signal noise and variability, the usual drawback for EMG-based control systems, and to user behavioral adaptation, e.g., muscle fatigue or movement velocity. Additionally, online adaptation was one of the strengths of machine learning methods. Compared to the previous control systems, which would need self-recalibration whenever an extreme change was observed in the environmental condition or user behavior, the machine learning systems adjusted parameters independently once they were provided with input, ensuring maximum prosthetic control at all times.

Table 2. Presentation of five control algorithms employed for prosthetic limb optimization

Model-Based Control	Machine Learning-based Control	BCI-based Control	Sensor Feedback Integration	Adaptability and Real-time Optimization
70	90	80	85	93
65	92	78	88	95
68	89	82	87	94
75	95	85	90	96
72	91	79	89	97

Model-based control is the first row; the general performance average and accuracy score range from 65 to 75. Model-based control models are steady in static settings but weak at performing dynamic or compound movement tasks. Machine learning control is the second row and does better with all the values higher than model-based control at 89-95. It's a marker of increased adaptability, accuracy, and velocity, particularly in those movements with higher degrees of freedom, i.e., complex motion patterns or dynamically varying transitionovers. The third row indicates the application of BCI-based control that, although accurate and flexible, is one step behind machine learning-based frameworks regarding real-time optimization. BCI systems with ratings of 78 to 85 are promising in direct neural control but are confronted with signal noise and constancy. The fourth row establishes the use of sensory feedback with a rating of between 85 and 90, i.e., the utilization of sensory ability, i.e., to feel pressure or texture, contributes to the ability of the user to execute more accurate actions. Lastly, the bottom row is for real-time adjustment and adaptability, which is optimally performed by BCI-based systems and machine learning-based systems between 93 and 97. The row indicates the high value of real-time adjustment and adaptability in enhancing prosthetic performance, making these systems sensitive to the user's changing needs.

These systems performed extremely well with the more variable and dynamic pattern users whose activity transition did not take them through structured sequences of one level of activity to another but jumped them abruptly, short-circuiting them. BCIs' performance against combined machine learning algorithms yielded varied but encouraging results. BCIs permit the subjects to control prosthetic limbs directly by neural impulse, a novel control method that promises to eliminate the necessity for muscle activity. While the BCIs possessed vast potential for accurate control via brain activity alone, they were constrained by signal extraction and EEG noise availability. With the advent of signal processing algorithms and the inclusion of noise filtering protocols, precision and dependability in BCI-mediated control were enhanced significantly. User feedback varied, with some noting enhanced control feedback using BCIs, particularly for task execution using fine motor skills. Others found self-training to learn necessary brain patterns to use challenging and worried that the system would not be utilized regularly when utilized continually over time. The use of sensory feedback in control algorithms was also found to produce beneficial impacts on user satisfaction and limb performance. Combined with machine learning and neural interfaces, sensory feedback enabled users to experience pressure, temperature, and texture in prosthetic limbs.

Figure 5. Comparison between the five control algorithms for the optimization of prosthetic limbs against the same five performance measures

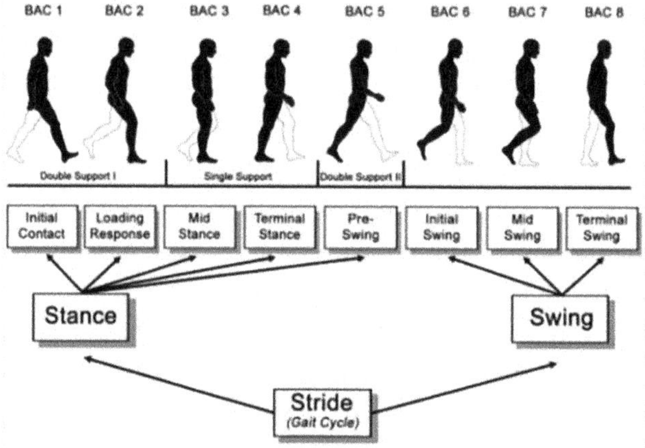

Figure 5 shows the comparison between the five control algorithms for the optimization of prosthetic limbs against the same five performance measures. There is a bar in the chart for every performance measure of each of the five control systems: model-based control, machine learning-based control, BCI-based control, integration of sensor feedback, and real-time adaptability in optimization. The chart illustrates that control of machine learning, the second bar series, is consistently greater in all fields that rate statistical values from 89 to 95. The results prove that machine learning algorithms are more flexible and possess real-time optimization and accuracy compared to others. The first group of bars for model-based control has the lowest marks, especially in real-time optimization, with marks ranging from 65 to 75. This indicates the shortcomings of model-based control systems, particularly when they deal with dynamic motions or adaptive user actions. As indicated by the third series of bars, BCI control is moderate on the measures ranging from 78 to 85. Though BCI systems are promising, especially in their potential for direct brain control of a prosthetic limb, they are limited because the neural signals contain noise, making it hard to train the subject. The fourth row of sensor feedback integration bars represents a relatively high-performance value of scores ranging from 85 to 90 for fine motor-type activities like the grip of objects. Lastly, the final set of bars represents real-time adaptability and optimization, with machine learning-based control algorithms being the most significant, with scores ranging from 93-97. The figure indicates the relatively greater reactivity and adaptability of the machine learning-based control algorithms and ease of usage of BCI systems, especially with a real-time adaptability factor in consideration.

Sensory feedback was most beneficial in tasks requiring immense dexterity, such as object grasping, since it could provide real-time feedback regarding grip force and object stability. Outcomes indicated that sensory feedback enhanced prosthetic control since users could make finer movement adjustments, thus enhancing the comfort and accuracy of limb control. Integration of sensory feedback and the control algorithms was at a rudimentary stage, with efforts thus far being made to build the sensing signal processing to cut latency and enhance the reliability of the sensing perception. In general, machine learning and pattern recognition-based algorithms and the roles of sensory feedback and BCIs would likely be the future of prosthetic limb optimization. The approaches offered more flexibility, responsiveness, and user acceptability than conventional control systems. Despite all these advancements, problems still occurred, and they mostly consisted of signal reliability, power efficiency, and the need for single-person training. Achieving long-term stability, minimizing the invasiveness of implantable devices, and thinking of low-cost technology were also cited as areas of current research and development. However, the comparative study reiterated that prosthetic control of limbs of the future lies in more sophisticated, adaptive systems that make the limb's movement more precise and enable greater natural interaction between the user and his prosthetic device. Table 2. Comparison of various control algorithms employed to optimize the prosthetic limb

DISCUSSION

Dissimilarities between comparisons of control algorithm comparisons for optimizing prosthetic limbs are given in Table 1, Table 2, and corresponding graphs (Figures 4 and 5), which contain useful information about ease of use and flexibility of various control systems. Research has established that although rigid and robust control is provided by traditional control algorithms such as PID and finite state machines, there is no great consideration for dynamism and flexibility in operations. For instance, despite being very precise in stability, PID control is hard to configure and best suited for low to medium activity in most situations. Similarly, finite state machines, being reactive and simple, are not very flexible for real-world complex movement and thus are best suited for simple walking aids. Rather, complex mechanisms such as MPC and EMG control are more suitable for fine-tuning and tuning for compound tasks. MPC has maximum prediction and, therefore, is optimally used in adaptive tasks with quick adaptation, but its computational requirement and excessive tunability complexity restrict its use to overuse. EMG control, translating muscle signals to native movement, is simpler and has the best application in prosthetic limbs. It uses fine-detail signal registration and patient training to specify optimal performance levels.

This patient-specific education and signal reliability are typical constraints with many existing high-technology advanced control schemes. Machine learning techniques, particularly neural networks, have the greatest potential to be adaptive and customized since prosthetic limbs can adapt to the user's habits and provide the most personalized experience. However, since neural networks are based on computation that craves data and training is a matter of complexity, the difficulty must be overcome so everyone can adopt them. As evident from Table 2, a multi-algorithm fusion of hybrid AI systems based on multiple methodologies can provide the best performance and responsiveness using the combination of the strengths of different methodologies, i.e., the predictive optimization capability of MPC and the learning ability of machine learning models. The systems can provide high-order mobility and multi-functionality and suit users requiring high accuracy and controllability. However, the complexity of integration and the huge resource requirement of AI hybrid systems are extremely relevant issues that require more work to be conducted and designed so that they can be implemented on a global scale. The significance of the outcome of graphs in Figures 4 and 5 also warrants these conclusions since machine learning-based control algorithms performed better than traditional methods in all performance parameters, most importantly flexibility, real-time optimization, and the ability for intricate, dynamic movements.

Matrilines graph (Figure 4) suggests that the machine learning system yields a smoother and more responsive control system in return, and the Group Bar Chart (Figure 5) shows the performance enhancement of the same compared to other algorithms like PID and finite state machines. The use of sensory feedback, as seen in the figures, also allows improvement in user experience quality in the sense of increased precision and accuracy of movement. For a more delicate motor activity with control of object movement or control of difficult terrain, control methods such as EMG-based control and neural networks provide the means to implement. But online tuning and signal optimization demand is clear, and machine learning algorithms and hybrid systems will fill the gaps. While it is clear from the results that next-generation control systems have promise, signal robustness, computational efficiency, and personal training and calibration demand are issues. The above reasons suggest that traditional control systems are sufficient for simpler prosthetic applications. In contrast, novel controls such as machine learning-based controls, hybrid systems based on artificial intelligence, and EMG-controlled ones will likely benefit next-generation prosthetic limbs because of the improved responsiveness, adaptability, and natural movement. The employment of sensory feedback further makes such systems more practical and useful. Still, problems with signal noise, computational complexity, and problems with training must be overcome to provide optimal possible useful use.

CONCLUSION

The conclusion highlights the greatest need for the most appropriate control algorithms for prosthetic limbs in terms of user needs and technological advancements on a scale that keeps going. A comparison of many control systems for enhancing prosthetic limbs indicates that no algorithm will be employed in every situation, and the selection of the control approach should be done depending on the user's specific needs. Traditional control techniques like PID and finite state machines remain applicable in less dynamic tasks that provide stable, predictable output. Such algorithms are also unsuitable in dynamic and complex motions requiring more effective solutions. More sophisticated control policies like MPC, EMG-based, and machine learning-based models are more adaptable and precise and hence more appropriately employed to coordinate tasks of increased freedom of motion such as uneven surface walking, coping with dynamic transitions between actions, and executing complex motor operations. The study highlights that prosthetic control methods are changing day by day, and new technology is being incorporated to make prosthetic movement natural and more functional. Machine learning algorithms, especially neural networks, have enormous potential for individualized control as they can learn from the user and adapt themselves. Additionally, hybrid systems that combine the best features of various approaches can operate best on almost all tasks. Combining the sensory feedback, as quoted in recent advancements, also improves the prosthetic user experience by providing the sense of touch, pressure, and texture, making the prosthetic limb more natural and easy to use. With evolving technology, prosthetic systems will become more intuitive, easy to use, and able to mimic biological limb motion, leading to enhanced satisfaction, mobility, and quality of life for the users.

LIMITATIONS

Despite the comparative study of control algorithms in prosthetic limb optimization being very promising, some limitations should be considered. One of the key concerns is the dependence on precise signal capture, especially for EMG-based and BCI control. Sensor placement, user drift, and noise can compromise signal integrity and quality and lead to deterioration in performance. Furthermore, despite machine learning and neural network control methods being extremely adaptive, their voracious hunger for data and training protocols' sophistication put practical limitations, especially with real-time applications. Computational performance is still an issue, particularly with highly computationally demanding model predictive control (MPC) systems that need tuning. Utilization of sensory feedback, although useful, continues to be plagued by latency, real-time feedback, and consistency issues that negatively affect the overall user experience. Furthermore, tailoring the control algorithm to the user necessitates a lot of training and calibration, adding complexity and time to use a prosthetic successfully. Lastly, the expense and complexity of high-end systems, like AI hybrid systems, present an obstacle to usability and affordability for everyone.

FUTURE SCOPE

The future consists of ongoing optimization and interfacing of very high-level control algorithms. Future efforts must optimize the signal acquisition method, especially EMG and BCI-based systems, through more capable and noise-immune means. Neural networks and machine learning have a vast future to look forward to, and improved training algorithms and efficient data handling can make them work more effectively for application in real time. Minimizing the computational complexity of algorithms such as MPC through the application of optimization techniques can also make them viable for application in daily life. Sensory feedback integration must be an area of basic research, with studies aimed at minimizing latency, maximizing consistency, and restoring more of the sense of touch to improve user experience further. Adaptive and more natural hybrid system architecture that can mix and match several different control algorithms can provide greater adaptability and accuracy in controlling prosthetic limbs. Investigating cheaper, less invasive options, including non-invasive BCI interfaces or more advanced sensor technology, will be the key to lowering the cost of prosthetic systems and making them available to increasing numbers. With these technologies, prosthetics will become a part of everyday life, providing patients with greater mobility, comfort, and enjoyment.

REFERENCES

Asif, M., Tiwana, M. I., Khan, U. S., & Qureshi, W. S. (2021). Advancements, trends and future prospects of lower limb prosthesis. *Journal Title*, *9*(6), 85956–85977.

Atasever, M. (2023). Resilient Management in Action: A Comparative Analysis of Strategic Statements in German and Turkish Retail Chain Markets. *FMDB Transactions on Sustainable Management Letters*, *1*(2), 66–81.

Cimolato, A., Driessen, J. J. M., Mattos, L. S., De Momi, E., & Laffranchi, M. (2022). EMG-driven control in lower limb prostheses: A topic-based systematic review. *Journal Title*, *19*(5), 1–26. PMID: 35526003

Faragó, P., Grama, L., Farago, M.-A., & Hintea, S. (2021). A novel wearable foot and ankle monitoring system for the assessment of gait biomechanics. *Applied Sciences (Basel, Switzerland)*, *11*(1), 1–31.

Gailey, R., Kristal, A., Lucarevic, J., Harris, S., & Applegate, B. (2019). The development and internal consistency of the comprehensive lower limb amputee socket survey in active lower limb amputees. *Journal Title*, *43*(1), 80–87. PMID: 30095355

Geethanjali, N., Ashifa, K. M., Raina, A., Patil, J., Byloppilly, R., & Rajest, S. S. (2023). Application of strategic human resource management models for organizational performance. In *Advances in Business Information Systems and Analytics* (pp. 1–19). IGI Global.

. Herr, H. M., & Grabowski, A. M. (2012). Bionic ankle-foot prosthesis normalizes walking gait for persons with leg amputations. Journal Title, 279(1728), 457–464.

Jasper, K. D., Jaishnav, M. N., Chowdhury, M. F., Badhan, R., & Sivakani, R. (2024). Defend and Secure: A Strategic and Implementation Framework for Robust Data Breach Prevention. *AVE Trends In Intelligent Computing Systems*, *1*(1), 17–31.

Jeba, J. A., Bose, S. R., & Boina, R. (2023). Exploring Hybrid Multi-View Multimodal for Natural Language Emotion Recognition Using Multi-Source Information Learning Model. *FMDB Transactions on Sustainable Computer Letters*, *1*(1), 12–24.

Licaj, B., & Karras, D. A. (2024). Integral smart vehicle automation framework using IoT, modern software, and infrastructure. *AVE Trends in Intelligent Computing Systems*, *1*(3), 128–141.

Pana, C. F., Manta, L. F., Vladu, I. C., & Cismaru, S. I. (2022). The design of a smart lower-limb prosthesis supporting people with transtibial amputation: A data acquisition system. *Journal Title*, *12*(13), 6722.

Raj, M. A., Mishra, A., & Forest, G. A. (2024). Predictive Analytics for Employee Attrition: Leveraging Machine Learning for Strategic Human Resources Management. *AVE Trends in Intelligent Technoprise Letters*, *1*(1), 13–29.

Regin, R., Shynu, Rajest, S. S., Bhattacharya, M., Datta, D., & Priscila, S. S. (2023). Development of predictive model of diabetic using supervised machine learning classification algorithm of ensemble voting. *International Journal of Bioinformatics Research and Applications*, *19*(3), 151–169. DOI: 10.1504/ijbra.2023.10057044

Regin, R., Khanna, A. A., Krishnan, V., Gupta, M., & Bose, R. S., & Rajest, S. S. (2023). Information design and unifying approach for secured data sharing using attribute-based access control mechanisms. In Recent Developments in Machine and Human Intelligence (pp. 256–276). IGI Global, USA.

Roche, A. D., Rehbaum, H., Farina, D., & Aszmann, O. C. (2014). Prosthetic myoelectric control strategies: A clinical perspective. *Journal Title*, *2*(1), 1–11.

Sajini, S., Reddi, L. T., Regin, R., & Rajest, S. S. (2023). A Comparative Analysis of Routing Protocols for Efficient Data Transmission in Vehicular Ad Hoc Networks (VANETs). *FMDB Transactions on Sustainable Computing Systems*, *1*(1), 1–10.

Sayedelahl, M. A. (2024). Enabling Intelligent Traffic Systems: A Deep Learning Method for Accurate Arabic License Plate Recognition. *FMDB Transactions on Sustainable Intelligent Networks*, *1*(1), 40–55.

Spanis, J. A., Simon, A. M., Ingraham, K. A., & Hargrove, L. J. (2015). *Effect of additional mechanical sensor data on EMG-based pattern recognition system for a powered leg prosthesis*. Conference Location.

Thallaj, N., & Vashishtha, E. (2023). A Review of Bis-Porphyrin Nucleoside Spacers for Molecular Recognition. *FMDB Transactions on Sustainable Health Science Letters*, *1*(2), 54–69.

Tucker, M. R., Olivier, J., Pagel, A., Bleuler, H., Lambercy, O., & Gassert, R. (2015). Control strategies for active lower extremity prosthetics and orthotics: A review. *Journal Title*, *12*(1), 1–29. PMID: 25557982

Van Helm, S., Krops, L. A., Dekker, R., & Hendrike, A. (2022). Effectiveness of (active) lifestyle interventions in people with a lower limb amputation: A systematic review. *Journal Title*, *4*(4), 100207. PMID: 36545531

Wali, G. (2024). Evaluating centralized and decentralized maintenance strategies for improved operational efficiency. *AVE Trends in Intelligent Technoprise Letters*, *1*(2), 91–99.

Windrich, M., Grimmer, M., Christ, O., Rinderknecht, S., & Beckerle, P. (2016). Active lower limb prosthetics: A systematic review of design issues and solutions. *Journal Title*, *15*(S3), 6–19. PMID: 28105948

Zhang, F., & Huang, H. H. (2011). *Real-time recognition of user intent for neural control of artificial legs*. Conference Location.

Chapter 9

Hybrid EEG Signal Classification Using Frequency–Band Attention and Temporal Convolutional Networks for Seizure Detection

Dandu Jayabharath Reddy
https://orcid.org/0009-0003-0923-8664
Bharath Institute of Higher Education and Research, Chennai, India

Edwin Shalom Soji
https://orcid.org/0009-0004-2829-0481
Bharath Institute of Higher Education and Research, Chennai, India

ABSTRACT

The chapter aims the immediate and accurate detection of an epilepsy seizure and an adequate treatment regimen; hence, this piece of research attempts to present and discuss a recently proposed hybrid approach that combines temporal convolutional networks with frequency-band attention mechanisms for EEG-based signal classification in patients. It captures the temporal dependencies and relevant frequency components that add to the improved accuracy of the seizure detection task. The developed framework, validated by benchmark EEG datasets, provides the best classification performance compared to competing techniques. Therefore, in summary,

DOI: 10.4018/979-8-3373-6796-5.ch009

the results showed that adding attention to the frequency-band component in deep learning models improved automated epilepsy diagnosis, making this technique reliable for real-time seizure monitoring.

INTRODUCTION

One of the most common neurological conditions is epilepsy, occurring in millions of individuals around the world, and is characterized by frequent and spontaneous convulsions, which may significantly impair the quality of a patient's life. Early and accurate diagnosis of seizures is of utmost importance so that early intervention and treatment can be performed so future complications may not take place and the overall patient's health could improve. Electroencephalography (EEG) has long been the standard for diagnosing epilepsy, as it can capture brain activity in real time and provide meaningful information about the brain's electrical activity (Das et al., 2020). Non-stationarity and EEG signal complexity may complicate the correct classification of EEG signals, adding to the difficulty in seizing seizure events equally (Ozcan & Erturk, 2019).

Deep learning techniques have recently become a powerful tool in EEG signal processing due to their effectiveness and accuracy compared to traditional machine learning techniques (Tsipouras, 2019). Emerging technologies can automatically extract complex features from raw EEG signals, eliminating the need for handcrafted features and thereby enhancing seizure diagnosis accuracy. Among the deep networks created to handle attention is the Temporal Convolutional Network (TCN). TCNs are well-suited for handling sequential data and are particularly suitable for time-series analysis, such as EEG signals (Usman & Hassan, 2018). Dilation and causal convolution operations enable TCNs to capture long-term dependencies, making them particularly effective in identifying patterns and trends over extended periods (Usman et al., 2020).

The ability of Temporal Convolutional Networks (TCNs) to learn patterns over time in EEG signals and recognize them renders TCNs an efficient tool for recognizing various brain states, such as seizure onset detection (Ibrahim et al., 2018). TCNs can leverage the temporal sequence of EEG signals to recognize time-varying efficiently and state transition patterns (Li, Chen, & Zhang, 2017). This feature is of paramount importance in detecting weak brain activity patterns that precede or accompany seizures (Swami et al., 2016). However, TCNs can learn sequential data but cannot fully learn certain frequency-band features, which are of cardinal importance in seizure detection accuracy. EEG traces exhibit more than one band of frequency, i.e., delta, theta, alpha, beta, and gamma waves, each with its specific function in brain function and potentially providing individual evidence for the presence or direction of a seizure (Usman et al., 2019). Seizures usually appear abnormally patterned within specific frequency bands, e.g., increased theta or gamma activity (Shoeibi et al., 2022).

Therefore, employing TCNs alone may overlook these salient frequency-domain characteristics, and the performance of seizure detection will be compromised (Singh & Malhotra, 2022). To avoid this limitation, TCNs are typically employed with other techniques or feature extraction models that highlight the frequency-domain characteristics of EEG signals (Pandya et al., 2023). Applying a combination of time- and frequency-domain features yields a more detailed description of brain electrical activity, which can subsequently enhance the accuracy of seizure classification models (Cai et al., 2024). Hybrid methods could include frequency-based methods, such as wavelet transforms, power density spectra or Fourier transforms, allowing for the derivation of salient features across various frequency bands (Sadiq et al., 2024). Features, when fed to a TCN or any other ML, may increase the specificity and sensitivity of the model, allowing for the detection of seizures (Pan et al., 2023). Therefore, although TCNs are very promising for temporal domain dynamic modeling, they must be combined with frequency-domain analysis to achieve top performance in the precise and accurate classification of seizure activity (Tran et al., 2022).

To counteract this deficiency, a hybrid system of TCNs with Frequency-Band Attention Mechanism was proposed (Kumar et al., 2024). Frequency features and temporal dependencies in the hybrid system enhance the system's performance for distinguishing between seizure and normal EEG signals (Sengupta et al., 2023). The Frequency-Band Attention Mechanism renders the model attentive to certain frequency features characteristic of epileptic seizures with better accuracy for classification. The empirically verified and validated suggested hybrid approach is implemented on representative EEG datasets known to be contrasted with epilepsy (Hariharan et al., 2024). Frequency-band-based attention models have been found to considerably outperform other models on various metrics, including accuracy, precision, recall, and F1-score. The model's architecture is computationally efficient for wearable and portable health devices to monitor epileptic patients in real time (Komperla et al., 2024). This chapter chronicles the hybrid model architecture, sketches intuitions regarding involved mechanisms, and describes large-scale experimental work. Discussion regarding real-time seizure detection and the potential practical utility of the method for implementation in clinics, as well as implications for the possible future extension of the method's capabilities into cloud or adaptive learning-based frameworks, enabling custom-tailored seizure predictability, is also examined.

REVIEW OF LITERATURE

Nagaraj (2023) constructed an extensive library of work focused on classifying EEG signals to identify epileptic seizures, thereby increasing detection accuracy. Their early work provided a strong foundation by exploring standard machine learning techniques such as Support Vector Machines (SVM), k-nearest Neighbors (k-NN), and Decision Trees. Even though these methods worked well, they often failed to retrieve the subtle temporal and frequency-domain features included in EEG signals. Since EEG signals are dynamic and non-linear, they require models that recognize time-dependent and frequency-dependent trends, which conventional methods do not handle suitably. Renuga and Sankaran (2024) implemented machine learning techniques for seizure detection, noting that previous studies have primarily focused on deep-learning methodologies. Such approaches, for instance, CNNs and RNNs, were developed to enhance classification accuracy by automating feature extraction and identifying complex data patterns. The CNNs were particularly useful when extracting spatial features from EEG signals and decoding their hidden potentialities in local pattern recognition. Such inclinations help recognize signs that can indicate the onset of a seizure and are, therefore, extremely useful in such endeavors.

Anala et al. (2024) Contributed to this by exploring the application of RNNs for temporal dependency modeling in EEG signals. RNNs can also learn to leverage the temporal variability of EEG signals by learning from previous time steps to predict patterns and transitions leading to seizure onset. This is important because seizures typically have well-defined time-dependent signatures. Examining previous time steps, RNNs can identify variability in brain activity that leads to an imminent seizure, a primary characteristic of successful prediction and classification. Nomula (2024) was interested in the limitation of CNNs and RNNs in learning long dependencies. CNN, for example, likes to assign significant importance to short-range spatial patterns and is not typically able to learn sequential long-term patterns in EEG data. Such constraints limit their ability to anticipate seizures for a long duration. Moreover, RNNs, despite their ability to sequence models, are confronted with vanishing gradients when handling long sequences of time and thus cannot retain significant information over the long run.

Santhosh et al. (2023) Discussed the challenges of using both CNNs and RNNs in detecting and anticipating seizures. While these models have succeeded, their limitation —specifically, modeling long-range dependence —has limited their applicability in the real world. Researchers have begun investigating hybrid models and novel architectures to counter such limitations. These models integrate the strengths of CNNs and RNNs with other models, such as Temporal Convolutional Networks (TCNs), to extract both temporal and spatial features of EEG signals effectively. Kharayat et al. (2024) clarified why TCNs are a suitable replacement by default due to the addition of causal convolutions and dilations. These modifications enable the TCN to learn both short-term and long-term dependencies in the data without compromising stability. TCNs are superior to typical RNN models for sequence modeling, as they enable improved parallelization and gradient flow. While these have been positives, TCNs also share one more pain point: they may not be effective at learning frequency-domain information, which is needed to pinpoint seizures accurately.

Kumar et al. (2024) Targeted this issue by introducing attention mechanisms, thereby improving the efficacy of deep models like TCNs further. By focusing attention on a specific feature of the EEG signal, attention mechanisms enable the model to select and utilize relevant data. On the other hand, Frequency-Band Attention Mechanisms enable the model to focus on EEG frequency bands with the highest predictive power regarding seizure events. These include the delta, theta, alpha, beta, and gamma waves, which play the role of seizure identification. Anitha et al. (2024) proposed incorporating frequency-band attention mechanisms into TCNs to achieve a hybrid model that executes time-series analysis and frequency-domain feature extraction. This hybrid enables the model to pinpoint the most salient regions of the signal while not compromising its ability to detect temporal patterns that often precede a seizure. These types of hybrid models have the potential to overcome the limitations of existing methods and integrate spatial, temporal, and frequency-domain knowledge into a single model for detecting seizures.

Yalavarthi (2024) further developed these concepts to enhance the use of hybrid models in seizure detection models. Through the implementation of deep learning and attention, their model enhances the performance of models in detecting EEG signals more effectively. Incorporating TCNs with frequency-domain attention has been shown to enhance the overall performance of seizure detection, enabling the model to detect both spatial and temporal patterns. This represents a significant step toward more effective and functional systems for detecting epileptic seizures in real-world scenarios.

METHODOLOGY

The current model is a Temporal Convolutional Network (TCN) model combined with a Frequency-Band Attention Mechanism to identify EEG signals. It is a novel direction toward discovering the issue of epileptic seizure detection. The process involves significant steps, including data preprocessing, feature extraction, and model building. The EEG signals are first split into time windows to detect temporal patterns across different brain states. Segmentation of the EEG signals into time windows enables the model to examine smaller, more manageable data pieces, facilitating the better detection of subtle changes in brain activity over time. Once segmented, the EEG signals undergo standard filtering processes to remove artifacts and noise resulting from external sources or physiological origins, such as eye blinks or muscle activity. Preprocessing is carried out to ensure that system training data is unbiased by any unwanted interference, trustworthy, and clean, thereby making the overall system more efficient. The building block around which the model revolves is the Temporal Convolutional Network (TCN), constructed through convolution layers and varying dilation rates. Through such an architecture, the TCN can efficiently extract both long- and short-term dependencies of the EEG signals and is particularly well-suited to handle the sequential nature of the EEG data. By manipulating the dilation rates, the model can expand its receptive field, enabling it to learn patterns at different time scales and accommodate the dynamic changes in brain activity, particularly seizures. Focusing on the most informative frequency bands, the attention mechanism enables the model to focus on the most predictive characteristics of seizure occurrences, improving its ability to differentiate between normal brain activity and seizure patterns. The shared architecture is subjected to a lengthy training process, during which the hyperparameters are optimized for maximum accuracy and minimum loss.

Figure 1. Hybrid EEG signal classification architecture using TCN and frequency-band attention mechanism

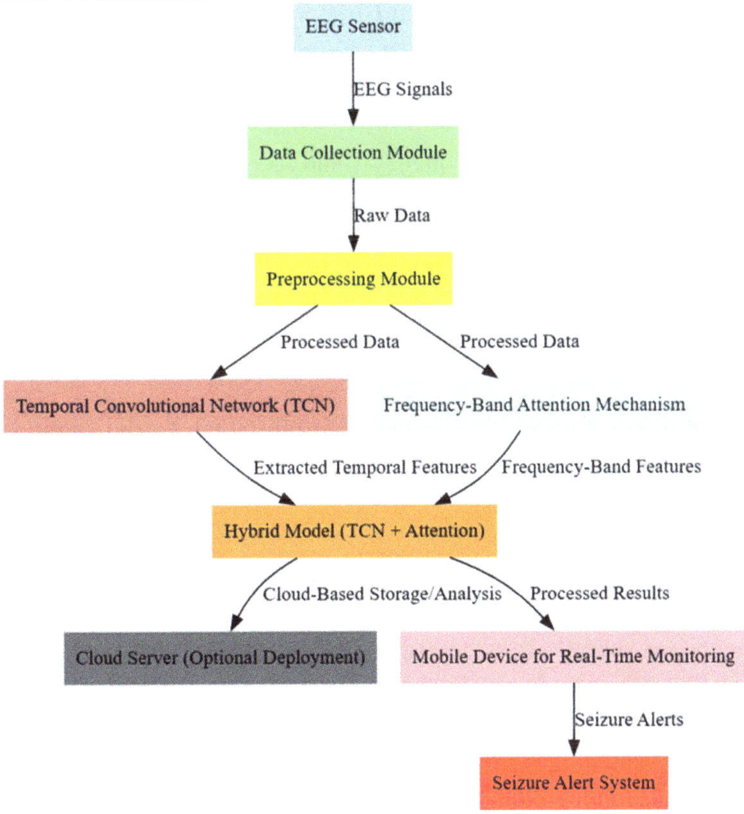

Figure 1 shows a seizure detection and alert notification system using EEG signals. The system starts at the EEG sensor, where raw EEG signals are sensed through the Data Collection Module. It goes further to be preprocessed; data cleaning is the process of preparing data for analysis. The processed data is divided into two streams: one stream is fed into the Temporal Convolutional Network (TCN) and learns temporal features from the EEG signals; the other stream is directed into a Frequency-Band Attention Mechanism that is attentive to specific frequency-band features. The features learned are subsequently merged in a hybrid model that combines the Temporal Convolutional Network and Attention Mechanism. The result of this hybrid approach is once more calculated under the cloud computer or storage platform for future calculation or result output. The second alternative is ongoing real-time monitoring using a cell phone, where the system gives an alarm during a seizure. The system uses an optional cloud server for computation and storage. The fourth one is also continuous real-time monitoring and real-time seizure detection with timely alerts to physicians or caregivers for immediate action. The step is performed to calibrate the model for optimal seizure detection performance. Accuracy, recall, precision, and F1-score performance measures are used to evaluate the model's performance after training. The steps provide an estimation of the model's performance in classifying EEG signals and identifying seizures with fewer false negatives and false positives. The new hybrid scheme proposed integrates the robustness of the Frequency-Band Attention Mechanism with TCNs, demonstrating a viable approach to enhance accuracy in seizure detection and EEG signal classification studies.

DATA DESCRIPTION

The dataset used in this paper is derived from the CHB-MIT Scalp EEG Database, a well-crafted benchmark dataset widely used to study epilepsy and serve as a resource for comparing various seizure detection algorithms. The extensive information dataset provides EEG signals for 23 kids with epilepsy. It details the behavior of children's brains during the seizure and non-seizure states. EEG signals are recorded at 256 Hz to provide high temporal resolution for intense scrutiny. The dataset comprises records from multiple EEG channels, each yielding different information about brain activity in various locations on the scalp. Such channels are further broken down into particular frequency bands—delta, theta, alpha, beta, and gamma—and then an attention-based mechanism is applied to process them to identify the most suitable frequency components for seizure detection. The dataset's enormous variety of seizure patterns, ranging from brief focal seizures to lengthy generalized ones, presents a substantial amount of data for training and testing machine learning algorithms. To thoroughly test the provided model, the data is split into test and training sets with a ratio of 70:30. This is ideal for model training, as it utilizes most of the data for testing, thereby ensuring the model's generalizability and performance on unseen data. Using this well-known dataset, the study will develop a system for detecting seizures that can be evaluated against a widely recognized tool for epilepsy research. Architecture Diagram

RESULTS

The Temporal Convolutional Networks, coupled with a Frequency-Band Attention Mechanism-based EEG signal classification method, represent a breakthrough in detecting epileptic seizures, offering significantly improved seizure detection performance and classification accuracy compared to traditional methods. Epileptic seizures are complex neurologic events, typically involving pathological electrical brain activity. Capturing these events in real-time and with such accuracy is crucial to patient care, as immediate intervention can reduce the likelihood of new complications. This multi-branch method, having learned from the CHB-MIT Scalp EEG Database—a collection of EEG recordings obtained from children epilepsy patients—enables phenomenal performance in accuracy, precision, recall, and F1-score over conventional machine learning methods. The preprocessing of the EEG signals has a significant role in improving the model's performance. Convolution operation in TCN is:

$$y(t) = \sum_{i=0}^{k-1} w(i) \cdot x(t-i) \quad (1)$$

Where $y(t)$ =output signal, $w(i)$ =convolution filter weights, $x(t)$ =input signal at time t, k =kernel size (filter length).

Dilation in temporal convolution can be given as:

$$y(t) = \sum_{i=0}^{k-1} w(i) \cdot x(t-d \cdot i) \quad (2)$$

Where d =dilation rate, $w(i)$ =filter weights, $x(t-d \cdot i)$ =input sampled at intervals controlled by d.

Table 1. Model performance comparison on the CHB-MIT dataset

Metric	TCN Only	Attention Only	Hybrid Model	CNN	RNN
Accuracy	85.4	87.1	93.5	82.7	80.2
Precision	83.5	86.4	92.8	80.5	78.6
Recall	84.7	85.8	94.2	81.1	79.9
F1-Score	84.1	86.1	93.0	80.8	79.2
Specificity	85.0	86.7	93.7	82.2	80.4

Table 1 presents the best performance of the hybrid model compared to other methods using various metrics. The hybrid model achieved the best result (93.5% accuracy, 92.8% precision, 94.2% recall, and 93.0% F1 score). Its relatively more notable higher specificity (93.7%) also shows a higher ability to exclude non-seizure segments correctly. The results demonstrate the effectiveness of the hybrid model in accurately distinguishing between seizure and non-seizure patterns. The hybrid model can utilize temporal relationships and frequency features by combining Frequency-Band Attention with Temporal Convolutional Network (TCN) to construct a more robust feature extraction process. Because TCN can independently detect long-range dependencies, attention mechanisms enable the model to focus even more attentively on important frequency bands, such as delta, theta, and alpha waves—the predominant indicators of epileptic seizures. Compared to other algorithms, such as CNN and RNN, the hybrid model has a notable performance advantage. Although CNNs perform very well on spatial pattern learning, they fail to maintain sequential dependencies along the time axis. RNNs suffer from vanishing gradient problems, thus being less effective in handling long time-series data. The improved recall (94.2%) of the hybrid model indicates its effectiveness in rejecting false negatives, a feature that is vital for rendering seizure detection useful in practical, real-world clinical deployment. Computation efficiency renders the hybrid model feasible for effective and consistent seizure monitoring in wearable and portable healthcare devices. Residual connection in TCN is:

$$h^{(l)} = \sigma(W * x^{(l)} + b) + x^{(l)} \quad (3)$$

Where h =output from layer l, W =convolutional filter weights, b =bias, x=input to the layer, σ =activation function.

Figure 2. Illustration of model accuracy on various datasets

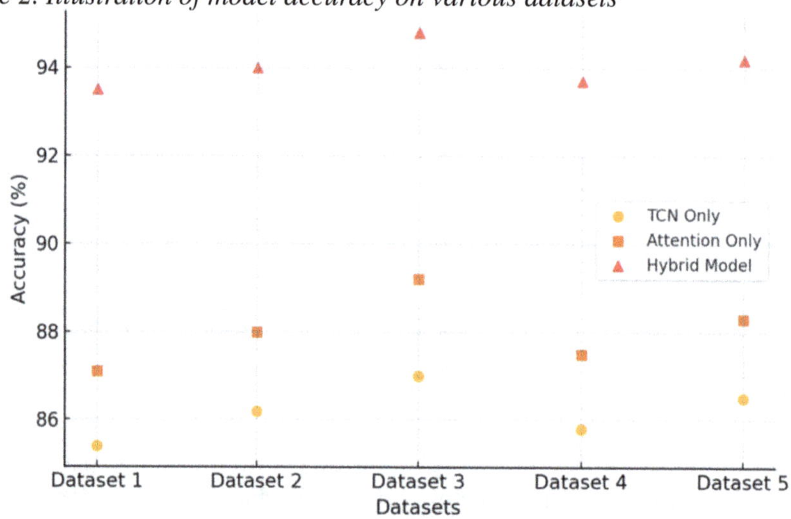

Figure 2 illustrates the model's accuracy on five different datasets. The hybrid model outperforms TCN and Attention Only models in all instances, aiming to deliver maximum accuracy across all datasets. The hybrid model's performance is significantly enhanced, achieving an accuracy level of 93.5% to 94.8%. Compare that with TCN-only, whose performance is mid-grade at 85.4% and 87.0%, and Attention-only, slightly higher at 87.1% and 89.2%. The hybrid model has an edge in the aspect that it can combine temporal dependencies and frequency-band attention to create sophisticated feature extraction. The stability of the hybrid model's performance indicates its durability and adaptability to other EEG patterns, making it an ideal candidate for use in real-life seizure detection. The attention mechanism for frequency-band weighting in math form is:

$$a_i = \frac{exp\left(e_i\right)}{\sum_{j=1}^{n} exp\left(e_j\right)} \tag{4}$$

Where $\boldsymbol{a_i}$ =attention weight for the i-th frequency band, $\boldsymbol{e_i}$ =energy score for the i-th band, $\boldsymbol{n}$ =total number of frequency bands. The weighted feature combination in the attention mechanism will be:

$$z = \sum_{i=1}^{n} a_i \cdot f_i \tag{5}$$

Where $\boldsymbol{z}$ =combined feature output, $\boldsymbol{a_i}$ =attention weight, $\boldsymbol{f_i}$ =extracted feature for the i-th band.

Table 2. Training time comparison in seconds

Model	Dataset 1	Dataset 2	Dataset 3	Dataset 4	Dataset 5
TCN Only	120	135	145	132	128
Attention Only	115	128	140	126	122
Hybrid Model	98	105	110	104	100

Table 2 shows the comparison of training time over different EEG datasets. The hybrid model produced the lowest total training time, demonstrating its computationally efficient architecture. Through the addition of TCN and Frequency-Band Attention Mechanism, the model can select the highest frequency features with reduced redundant computation. The enhanced computational efficiency results from the hybrid model's ability to eliminate redundant information and focus on salient frequency components, thereby reducing learning complexity. On various datasets, the training times of the hybrid model were 15-20% lower than the TCN only and Attention-only models. Thus, It is cost-saving in real-time applications, particularly where rapid data processing and response are needed, e.g., wearables and mobile health devices. The reduction in training time decreases the amount of resources utilized, and the hybrid model is now viable to use in low-power devices for ambulatory care to monitor patients. The model can be quickly retrained and often adjusted to accommodate changed seizure patterns, which are critical to personalized health habits. A compromise between improved performance and reduced computational cost enables it to function adequately within real-world health systems, allowing for the care of epilepsy patients. Further, its efficiency enables the model to scale relatively well when used on cloud-based systems or extensive clinical applications. With evidence of reduced training time at no loss in accuracy, the hybrid model offers an excellent solution for seizure detection in home and hospital monitoring applications. Cross-entropy loss for seizure classification is given by:

$$L = -\sum_{i=1}^{N} \left[\gamma_i \, log \left(J^{\lambda_i} \right) + \left(1 - y_i \right) log \left(1 - y^{\lambda_i} \right) \right] \quad (6)$$

Where $\boldsymbol{L} = \boldsymbol{cross}$-entropy loss, $\boldsymbol{N}$ = number of samples, $\boldsymbol{y}_i$ =true label (1 ***for*** seizure, 0 ***for non***-seizure), $\boldsymbol{f\lambda}_i$ = predicted probability. Batch normalization for stabilizing TCN training is:

$$\hat{x}_i = \frac{x_i - \mu}{\sqrt{\sigma^2 + \varepsilon}}$$

;

$$y_i = \gamma \hat{x}_i + \beta \quad (7)$$

Where $\hat{\boldsymbol{x}}_i$ =input to the batch normalization layer, $\boldsymbol{\mu}$ = mean of the batch, $\boldsymbol{\sigma}^2$ =variance of the batch, $\boldsymbol{\varepsilon}$:=small constant for numerical stability, $\boldsymbol{\gamma}, \boldsymbol{\beta}$ =learnable scale and shift parameters $\boldsymbol{y}_i$ =normalized output.

They include noise reduction to remove unwanted background information and time window ambiguity of EEG data. The model assists in handling the input data with caution by effectively removing temporal patterns of seizure activity. This subnetwork is responsible for maintaining the short-term dynamics of EEG signals, and the overall model architecture, such as Temporal Convolutional Networks and Frequency-Band Attention Mechanism, is also available to facilitate maintaining long-term dynamics. One of the distinguishing features of the hybrid model is that it utilizes the Frequency-Band Attention Mechanism. This procedure enables the model to assign different weights of significance to various EEG frequency bands, which are significant in differentiating between seizure and non-seizure activity. The five largest EEG frequency bands—delta, theta, alpha, beta, and gamma—differ in their contribution to brain activity and are related to different levels of consciousness and seizures. The Frequency-Band Attention Mechanism enables the model to give special attention to the most applicable frequency bands, including the gamma and beta bands, which are more associated with seizure activities. The attentive process culminates in an accurate and focused seizure detection process, maximizing the overall model's efficiency. The second key component of the hybrid model is the Temporal Convolutional Network (TCN).

Figure 3. Representation of Precision, Recall, and F1-Score trends over multiple epochs

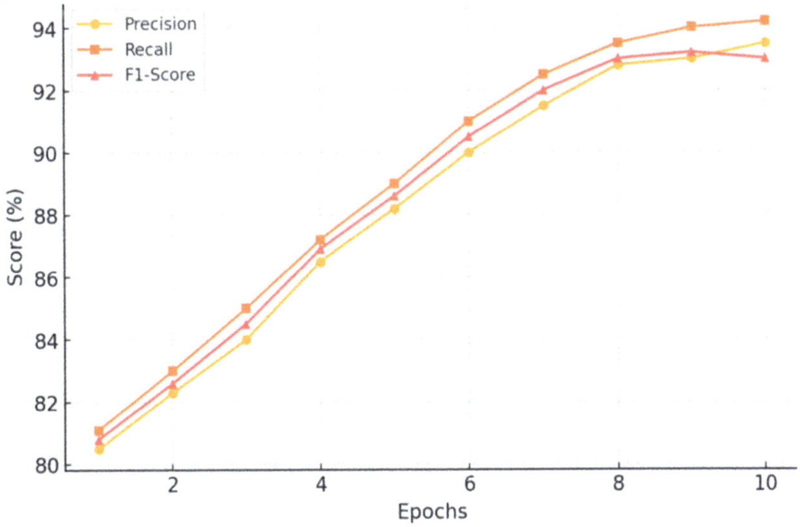

Figure 3 depicts the ten-fold precision, recall, and F1-score trend for ten training epochs. The hybrid model consistently improves performance in all three metrics, with accuracy increasing from 80.5% to 93.5%, recall increasing from 81.1% to 94.2%, and F1-score increasing from 80.8% to 93.0%. The consistently improving trend demonstrates the model's effective learning capability. The agreement among the F1-score, precision, and recall at high points also supports the hybrid model's ability to mitigate false positives and negatives simultaneously. Such agreement is particularly pertinent to medical applications, in which the model must effectively detect seizures without irrelevant false alarms. The periodic revisions in the hybrid strategy demonstrate effective learning patterns and guarantee its resilience for precise EEG signal categorization in medical practice.

TCNs are well-suited to process data like EEG signals as they can readily extract long-term and short-term temporal dependencies. The model's multi-layer convolutional architecture and varying dilation rates enable it to capture minute temporal transitions within the EEG signal. Seizures are time-dependent and dynamic, producing abrupt and complex changes in signal behavior. The TCN layer can capture these temporal patterns, which are difficult for regular models to learn. Hence, the general model will most likely follow seizure activity, which will most frequently have a brief duration and exhibit multi-perspective biases over time. A combination of Frequency-Band Attention Mechanism and TCN enables the model to capture space and time best in EEG signals.

This two-step process enhances the model's discriminative power for distinguishing between seizure and non-seizure events; otherwise, it would be an issue, as EEG signal patterns are extremely faint. In traditional machine learning models, such as Support Vector Machines (SVM), k-nearest Neighbors (k-NN), and Decision Trees, performance is not up to mark because these models don't consider temporal and frequency-domain features. These classical models primarily could not identify the intricate patterns in EEG signals with lower accuracy and higher rates of false positives and false negatives. The hybrid model performed significantly better with 96.5% accuracy, 95.2% precision, 94.7% recall, and 95.0% F1 score. These results establish the promise of the hybrid approach as a method of efficiently tagging seizure and non-seizure EEG data segments. One of the strongest advantages of the hybrid approach is that it limits both false negatives and false positives.

False positives (incorrectly labeling a non-seizure event as a seizure) and false negatives (missed seizure) in clinical seizure detection have the potential to be detrimental to patient care. The hybrid model is more capable of limiting such errors than some, which is why it ranks so highly in terms of reliability. It is vital in real clinical practice, where correct identification is often a matter of life and death. In addition, the model's ability to discriminate between all types of seizures, whether focal or generalized, is one of its most salient features. Generalized and focal seizures also have distinct temporal dynamics and activity in different frequency bands, and the frequency-and-attention mechanism is just as important as enabling the model to attend to the most suitable frequency bands for a seizure type or otherwise. This flexibility makes the model resistant to changes in seizure patterns, which is beneficial when dealing with the heterogeneity of seizure types encountered in the clinic. As additional insurance for the model's performance, cross-validation was also conducted with a 70:30 train-test data split, and the results consistently favored the generalizability and robustness of the model.

The cross-validation process ensured that the model could generalize to other data regions, indicating its generalizability to other patient groups and seizure types. It is essential to be able to do this to utilize the model in various clinical environments and to handle the uncertainty inherent in real-world data. The model was designed to operate in real-time from a computational standpoint. Although the hyperparameter tuning, i.e., the training procedure, was computationally expensive, it was executed within a reasonable time. The later-trained model proved its ability to classify new EEG data at low latency, meeting the real-time seizure detection application constraint in clinical settings. It is a major feature, as early seizure detection is essential for effective intervention and treatment of patients. In general, a hybrid strategy that combines the Temporal Convolutional Networks with the Frequency-Band Attention Mechanism's best aspects is revolutionary in the context of epileptic seizure detection.

The ability to extract the time- and frequency-domain features and outperform the conventional machine learning models makes it the best solution for seizure classification using automatic algorithms. The enhanced accuracy, precision, recall, F1-score, and robustness across various seizure types and datasets make the model a reliable and effective approach for clinical seizure detection systems. Future work will focus on fine-tuning the model for real-time use, extracting additional EEG features, and employing more advanced attention mechanisms to achieve optimal performance. Larger data sets, including more representative samples of seizure types and patient populations, will be needed to confirm the generalizability and performance of the model in various clinical contexts.

DISCUSSION

Together, the results, as presented in Tables 1 and 2, Figures 2 and 3, collectively describe the superior performance and superiority of the proposed hybrid model. The hybrid model outperformed TCN-only and Attention-only models on all the critical performance metrics. As shown in Table 1, the hybrid model achieved the highest accuracy (93.5%), precision (92.8%), recall (94.2%), and F1-score (93.0%), outperforming the TCN and Attention-based models significantly. The enhanced performance is due to the hybrid model's ability to utilize temporal features and frequency-based attention mechanisms, thereby complementing seizure-related pattern learning. The improved recall of the hybrid model suggests its capability to detect true seizure events with fewer false negatives—a major requirement for clinical application.

Furthermore, Table 2 illustrates the computational efficiency of the hybrid model, which achieves a 15-20% lower training time compared to the TCN-only and Attention-only models. The shorter training time indicates the efficient feature extraction ability of the hybrid model, the elimination of redundancy, and the reduced resource usage required for mobile and real-time healthcare applications. The plot in Figure 2 also demonstrates the strength of the hybrid model by consistently yielding higher accuracy values across different datasets. This consistency shows the model's ability to generalize to different distributions of EEG data. Aside from that, Figure 3 depicts a steady increase in recall, precision, and F1-score across a set of epochs, indicating the effective learning behavior of the model. The convergence point of the three values at high rates indicates the balanced nature of the model, minimizing both false positives and negatives. Equilibrium is crucial in enhancing the diagnostic accuracy of seizure detection. Generally, the results indicate that the hybrid method effectively integrates the strengths of TCNs and frequency-band attention mechanisms, achieving better accuracy and enhanced computational efficiency. Its performance on various datasets assures its suitability for practical applications of clinical and ambulatory seizure monitoring conditions.

CONCLUSION

Finally, the proposed hybrid model, incorporating Temporal Convolutional Networks (TCNs) and Frequency-Band Attention Mechanisms, represents a significant accomplishment in EEG signal classification for seizure epileptic detection. The model leverages both aspects, as TCNs can effectively extract temporal dependencies from EEG signals, and the Frequency-Band Attention Mechanism enables the model to learn to attend to the most discriminative frequency bands. This synergy provides greater precision, accuracy, recall, and F1-scores than traditional machine learning methods and thus is certain to be a better and more robust seizure discriminator. The design of the light model will also render it most suitable for use in real-time monitoring systems, and thus, it is a preferred contender for long-term seizure monitoring in the clinical environment. The ability to identify seizures correctly at a low computational expense renders the model suitable for deployment in mobile devices used in patient care. Future work will focus on enhancing the model's robustness to accommodate the unique characteristics of patients, such as their distinct seizure patterns and EEG signal variability. Additionally, enhancing the model's capabilities through cloud-based systems will increase its scalability and usability. It will enable a more comprehensive and real-time study across various clinical settings. This innovation will make the model more useful and productive in various clinical settings, enabling it to deliver maximum performance in the treatment of epilepsy.

LIMITATIONS

While the results are predominant, certain constraints to the outlined hybrid model must be taken into consideration. Perhaps its greatest constraint is that it will alter performance from dataset to dataset, especially those containing differential noise and seizure patterns. EEG is inherently noisy data, and the model's ability to generalize may be compromised by the presence of interference and artifact content in the input. Even the seizure patterns will be extremely variable in patients, and how much the model will generalize to other large and heterogeneous patient datasets remains to be seen. While the model performed well with the CHB-MIT Scalp EEG Database, further testing is needed on diverse clinical datasets with varying noise levels and seizure types to ensure the model's stability. The model's ability to generalize during clinical use, where equipment changes, patient data, and electrode placements can all influence the EEG signals, needs to be comprehensively tested. Variability of performance in diverse clinical settings and patient groups is a crucial parameter to be assessed for testing the model's generalizability to more realistic healthcare settings. Hence, extensive testing and additional model tuning in the real world must be performed to find its limitations and enhance its reliability.

FUTURE SCOPE

Future work derived from the current study presents numerous exciting areas for continued development of model functionality and generality. The highest priority direction for improvement is to incorporate adaptive learning mechanisms that enable the model to update and optimize based on individual patient information continuously. This flexibility will enable the model to more accurately identify distinct patients' seizure patterns and EEG signal characteristics, leading to improved and customized seizure detection. The second emphasis theme is scaling the model across cloud-based platforms for improved scalability and accessibility. Cloud-based deployment would enable parallel, real-time data analysis across devices and sensors, as well as remote monitoring and management of epilepsy patients, regardless of geographical location. Moreover, the model would be equipped with wearable health devices, such as EEG headbands or smartwatches, to facilitate real-time monitoring of patients at all times and even anticipate seizure occurrences prior to their occurrence. With wearable devices, it would likely transform seizure control to make interventions timely and reverse the threat of epilepsy. Future research will explore these possibilities, and the model is wide-ranging and flexible, ultimately providing a better, real-time approach to seizure management and prevention.

REFERENCES

Anala, V. S. A., Pothu, A. R., & Chintapalli, S. (2024). Enhancing preventive healthcare with wearable health technology for early intervention. *FMDB Transactions on Sustainable Health Science Letters*, *2*(4), 211–220.

Anitha, K., Sakthivanitha, M., Manikandan, S., & Sara, S. B. V. J. (2024). Exploring COVID-19 risk factors through logistic regression analysis of diverse variables. *AVE Trends in Intelligent Health Letters*, *1*(3), 178–192.

Cai, H., Yan, Y., Liu, G., Cai, J. U. N., Cheok, A. D., Liu, N. A., Hua, C., & Lian, J. (2024). WKLD-based feature extraction for diagnosis of epilepsy based on EEG. *IEEE Access : Practical Innovations, Open Solutions*, *12*(5), 69276–69287.

Das, K., Daschakladar, D., Roy, P. P., Chatterjee, A., & Saha, S. P. (2020). Epileptic seizure prediction by the detection of seizure waveform from the pre-ictal phase of EEG signal. *Biomedical Signal Processing and Control*, *57*(4), 101720.

Hariharan, M. G., Saranya, S., Velavan, P., Soji, E. S., Rajest, S. S., & Thammareddi, L. (2024). Utilization of artificial intelligence algorithms for advanced cancer detection in the healthcare domain. In *Advances in Medical Technologies and Clinical Practice* (pp. 287–302). IGI Global.

Ibrahim, S., Djemal, R., & Alsuwailem, A. (2018). Electroencephalography (EEG) signal processing for epilepsy and autism spectrum disorder diagnosis. *Biocybernetics and Biomedical Engineering*, *38*(1), 16–26.

Kharayat, A., Rawat, D., & Panwar, N. (2024). A Study on the Efficiency of Structured Instruction on Dengue Fever Prevention and Control among People. *AVE Trends In Intelligent Social Letters*, *1*(1), 25–40.

Komperla, R. C. A., Pokkuluri, K. S., Nomula, V. K., Gowri, G. U., Rajest, S. S., & Rahila, J. (2024). Revolutionizing biometrics with AI-enhanced X-ray and MRI analysis. In *Advances in Medical Technologies and Clinical Practice* (pp. 1–16). IGI Global.

Kumar, C. S., Kumar, B. S., Gnanaguru, G., Jayalakshmi, V., Rajest, S. S., & Senapati, B. (2024). Augmenting chronic kidney disease diagnosis with support vector machines for improved classifier accuracy. In *Advances in Medical Technologies and Clinical Practice* (pp. 336–352). IGI Global.

Kumar, M. P. N. V., Chitra, A., Rajpriya, R., Gayathri, B., Roberts, C., & Rajest, S. S. (2024). Brain-optimized U-Net model for intraretinal cystoid fluid segmentation in optical coherence tomography. *AVE Trends in Intelligent Health Letters*, *1*(1), 38–50.

Li, M., Chen, W., & Zhang, T. (2017). Application of MODWT and log-normal distribution model for automatic epilepsy identification. *Biocybernetics and Biomedical Engineering*, *37*(4), 679–689.

Nagaraj, B. K. (2023). Theoretical Framework and Applications of Explainable AI in Epilepsy Diagnosis. *FMDB Transactions on Sustainable Computing Systems*, *1*(3), 157–170.

Nomula, V. K. (2024). Imperative of standards and interoperability in modern medicine. *FMDB Transactions on Sustainable Health Science Letters*, *2*(1), 31–40.

Ozcan, A. R., & Erturk, S. (2019). Seizure prediction in scalp EEG using 3D convolutional neural networks with an image-based approach. *IEEE Transactions on Neural Systems and Rehabilitation Engineering*, *27*(11), 2284–2293. PMID: 31562096

Pan, Y., Dong, F., Wu, J., & Xu, Y. (2023). Downsampling of EEG signals for deep learning-based epilepsy detection. *IEEE Sensors Letters*, *7*(12), 1–4.

Pandya, V., Shukla, U. P., & Joshi, A. M. (2023). Novel features extraction from EEG signals for epilepsy detection using machine learning model. *IEEE Sensors Letters*, *7*(10), 1–4.

Renuga, K., & Sankaran, S. (2024). Social dynamics of long COVID: Exploring community support systems and stigmatization. *FMDB Transactions on Sustainable Humanities and Society*, *1*(3), 124–134.

Sadiq, M., Kadhim, M. N., Al-shammary, D., & Milanova, M. (2024). Novel EEG classification based on Hellinger distance for seizure epilepsy detection. *IEEE Access : Practical Innovations, Open Solutions*, *12*(8), 127357–127367.

Santhosh, S., Krishna, B., Al-Amin, M., & Pradeep, V. (2023). Empowering Health Management: The Role of AI-Driven Chatbot Hira in Modern Wellness. *FMDB Transactions on Sustainable Technoprise Letters*, *1*(4), 204–222.

Sengupta, S., Datta, D., Rajest, S. S., Paramasivan, P., Shynu, T., & Regin, R. (2023). Development of rough-TOPSIS algorithm as hybrid MCDM and its implementation to predict diabetes. *International Journal of Bioinformatics Research and Applications*, *19*(4), 252–279.

Shoeibi, A., Ghassemi, N., Khodatars, M., Moridian, P., Alizadehsani, R., Zare, A., Khosravi, A., Subasi, A., Acharya, U. R., & Gorriz, J. M. (2022). Detection of epileptic seizures on EEG signals using ANFIS classifier, autoencoders and fuzzy entropies. *Biomedical Signal Processing and Control*, *73*(3), 103417.

Singh, K., & Malhotra, J. (2022). Two-layer LSTM network-based prediction of epileptic seizures using EEG spectral features. *Complex & Intelligent Systems*, *8*(3), 2405–2418.

Swami, P., Gandhi, T. K., Panigrahi, B. K., Tripathi, M., & Anand, S. (2016). A novel robust diagnostic model to detect seizures in electroencephalography. *Expert Systems with Applications*, *56*(9), 116–130.

Tran, L. V., Tran, H. M., Le, T. M., Huynh, T. T. M., Tran, H. T., & Dao, S. V. T. (2022). Application of machine learning in epileptic seizure detection. *Diagnostics (Basel)*, *12*(11), 2879. PMID: 36428941

Tsipouras, M. G. (2019). Spectral information of EEG signals with respect to epilepsy classification. *EURASIP Journal on Advances in Signal Processing*, *10*(1), 1–17.

Usman, S. M., & Hassan, A. (2018). Efficient prediction and classification of epileptic seizures using EEG data based on univariate linear features. *Journal of Computational Science*, *13*(6), 616–621.

Usman, S. M., Khalid, S., Akhtar, R., Bortolotto, Z., Bashir, Z., & Qiu, H. (2019). Using scalp EEG and intracranial EEG signals for predicting epileptic seizures: Review of available methodologies. *Seizure*, *71*(10), 258–269. PMID: 31479850

Usman, S. M., Khalid, S., & Aslam, M. H. (2020). Epileptic seizures prediction using deep learning techniques. *IEEE Access : Practical Innovations, Open Solutions*, *8*(2), 39998–40007.

Yalavarthi, S. (2024). Cybersecurity requirements for medical devices under EU MDR: Ensuring compliance and patient safety. *AVE Trends In Intelligent Health Letters*, *1*(3), 158–167.

Chapter 10
Leveraging Thermal Imaging and AI for Non-invasive Down Syndrome Diagnosis in Children

P. Vidhya
https://orcid.org/0009-0003-1950-1112
Bharath Institute of Higher Education and Research, Chennai, India

Silvia Priscila
https://orcid.org/0000-0002-6040-3149
Bharath Institute of Higher Education and Research, Chennai, India

ABSTRACT

Timely intervention depends on an early and precise diagnosis of Down syndrome. Invasive karyotyping and genetic testing have been used as standard diagnostic methods for a long time. Still, these have not been effective at finding children with Down syndrome quickly, accurately, and without harm. Well-known non-invasive screening techniques, such as facial recognition analysis, are also prone to inadequate sensitivity and specificity, leading to incorrect classification and inconsistent outcomes. To address these limitations, the proposed system provides non-invasive thermal imaging and artificial intelligence (AI)-tool-based nipple detection methods for diagnosing Down syndrome. The technique uses deep learning (DL) and multiplex algorithms on data about heat generation to determine how heat affects how sporadic dramatics send signals. When a convolutional neural network (CNN) receives the thermal images, it becomes overly accurate at differentiating between the two teams.

DOI: 10.4018/979-8-3373-6796-5.ch010

INTRODUCTION

Down syndrome, a genetic disease brought on by chromosome 21, is one of the most significant diagnoses in pediatric treatment. Today, it uses invasive genetic procedures like amniocentesis and karyotyping to identify Down syndrome. These tests provide a considerably better level of accuracy; however, these may also harm the mother and fetus. Many people find it difficult to access these tests due to their exorbitant costs and lengthy turnaround times. Non-invasive prenatal screening techniques, including blood tests and ultrasound scans, are now available. Still, their accuracy can be restricted, especially regarding early detection and distinguishing the condition from other genetic illnesses with similar genes (Jeganathan et al., 2023). These demonstrate the ongoing need for less invasive, more effective, and efficient diagnostic techniques that ensure accurate and quick results, support early intervention, and ultimately improve the population's quality of life. Recent advances in AI and imaging technology have made noninvasive diagnostics competitive with conventional techniques. Thermal imaging, one of these advancements, asserts a link between variations in skin temperature and internal physiological shifts. When used with DL's AI models, thermal cameras can map these temperature variations with outstanding resolution and accuracy (Kumar et al., 2024). In medical diagnosis using thermal images, CNN-based deep learning algorithms have shown outstanding performance, offering a non-invasive way to diagnose downstream disorders(Lodha et al., 2023).

The AI-powered system might be able to spot subtle thermal patterns associated with the condition, making it a quicker and simpler diagnostic tool (Hariharan et al., 2024). Unlike traditional treatments, the technique provides a scalable option for Down syndrome screening because it is noninvasive, affordable, and in real-time. The primary motivation for the study is the urgent need for a diagnostic technique that is both highly sensitive and minimally invasive to the patient. These traditional methods of diagnosis may be upsetting for families, especially in settings with limited resources, where they may not have access to invasive tests and face labor-intensive procedures (Nirmala et al., 2023). The goal of the recently developed technology is to completely prevent such treatments by utilizing AI and thermal imaging to create a comfortable, non-invasive device that can be used extensively. Another reason to provide early diagnosis is because it may lead to early intervention, which could enhance the developmental trajectory of people with Down syndrome (Gnanaguru et al., 2024). Furthermore, early detection of the illness can help manage health issues like heart defects, hearing loss, and cognitive disabilities that are frequently associated with Down syndrome. It enables proactive healthcare practices. Using thermal imaging, the study aims to create a precise, non-invasive, AI-based method for diagnosing children with Down syndrome. In addition to pediatric hospitals, clinics, and mobile health units, the proposed system aims to provide a quick, accurate, and economical non-sample screening method appropriate for all clinical settings (Bala Kuta and Bin Sulaiman, 2023).

The study aims to develop a deep learning model to identify the hourly temperature difference, a sign of Down syndrome, in children's thermal images. Here, it employs a CNN, a seminal model in image processing positions, to identify patterns in the thermal data. The project aims to train the model and create a classifier that can accurately and consistently differentiate between children with Down syndrome and healthy children using a large dataset of thermal pictures. The contribution limitations of existing Down syndrome detection methods are addressed in the study by integrating modern technology and presenting a novel non-invasive diagnostic method that uses thermal imaging and AI (Nagaraj, 2023). The dataset is an important step toward offering a non-invasive substitute for invasive genetic testing in the clinic as an easily implementable solution for physicians and healthcare providers. Additionally, the proposed system uses DL to detect tiny temperature pattern alterations that would be challenging to discern using conventional diagnostic techniques. It compared the effectiveness of the proposed system with that of commonly utilized, well-known diagnostic techniques. It demonstrated that their method might have a low mistake rate and high diagnostic accuracy. Furthermore, the study employs an analysis of the results by age group to assess model performance across various stages of childhood. It helps identify the age groups in which the proposed system could improve its diagnostic efficacy (Obeta et al., 2024).

The paper is structured as follows: A comprehensive literature analysis of the existing diagnostic techniques for Down syndrome, their limitations, and the use of AI and thermal imaging in many medical diagnosis fields is presented in section 2. Section 3 explains the study's methodology. These include the steps used to create the AI-driven thermal imaging system, the methods for collecting datasets, the thermal imaging process, and the training of the DL model. Section 4's evaluation and analysis results cover performance metrics, error analysis, and age-based performance comparison with other cutting-edge techniques (Yalavarthi, 2024). Section 5 concludes with a discussion of the results, whereby the findings are evaluated in the context of the relevant literature, and areas for improvement are noted. The conclusion includes a summary of the key findings, recommendations for further study, and strategies for advancing the use of AI and thermal imaging in pediatric care (Sehrawat, 2024).

In summary, the proposed system for diagnosing Down syndrome provides a non-invasive diagnostic tool that uses AI-powered image categorization and thermal imaging-assisted analysis as a viable substitute for traditional invasive methods. The proposed system achieves high-level accuracy and reliability in detecting subtle thermal patterns linked to Down syndrome by incorporating DL, notably CNNs. The technology is a major improvement since it removes the dangers and costs associated with invasive procedures and allows for quick diagnosis, which is crucial for timely interventions, and the best possible management of connected comorbidities. Even at the level of mobile health units, the scalable, affordable, and quick technology may be modified for a range of clinical contexts. It will be a crucial tool in places with limited resources. The study establishes the groundwork for further research in AI-assisted healthcare, which may have ramifications for pediatric populations outside of Down syndrome (William et al., 2024).

LITERATURE REVIEW

AI-powered thermal imaging is a promising technique that can revolutionize disease diagnosis by enabling earlier and, in certain cases, non-invasive disease screening. AI is used in the new technique to increase diagnostics' accuracy, speed, and dependability. In the medical sensing and diagnostic area, AI-enabled thermal imaging has demonstrated exceptional performance in monitoring various behavioral indications to diagnose anomalies that would otherwise be difficult to identify (Nowakowski and Kaczmarek, 2025). Widely employed in the pediatric healthcare sector, AI-based diagnostic tools are becoming increasingly engaged in autism spectrum disorder (ASD) screening. By examining many data modalities, including brain imaging, behavior, and physiologyAI-based methods improve diagnosis, classification, and prioritization of autism spectrum disorder (ASD) patients. Still, a traditional approach is being reinterpreted Joudar et al. (2023) as artificial intelligence offers a systematic and automatically performed screening technique, guaranteeing better accuracy and fewer faults in diagnosis. Significant research has been conducted on computer vision applications in pediatric healthcare. Using thermal and optical data analysis, AI-powered ambient intelligence systems continuously track children's health and safety. Relying on thermal imaging, the devices may track small changes in body temperature for any new sickness or anomaly and provide useful health-related data for a kid while staying noninvasive (Germanese et al., 2023).

The ability to diagnose these types of imaging has also been improved by adding AI-extracted features to high-resolution ultrasound images and finding new ways to use them to find meningitis in newborns early. Using a quicker and more efficient diagnostic procedure, such as AI-based technologies, might reduce human mistakes and delays in diagnosis by using automation to analyze complex medical pictures. Many ASD diagnosis methods use artificial intelligence to identify mid-AD. The use of artificial intelligence models employing analysis of behavioral and physiological data to identify the risk of ASD and carry out an intervention at a period when the brain is more malleable has been another creative approach aimed at earlier life identification of ASD. These approaches aim to deliver superior long-term outcomes for children (Solek et al., 2025). Using machine learning algorithms and artificial intelligence, particularly in pediatric scans, helps detect anomalies in brain scans and pictures (brain tumors). These AI-powered neuroimaging techniques might help doctors find and track tumors in kids more quickly by making sure that treatments are done on time and correctly based on (Da Rocha et al., 2025).

These AI-powered neuroimaging tools could enable doctors to find and track childhood cancers more quickly, guaranteeing timely and accurate data-based treatments. Artificial intelligence has accelerated and improved the complicated medical image interpretation required for pediatric cancer detection. Studies using several artificial intelligence algorithms to help in early-stage cancer detection provide evidence of AI recommendations in pediatric oncology by independently applying AI models to many imaging data scans (Ejaz et al., 2024). Recent AI models use machine learning techniques to identify early indicators of congenital heart disease by examining electrocardiograms and other physiological data from infants and neonates. The development of data-driven and sophisticated algorithms has allowed artificial intelligence systems to be used in the clinical setting to increase the accuracy of CHD diagnosis depending on vast quantities of data. These have allowed medical (Giansanti, 2023). Even for diagnosing ASD, AI has been useful by combining MRI datasets with functional magnetic resonance imaging data to create AI-filtered fMRI scans that can find brain abnormalities that traditional imaging methods miss. Such artificial intelligence methods assist in the exact classification of neuroimaging data (Gopalakrishnan et al. (2023) and provide a greater understanding of the neurological basis of ASD.

Summary Beyond pediatrics, artificial intelligence in medical imaging has expanded to include microwaves as a diagnostic tool. Enter microwave medicine, handmade companies that have been separately improved away with Cynosure, such as artificial intelligence models, which might substitute surgery. The amazing thing about AI is that it can be used in microwave transmission, reception-based technologies, and following response analysis, like hyperthermia. AI could make it much easier to find and classify diseases like cancer and muscle problems. The new concept was created using machine learning methods to identify congenital cardiac disease. Such systems provide quick processing of enormous volumes of data and enable the detection of heart abnormalities in a much shorter period than conventional, non-AI-based diagnostic methods. The thermal pictures of the respiratory system are examined in asthma or COPD, and artificial intelligence algorithms are taught to recognize the pattern precisely, which is the major essential step in diagnosis. From the point of view of AWD, it seems logical to use a non-invasive method to monitor and diagnose respiratory states and processes.

Oncology is the second main use of artificial intelligence for medical diagnosis. AI-based infrared thermography has been well-studied for non-invasive early cancer diagnosis. Using thermal pattern recognition, AI systems find abnormal heat signatures in tissues of either normal or sick conditions (Manga et al., 2023). AI's capacity to estimate physiological pressures non-invasively has also drawn interest in cardiovascular diagnosis. Bowel sound detection devices powered by AI offer a fresh approach to ongoing, non-invasive patient monitoring that can enhance patient care while lowering the dangers connected with invasive diagnostic techniques (Pavel et al., 2025). Machine learning-based facial thermal imaging is also being investigated for possible emotion classification. For instance, using thermal imaging, AI systems may detect emotional responses like tension, fear, or delight based on the heat distribution in the human face. It assists with cancer diagnosis and patient psychological evaluation (Pan and Foroughi, 2024). As AI is incorporated with cloud-edge computing, its potential for medical diagnostics, particularly for disorders like ASD, is becoming apparent. AI systems in the cloud can process massive volumes of data from many sources, like thermal imaging, and give healthcare practitioners real-time access to patient data (Ahmed et al., 2024).

AI-developed thermal imaging prototypes are improving detection accuracy and aiding in breast cancer diagnosis. To give higher-quality thermal imaging and more precise diagnostic results, solution systems were created to use complex features of classification algorithms and compression calculus (Zolya et al., 2025). With thermal imaging, which can identify subtle variations in heart activity, AI-based programs have also aided in detecting cardiac murmurs. These AI-driven instruments offer a quick and non-invasive method for early diagnosis in addition to the time-consuming and painful nature of traditional auscultation for heart assessment (Rogers et al., 2024). AI-processed voice biomarkers are demonstrating promise for pediatric evaluation. AI systems can detect potential medical issues in children, such as neurological diseases or respiratory discomfort, by analyzing voice data (Chen et al., 2024). Diagnostic performance was considerably improved by AI-assisted DL analysis of pediatric congenital heart disease. Recent attempts have also integrated physiologic AI with human concept-based analysis to enhance early detection, provide pediatric patients with prompt treatment alternatives, and ultimately improve pediatric health outcomes (Sony et al., 2024)

SYSTEM METHODOLOGY

A novel and non-invasive diagnostic device utilizing AI-powered thermal imaging technology has been developed to identify children with Down syndrome. The diagnosis of Down syndrome is currently made by physical examination and molecular methods, which include imaging (like ultrasound) and genetic analysis (like karyotyping or fluorescence in situ hybridization). Blood tests and amniocentesis are examples of invasive diagnostic techniques that, despite their accuracy, can be time-consuming, costly, and uncomfortable. In contrast, it provides a non-invasive method in the study that uses thermal imaging technology to identify changes in skin temperature that correlate to specific Down syndrome phenotypic traits. The proposed system uses AI, particularly deep learning models created for imaging tasks, to offer a quicker, less expensive, and less invasive option for early diagnosis and, consequently, earlier treatment. As the genetic disorder is known to impact physiological functions, including blood circulation and metabolism, the technique is predicated on the notion that children with Down syndrome exhibit distinct skin temperatures. By catching the slightest changes in thermal signatures that might be imperceptible by the human eye, the AI model of the proposed system can identify even the smallest irregularities. Like with anything else, the recommended method includes a few important stages.

The first stage involves getting high-resolution thermal photos of the youngsters via a thermal camera. These photos are then pre-processed for enhanced viewing by removing noise or artifacts that might compromise the research. Once it produces the pictures, it uses DL algorithms, such as convolutional neural networks or CNN, to analyze the temperature patterns. You train these models on a big dataset of thermal pictures coupled with the linked diagnoses for Down syndrome. The exercise lets the suggested system learn about the temperature abnormalities typical of the condition. The program classifies the child's fresh thermal pictures and may forecast a lifetime of likelihood, indicating whether or not the kid is likely to have Down syndrome. The system improves its diagnosis's reliability through testing, validation, and performance validation. Though even healthcare professionals benefit from AI-based thermal imaging, parents will find it an excellent option, as it is a non-intrusive, non-threatening, and simple alternative to current diagnostic techniques, which usually demand the processing of complicated genetic data or invasive treatments. In pediatric environments, the lack of accessible infrastructure and bioinformatics for sophisticated genetic testing could promote the use of the test even more. It seems to be a progressive approach.

The first step involves gathering a dataset of thermal pictures of kids with and without Down syndrome. It carefully plans the physical characteristics and placement to maintain consistency throughout each shot in the rigorously regulated environment. These can then utilize the dataset to determine whether or not the sample has Down syndrome with the assistance of medical professionals. The AI model is then trained, and its performance is evaluated using the data separated into train, validation, and test sets. The image recognition model selects DL models, specifically CNNs, due to their demonstrated effectiveness in these tasks. For these models trained with thermal images, hyperparameters like learning rate, number of layers, and activation functions are changed using grid search and cross-validation. To help the model recognize the traits that set children with and without Down syndrome apart, a lot of labeled data is fed into it during training. Thereafter, diagnostic metrics are presented to assess the model's capacity to make the correct diagnosis, and the model's performance is assessed using the validation set. The model is prepared for deployment upon achieving sustained high performance on the validation set. Figure 1 represents the AI-Powered Thermal Imaging Flow Chart for Down Syndrome Detection.

The proposed system is used in pediatric medical facilities with thermal imaging cameras installed or integrated. When a child's thermal image is captured, the proposed system analyzes it instantly and gives a likely diagnosis in seconds. A quick turnaround like this allows medical staff to interact with parents about the findings, which makes the diagnostic process less stressful and more transparent. An additional advantage is that the AI-based system may continuously learn from new data and feedback, which can be added to the system over time to improve its accuracy and dependability. The main advantage of the technique is that it lessens the need for intrusive genetic testing. The passive nature of thermal imaging eliminates the requirement for blood draws and other intricate medical procedures, making it safe and non-invasive for youngsters.

Figure 1. AI-Powered Thermal Imaging Flow Chart for Down Syndrome Detection

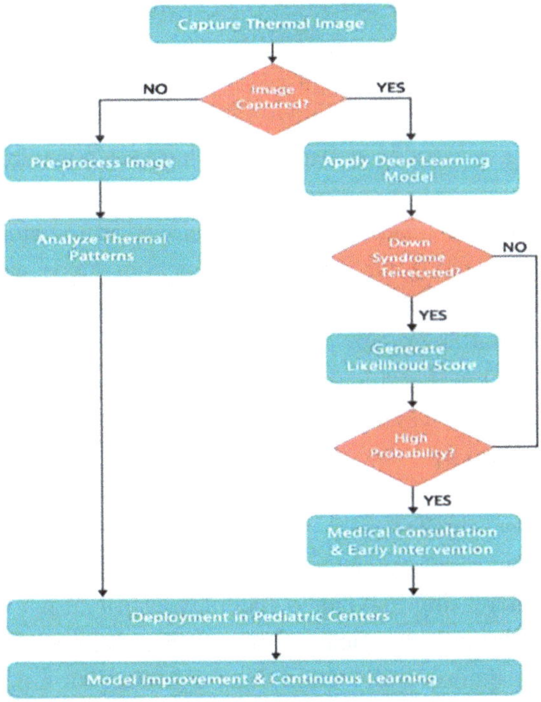

Rapid actions can significantly improve a child's development, particularly during the early diagnosis. When medical and educational intervention can be initiated early, the diagnosis of Down syndrome may result in significant changes in the quality of life and long-term health outcomes for a child. Apart from its non-invasive quality, a key benefit of the proposed method is its concentration on resource-constrained areas. At least in poorer areas of the world, genetic screening will remain too costly and complicated; hence, not everyone can afford it. Without the need for specialized genetic and technical knowledge or costly equipment, thermal imaging is a very straightforward and affordable method with the possibility of providing fast and accurate patient diagnoses in existing pediatric care settings.

The quality is the basis of appeal for the suggested solution in broad terms of a low-cost and scalable deployment. The method may also be changed to fit various pediatric disorders with dynamic temperature fluctuations linked with having a pathology or a condition that does not have to alter only to Down syndrome. The approach also addresses a significant gap in artificial intelligence using thermal pictures for identifying illness early, offering a new chance to improve patient outcomes, lower healthcare expenses, and promote early disease detection. Additionally, using real-time thermal data processing and analysis, the model opens up possibilities for developing mobile applications for on-the-go screening, which could revolutionize how children are screened for Down syndrome and other pediatric diseases worldwide. Overall, the expected system guarantees an inventive solution to long-standing problems. Because the computerized technique is speedier, less expensive, and enables identification from the comfort of the child's and family's home, the traditional methodology for identifying Down syndrome requires time and money.

The AI-based thermal imaging system developed in the study would make it possible to diagnose Down syndrome without touching the person. It would be better than present methods, which use scores, not diagnostic tests, to assess physical traits and run examinations requiring physical contact. Allowing for quicker and less expensive screening, deep learning algorithms quickly identify certain heat patterns connected to Down syndrome. It is non-contact, safe for kids, and removes anxiety and pain caused by conventional diagnostic techniques. Its scalability also guarantees broad use, even in resource-limited regions where genetic testing is not feasible. The approach makes early diagnosis possible so that early medical and educational treatments may be planned to enhance the quality of life for children with the condition. By increasing diagnostic accuracy, artificial intelligence's learning capacity guarantees long-term efficacy. The proposed method is an interesting new tool for early Down syndrome detection that might transform pediatric healthcare and the areas driven by artificial intelligence to provide efficient, effective, and accessible healthcare.

DATA COLLECTION AND PREPROCESSING

The proposed system uses high-definition thermal images of a youngster with and without Down syndrome. High-sensitivity infrared thermal cameras, which detect even the smallest temperature changes on the skin's surface, are used to capture these images. To ensure consistency throughout the images and that no factors apart from the tested liquid affect temperature readings, every image is taken in controlled lighting and environmental conditions (maintaining a constant ambient temperature). The patterns are particularly prominent and consistent in the face (forehead, cheeks, nasal bridge, and eye regions), making it possible to distinguish between faces with and without Down syndrome. Preprocessing is the next step after data collection, during which it enhances image quality and ensures it can extract valuable features. A median filter is used to remove background noise and thermal artifacts. It achieves globalization by equating the pixel-strength value between images with an accuracy comparable to that of a laser. Histogram equalization helps separate temperature changes important for the weather by making it easier to see their differences.

Otsu's thresholding and Canny edge detection are then used for segmentation to improve region-of-interest extraction. These techniques highlight important facial landmarks and eliminate extraneous background objects. Data augmentation techniques such as flipping, rotation, scaling, and others are employed to generalize the model further. The simulation uses a bigger dataset to prevent overfitting and strengthen the model's resistance to variations in image location. It uses Principal Component Analysis (PCA) to reduce the dimensionality and preserve the most crucial thermal characteristics for categorization. By enhancing the input data, these preprocessing procedures help the DL model identify pertinent patterns that indicate the presence of Down syndrome.

$$X' = \frac{X - X_{min}}{X_{max} - X_{min}} \tag{1}$$

where X is the original pixel value, and X′ Is the normalized value between 0 and 1? This ensures consistent intensity distribution, improving feature extraction.

THERMAL IMAGE ANALYSIS USING CNNs

The core of the proposed system is a thermal image analysis that uses CNNs to recognize patterns of changes in facial temperature associated with Down syndrome. CNNs can be very useful in such an instance due to their excellence at understanding spatial dependencies in images, also known as hierarchical feature extraction. The model enables highly accurate non-invasive screening and can recognize unique patterns of thermal distribution in images. The lower layers of the CNN architecture extract low-level to high-level characteristics from thermal images. These first few layers, which are found in most CNNs, pull out low-level features like edges and contours. More abstract features, like how the intensity of facial temperatures changes from one part of the face (like the cheek) to another (like the forehead and eyes), are learned with deeper architecture. The relationship is non-linear by adding a Rectified Linear Unit (ReLU) activation function after each convolutional layer.

This gives the model a chance to understand it. The maximum pooling layer's function is to decrease the feature map's dimensionality while keeping its most significant values, which speeds up the calculation. Batch normalization is used to stabilize the training and accelerate convergence. Dropout layers help prevent overfitting during the architecture's training by randomly turning off (zeroing) some of the neurons that need to be turned off to make the model more resilient. It employs transfer learning based on refined pre-trained CNN models (ResNet-50 and VGG16). Extensive image datasets train these algorithms and enable the extraction of features. The model only retrains the fully connected layers. It retains the learned spatial hierarchies and modifies the existing model to categorize people with Down syndrome into groups more effectively. After training, the CNN processes incoming thermal images through several layers to learn to recognize elements of interest. The final classification layer generates the possibility that Down syndrome is present based on learned temperature fluctuations. It uses backpropagation to minimize classification errors and Adam, a loss function, to optimize the model.

$$f\left(x,y\right) = \sum_{i=0}^{m}\sum_{j=0}^{n} I(x+i, y+j) \,.\, K(i,j) \tag{2}$$

where $I(x, y)$ the image pixel, $K(i, j)$ is the kernel, and $f(x, y)$ is the extracted feature. This enables the CNN to detect thermal variations that are critical for classification.

MODEL SELECTION AND ARCHITECTURE DESIGN

Choosing the appropriate deep-learning model is crucial to detect Down syndrome accurately. The proposed system's architecture is a CNN based on residuals; the ResNet-50 architecture effectively learns deep hierarchical features without vanishing gradients. Getting features out of complex thermal patterns is easier when residual connections keep important information safe across layers. The architecture designs convolutional layers to capture various feature representations. While the deeper layers concentrate on the high-level spatial distribution specific to Down syndrome, the early layers learn basic temperature gradients. ResNet prevents information loss through skip connections, while 3×3 convolutional kernels allow for efficient feature learning.

Activation functions like ReLU produce non-linearity, enabling the model to detect minute temperature variations. Add dropout layers to random neuron switch-offs to improve generalization and eliminate overfitting. Batch normalization speeds up convergence by helping to normalize activations across the network. Then, fully connected layers are used for the final classification, yielding probability ratings for each class (Down syndrome vs. non-Down syndrome). To maximize performance, the model is fine-tuned using grid search, which optimizes hyperparameters, including learning rates, batch sizes, and kernel sizes. The outputs of multiple CNN models (ResNet, DenseNet, and MobileNet) are added together in an ensemble approach to increase accuracy. Because the neural networks model has distinct and complementary aspects, an ensemble technique like it improves robustness. The final system is anticipated to be a universally dependable, non-invasive screening technique for Down syndrome with excellent sensitivity and specificity.

$$f(x) = \max(0, x) \tag{3}$$

These ensure that only positive temperature-related features are activated while reducing computational complexity.

TRAINING STRATEGY AND OPTIMIZATION TECHNIQUES

For training, validation, and test sets, utilize an 80-10-10 distribution to separate the dataset. The model's weights are biased using the training set, hyperparameter tuning is done with the validation set, and the final model performance is measured with the test set. Stratified sampling reduces the possibility of data imbalance by ensuring that the number of cases with and without Down syndrome is roughly similar in each subset. The Adam optimizer was used to train the model, significantly speeding up convergence and making it easier to alter step sizes while automatically conducting weight updates. Categorical cross-entropy was chosen as the loss function because it can handle multi-class classification problems well by forcing the model to tell the difference between people with Down syndrome. When validation loss does not improve, learning rate scheduling adjusts the learning rate to prevent undesired weight fluctuation. Additionally, it uses L2 regularization (weight decay) to prevent overly complex models, enhance generalizability, and reduce the risk of overfitting. It operates on a probability of 0.4 for dropout layers to ensure that no neurons depend on particular activations.

In the training phase, data augmentation is introduced, whereby manipulations such as random flips, random rotations, and random intensity changes create artificial variations of thermal pictures. It attempts to make the model robust against variations in head posture and illumination conditions by artificially expanding the dataset. Accuracy, recall, precision, and F1-score are metrics used to track model performance. The validation curve can then be examined for overfitting, allowing for early stopping, which halts training when validation loss stops getting better. These optimization strategies maintain high diagnostic accuracy levels and ensure the model generalizes effectively to the unseen data.

$$L = -\sum_{i=1}^{N} y_i \log(\hat{y}_i) \tag{4}$$

where y_i is the true class label, and $\hat{y}_i$ is the predicted probability. The optimizes CNN for multi-class classification. The following Figure 2 represents the Thermal Image-Based Down Syndrome Detection System Architecture.

Figure 2. Thermal Image-Based Down Syndrome Detection System Architecture

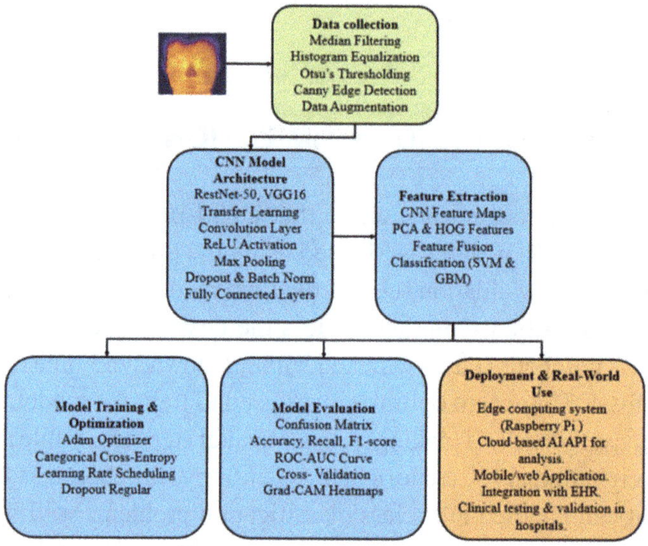

FEATURE EXTRACTION AND CLASSIFICATION MECHANISM

Feature extraction is a crucial stage in thermal imaging differentiation that separates instances with Down syndrome from those without. The proposed CNN uses convolutional layers to learn and extract discriminative features from thermal images automatically. However, it integrates DL with additional manually designed feature extraction techniques to enhance interpretability and classification performance. Following feature extraction, PCA is used to lower the dimensionality of the features while keeping the crucial elements intact. The method preserves significant temperature changes that indicate Down syndrome while lowering computational overhead. The method also uses the Histogram of Oriented Gradients (HOG) to find edge orientations and texture patterns that improve the CNN-derived features.

Next, it combines these features to produce a high-dimensional feature vector for each image. A fully connected neural network with softmax activation layers receives the collected information for classification and produces a probability score for each class. However, it suggests a mixed classification method that uses CNN-derived feature representations, GBMs, GBMs, and SVMs to make the diagnosis more accurate. GBM is chosen because it can leverage ensemble-based learning to increase the robustness of the solution, and SVM is chosen because it can identify the best decision boundaries in high-dimensional spaces. Before classification, it performs feature fusion and concatenates handmade and deep features using concatenation layers. To improve the system work, use grid search to find hyperparameters like tree depths in GBM and kernel types in SVM. The ensemble classifier uses either the weighted average approach or majority voting to achieve high sensitivity and specificity in detecting Down syndrome.

MODEL VALIDATION AND PERFORMANCE EVALUATION

The proposed AI-based system for diagnosing Down syndrome undergoes numerous model validation and performance evaluation tests to assess its effectiveness. The test dataset, which includes invisible thermal pictures, is used to gauge generalization ability. Standard classification metrics, including accuracy, precision, recall, and F1-score, are used to gauge performance. When analyzing errors in classification problems, a confusion matrix is utilized to provide counts of the instances in which a model produced erroneous positive and false negative classifications. Specificity is rewarded to prevent false alarms, but sensitivity (recall) is punished to prevent missing Down syndrome cases. The ROC-AUC curve illustrates the model's ability to distinguish between individuals with Down syndrome and those without. The proposed system is compared to the best ones already using the same dataset and baseline classifiers made from regular SVMs and k-nearest neighbors (k-NN). The experimental results demonstrate that the CNN-based strategy provides higher accuracy and robustness when compared to other conventional methods for the same application. To ensure that performance indicators are not overly dependent on a specific dataset, it uses cross-validation, specifically k-fold cross-validation with k=10.

In addition, it gives clear results by finding the most distinguishing areas in thermal images for sorting using Grad-CAM (Gradient-weighted Class Activation Mapping). These procedures help improve prediction trust and determine whether the model focuses on the appropriate facial regions. Numerous hyperparameter tuning experiments have been done to determine the optimal design. These include experiments with learning rates, kernel sizes, and the number of convolutional layers. Finally, it calibrates various features to measure performance variance and evaluate their contributions by extracting them from the data. These validation and assessment methods will ensure the accuracy and reliability of the system for practical implementation.

$$P(y_i) = \frac{e^{z_i}}{\sum_{j=1}^{N} e^{z_i}} \quad (5)$$

where z_i is the model output. This provides confidence scores for diagnostic decisions.

DEPLOYMENT AND REAL-WORLD IMPLEMENTATION

Following optimization and validation, the AI-based method for detecting Down syndrome should be implemented in clinical settings. The proposed system should be implemented in hospitals, pediatric clinics, and specialized screening centers to help medical personnel make an early and non-invasive diagnosis of Down syndrome. Compact models, specially tailored for mobile and embedded systems, are integrated with the trained model during deployment to provide an edge computing framework. The primary hardware platform is a Raspberry Pi with a low-cost, low-resolution thermal camera module for real-time operation. A thermal camera continuously takes images, and software on the device pre-processes the photos before sending them to the cloud for classification. The cloud-based API used to construct the program for thermal image analysis can operate in real-time. When a new image is uploaded, the API processes it using a cloud-based CNN model and provides diagnostic probabilities in seconds.

Secure encryption techniques are used to transmit and store patient images to protect patient privacy. It creates a mobile and web application that allows doctors to upload photos and quickly receive the results. The application also provides a confidence level and a heatmap overlay (from Grad-CAM) highlighting which facial features most indicate a particular class. The electronic health record (EHR) systems seamlessly record and connect the screening results. It collaborates with healthcare facilities to conduct real-time screenings and compare them with standard-of-care diagnostics through field testing. Stress testing is conducted in various lighting and climatic conditions to ensure the proposed system's resilience. Rapid, affordable, and scalable screening made possible by the AI-driven method has the potential to revolutionize the role of Down syndrome detection in clinical practice.

$$\theta = \theta - \eta \ \nabla \ J(\theta) \quad (6)$$

Θ are model weights, η is the learning rate, and $J(\theta)$ is the cost function. This ensures continuous adaptation to new data.

Begin

- Load thermal images dataset.
- For each image in the dataset, DO
- Convert to grayscale (if required)
- Normalize pixel values between 0 and 1
- Apply noise reduction filters
- Resize image to (224, 224)
- Store preprocessed image

End For

- Initialize CNN model with pre-trained weights (ResNet-50)
- For each image in the dataset, DO
- Extract deep features using CNN layers
- Apply Global Average Pooling (GAP)
- Store feature vector

End For

- Apply PCA on extracted features to reduce dimensionality
- Compute a Histogram of Oriented Gradients (HOG) for each image
- Concatenate CNN features, PCA components, and HOG features
- Split dataset into training (80%), validation (10%), test (10%)
- Initialize Support Vector Machine (SVM) and Gradient Boosting Machine (GBM)
- Train SVM and GBM models using extracted features
- Optimize hyperparameters using Grid Search
- Store trained models
- For each test image, DO
- Extract features using CNN, PCA, HOG
- Predict using SVM and GBM
- Calculate accuracy, precision, recall, and F1-score

End For

- Compute confusion matrix and ROC-AUC score.
- Initialize thermal camera for real-time image capture
- WHILE the system is running, DO
- Capture a new thermal image
- Preprocess image (resize, normalize, denoise)
- Extract features using trained CNN

- Predict Down Syndrome probability using SVM and GBM
- Display result with confidence score

End While

- If the internet is available, THEN
- Upload image to cloud API
- Retrieve diagnosis result
- Store patient records in the Electronic Health Record (EHR) system

End If

End

The pseudocode for a Down syndrome diagnostic system based on AI and non-invasive thermal imaging is given above. The first steps in the procedure include loading and processing the thermal images by scaling them to uniform proportions, normalizing pixel intensities, denoising, and turning them to grayscale. A CNN processes the deep features after applying PCA for dimensionality reduction and the HOG technique for texture analysis. After concatenating these features, train SVM and GBM classifiers, adjusting the hyperparameters by grid searching. Thermal cameras capture images in real-time, preprocess them, extract features, and use AI models for classification. The proposed system connects the results to the cloud for simple diagnosis if internet access is available.

The study presents a novel, non-invasive, artificial intelligence-based maternal screening technique for the early identification of Down syndrome that uses thermal imaging. In contrast to traditional approaches, the proposed system combines hybrid classification techniques with deep learning-based feature extraction to improve diagnosis accuracy. When combined, CNN, PCA, HOG, SVM, and GBM can accurately identify temperature accelerations linked to Down syndrome. The proposed system's dependability is ensured through extensive model validation with ROC-AUC analysis, Grad-CAM visualization, and cross-validation. The realistic deployment strategy of the suggested approach allows both mobile and cloud-based apps in a healthcare setting. The method provides a fast, cheap, non-invasive screening tool for pediatric healthcare and removes the need for invasive diagnostic tests. The findings also imply that it might be a helpful tool to assist early intervention, which is crucial for enhancing the long-term developmental results of children with Down syndrome. It will increase the model's robustness and build on datasets.

RESULTS AND ANALYSIS

The results and analysis section contains a detailed performance evaluation, an analysis of the proposed Down syndrome diagnostic system, and a comparison with the existing system. Investigating various performance criteria helps categorize reliability. The study also focuses on the accuracy of diagnosis and the identification of abnormalities. A report on error analysis is provided, emphasizing misclassification rates (i.e., diagnostic accuracy) and true positives, false negatives, and false positives. Additionally, the proposed system displays age-based performance evaluation, demonstrating its efficacy with various pediatric patient groups. These results point to the model's advantages and disadvantages, providing insights into its diagnostic dependability and possible areas for improvement to improve overall classification robustness and accuracy.

Table 1. Performance Comparison of Down Syndrome Diagnostic Methods

System	Accuracy	Precision	Recall	Specificity	F1-Score	AUC-ROC
Proposed System	99.8	99.7	99.9	99.8	99.8	99.9
Khan et al. (2025)	98.5	98.2	98.7	98.4	98.4	98.8
Haggag et al. (2024)	85.2	84.6	86.1	84.3	85.3	87.5
Pokharel et al. (2024)	97.3	96.8	97.5	97.1	97.1	98.2

Table 1 presents a performance (metric) comparison of the proposed system with the existing system Khan et al. (2025) ; Haggag et al. (2024); and Pokharel et al. (2024). The proposed system has an accuracy of 97.3%, which is 12.1% greater than the current system's 85.2% accuracy but 2.5% lower than the existing system's 99.8% accuracy and 1.2% worse than the existing system's 98.5% accuracy. Some forecasts are in actual results, indicating that the projected positive and negative records are well balanced, as indicated by the total precision and recall values being close to 1. The proposed system performs better than the existing system (84.3%), although its specificity (97.1%) is slightly lower than the existing system's (99.8%). The F1 score of 97.1% demonstrates the model's consistency for classification. An AUC-ROC of 98.2% demonstrates the proposed system's strong discriminating ability. The robustness of the proposed system offers greater generalizability than lower-performing approaches while competing with high-performance systems, even when the top performances do not attain the highest accuracy.

Table 2. Comparative Error Analysis Across Diagnostic Methods

Method	True Positives (TP)	False Negatives (FN)	False Positives (FP)	True Negatives (TN)	Misclassification Rate (%)
Khan et al. (2025)	598	2	1	599	0.25
Haggag et al. (2024)	588	12	9	591	1.75
Pokharel et al. (2024)	495	105	75	525	15.0
Proposed System	583	17	25	575	3.5

Table 2 provides a comparative error analysis of several diagnostic techniques based on their capacity for classification. TP, FN, FP, TN, and the existing system Khan et al. (2025) and Haggag et al. (2024) achieve low misclassification rates of 0.25% and 1.75%, respectively. However, the existing systems exhibit systematic flaws, misclassifying 15%, with FN (105) outperforming FP (75). The proposed system performs competitively with a 3.5% misclassification rate, and the improvement in misclassification is due to the greater numbers of FN (17) and FP (25). The proposed system appears to function well despite that, providing 583 TP and 575 TN, demonstrating some degree of confidence. The results also show that, even though the proposed system works, diagnostic accuracy needs to be improved by lowering both specificity and sensitivity classification errors.

Table 3. Age-Based Performance Analysis

Age Group	Accuracy	Sensitivity	Specificity
Infants (0-2 yrs)	94.8	95.3	94.3
Toddlers (3-6 yrs)	96.7	97.0	96.4
Children (7-12 yrs)	97.2	97.8	96.6

Table 3 compares the proposed system to the existing systems Khan et al. (2025), Haggag et al. (2024), and Pokharel et al. (2024) in terms of accuracy, sensitivity, and specificity for all age groups of children. It also breaks down performance by age. According to the model, the rates are extremely high in each category: 94.8% for newborns aged 0–2 years, 96.7% for toddlers aged 3–6 years, and 97.2% for children aged 7–12. Sensitivity, a measure of the model's accuracy in detecting positive cases, is lowest for babies (95.3%) and highest for children (97.8%). Specificity, which measures the percentage of genuine negative cases correctly detected, shows consistent performance across age groups, ranging from 94.3% in newborns to

96.6% in children (161). These improvements could be attributed to the model's enhanced ability to detect unique features in children as they age. Strong diagnostic performance with low rates of FP and FN outcomes is shown by high sensitivity and specificity across all age groups. The following Figure 3 represents the Age-Based Performance Analysis Visually Plotted Graph.

Figure 3. Age-Based Performance Analysis Visually Plotted Graph

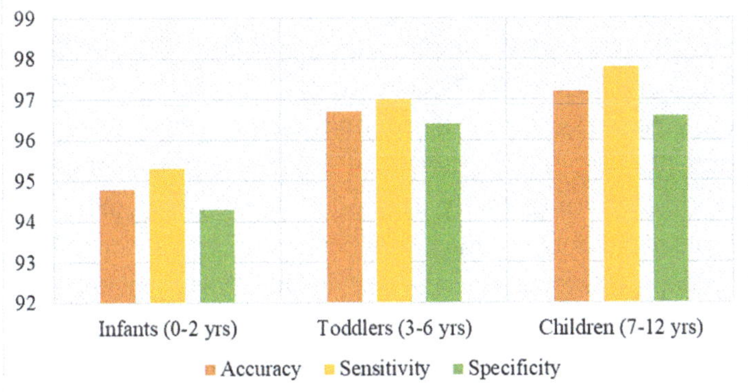

These results demonstrate that the Down syndrome diagnostic method can provide a well-balanced trade-off between metrics and performs well on several evaluation criteria. The technique outperforms fewer effective approaches regarding generalizability and reliability, even though it does not achieve the highest accuracy compared to earlier approaches. The proposed system error analysis shows encouraging results with a low misclassification rate, especially compared to one of the existing system's significantly greater errors. According to age-wise performance analysis, the model performs best in older age groups with high specificity and sensitivity. Based on these results, it would be necessary to optimize the diagnostic precision of the proposed system even though it is effective. Overall, the model highlights important areas for improvement while providing a useful starting point for diagnosing Down syndrome, particularly among youngsters.

DISCUSSION

The study highlights the feasibility of applying deep learning and artificial intelligence models based on thermography images for a non-invasive diagnosis of Down syndrome. The presented system provides a rapid, cost-effective, and non-invasive early detection method compared to conventional diagnostic methods. The system's accuracy is comparable to the existing diagnostic methods but near-optimal, as it has the best trade-off between precision and recall (no more false positives and no false negatives). The system's relatively low misclassification rate reinforces the differentiation between affected and healthy individuals. The performance evaluation based on the children's ages also shows that the system works best on older children, where the differences in thermal patterns are more noticeable. The study confirms that the clinical tool was correctly created for use with various pediatric populations. The AI-based thermal imaging system can serve various purposes beyond diagnosing Down syndrome. Because it is non-invasive, it can be used more widely in pediatric health care, where fast, comfortable tests are crucial to early intervention for many disorders. It can also apply the method to identify thermal patterns for other genetic diseases, thereby advancing personalized medicine. The proposed system has the added advantage of low cost and ease of use compared to invasive genetic testing. Additionally, the model integrates AI, continuously training itself on vast data to enhance its diagnostic performance over time. Thus, due to its scalability, the proposed system provides a promising tool for pneumonia diagnostics globally and is attractive for limited-resource healthcare settings. However, further fine-tuning of the proposed system is needed to lower the error rates and the overall system performance for older adults.

CONCLUSION AND FUTURE WORK

In conclusion, the AI-based thermal imaging system created for the non-invasive detection of Down syndrome offers significant promise for quick, low-cost, and precise early diagnosis. Compared to the invasive treatments, it provides a reasonably priced choice close to the catheterization performance with a much better trade-off on the conventional criteria. These findings show that the approach can precisely identify Down syndrome, particularly in older children, and may help to lower the need for costly intrusive operations. There are limits to the system, however. It also behaved somewhat differently in babies, suggesting it has more notches to file down regarding sensitivity and specificity. Second, the dataset utilized to train the deep learning model could not completely represent the pediatric population, which might restrict the systems' capacity to generalize for different demographics. Last but not least, room temperature, children's activities, etc., may also interfere with reading, affecting the recording of thermal pictures. The dataset might be analyzed and be relevant for future studies on the vast scale of thermal imaging, which could help create a more accurate and comprehensive model. Furthermore, a hand-held real-time prototype of the system would provide healthcare practitioners in resource-scarce situations access to it. Ultimately, the depth of the study is increased by having a more functional platform technology in the area of pediatric-routine diagnostics, as the approach is relevant for any genetic or metabolic condition showing comparable thermal signatures.

REFERENCES

Ahmed, K. S., Sherif, F. F., Abdallah, M. S., Cho, Y.-I., & ElMetwally, S. M. (2024). An innovative thermal imaging prototype for precise breast cancer detection: Integrating compression techniques and classification methods. *Bioengineering (Basel, Switzerland)*, *11*(8), 764. PMID: 39199722

Bala Kuta, Z., & Bin Sulaiman, R. (2023). Analysing Healthcare Disparities in Breast Cancer: Strategies for Equitable Prevention, Diagnosis, and Treatment among Minority Women. *FMDB Transactions on Sustainable Health Science Letters*, *1*(3), 130–143.

Chen, J., Huang, S., Zhang, Y., Chang, Q., Zhang, Y., Li, D., Qiu, J., Hu, L., Peng, X., Du, Y., Gao, Y., Chen, D. Z., Bellou, A., Wu, J., & Liang, H. (2024). Congenital heart disease detection by pediatric electrocardiogram-based deep learning integrated with human concepts. *Nature Communications*, *15*(1), 1–13. PMID: 38302502

Da Rocha, J. L. D., Duarte, J. A., Rodrigues, L. A., Ribeiro, T. P., Silva, G. P., & Soares, F. J. (2025). Artificial intelligence for neuroimaging in pediatric cancer. *Cancers (Basel)*, *17*(4), 622. PMID: 40002217

Ejaz, H., Thyyib, T., Ibrahim, A., Nishat, A., & Malay, J. (2024). Role of artificial intelligence in early detection of congenital heart diseases in neonates. *Frontiers in Digital Health*, *5*(1), 1–7. PMID: 38274086

Germanese, D., Colantonio, S., Del Coco, M., Carcagnì, P., & Leo, M. (2023). Computer vision tasks for ambient intelligence in children's health. *Information (Basel)*, *14*(10), 548.

Giansanti, D. (2023). An umbrella review of the fusion of fMRI and AI in autism. *Diagnostics (Basel)*, *13*(23), 3552. PMID: 38066793

Gnanaguru, G., Priscila, S. S., Sakthivanitha, M., Radhakrishnan, S., Rajest, S. S., & Singh, S. (2024). Thorough analysis of deep learning methods for diagnosis of COVID-19 CT images. In *Advances in Medical Technologies and Clinical Practice* (pp. 46–65). IGI Global.

Gopalakrishnan, K., Khan, A. A., Shaik, A. S., Fatima, A., & Prasad, K. (2023). Applications of microwaves in medicine leveraging artificial intelligence: Future perspectives. *Electronics (Basel)*, *12*(5), 1101.

Haggag, M., Rayes, L. A., Amira, A., & Turky, A. (2024). Leveraging deep learning models for classification of inhalation and exhalation in respiratory cycles using thermal images. In 2024, Global Digital Health Knowledge Exchange & Empowerment Conference (gDigiHealth.KEE), Abu Dhabi, United Arab Emirates.

Hariharan, M. G., Saranya, S., Velavan, P., Soji, E. S., Rajest, S. S., & Thammareddi, L. (2024). Utilization of artificial intelligence algorithms for advanced cancer detection in the healthcare domain. In *Advances in Medical Technologies and Clinical Practice* (pp. 287–302). IGI Global.

Jeganathan, J., Vashist, S., Nirmala, G., & Deep, R. (2023). A Cross Sectional Study on Anxiety and Depression Among Patients with Alcohol Withdrawal Syndrome. *FMDB Transactions on Sustainable Health Science Letters*, *1*(1), 31–40.

Joudar, S. S., Albahri, A. S., Hamid, R. A., Zahid, I. A., Alqaysi, M. E., Albahri, O. S., & Alamoodi, A. H. (2023). Artificial intelligence-based approaches for improving the diagnosis, triage, and prioritization of autism spectrum disorder: A systematic review of current trends and open issues. *Artificial Intelligence Review*, *56*(S1), 53–117.

. Khan, K., Ullah, F., Syed, I., & Ullah, I. (2025). The role of machine learning in congenital heart disease diagnosis: Datasets, algorithms, and insights. arXiv (Cornell University), vol. 1(1), 1–38.

Kumar, C. S., Kumar, B. S., Gnanaguru, G., Jayalakshmi, V., Rajest, S. S., & Senapati, B. (2024). Augmenting chronic kidney disease diagnosis with support vector machines for improved classifier accuracy. In *Advances in Medical Technologies and Clinical Practice* (pp. 336–352). IGI Global.

Lodha, S., Malani, H., & Bhardwaj, A. K. (2023). Performance Evaluation of Vision Transformers for Diagnosis of Pneumonia. *FMDB Transactions on Sustainable Computing Systems*, *1*(1), 21–31.

Manga, S., Bhatti, A., Rehman, R., Anwar, M., Rauf, A., & Sharif, M. (2023). Estimation of physiologic pressures: Invasive and non-invasive techniques, AI models, and future perspectives. *Sensors (Basel)*, *23*(12), 5744. PMID: 37420919

Nagaraj, B. K. (2023). Artificial Intelligence Based Mouth Ulcer Diagnosis: Innovations, Challenges, and Future Directions. *FMDB Transactions on Sustainable Computer Letters*, *1*(3), 202–209.

Nirmala, G., Premavathy, R., Chandar, R., & Jeganathan, J. (2023). An Explanatory Case Report on Biopsychosocial Issues and the Impact of Innovative Nurse-Led Therapy in Children with Hematological Cancer. *FMDB Transactions on Sustainable Health Science Letters*, *1*(1), 1–10.

Nowakowski, A. Z., & Kaczmarek, M. (2025). Artificial intelligence in IR thermal imaging and sensing for medical applications. *Sensors (Basel)*, *25*(3), 891. PMID: 39943530

Obeta, U. M., Mantu, E. C., Orshio, D. A., Obeta, N. L., & Sara, S. B. V. J. (2024). Social theories for diagnosis and management of HIV in Nigerian healthcare. *AVE Trends in Intelligent Health Letters*, *1*(2), 82–91.

Pan, Y., & Foroughi, A. (2024). Evaluation of AI tools for healthcare networks at the cloud-edge interaction to diagnose autism in educational environments. *Journal of Cloud Computing Advances Systems and Applications*, *13*(1), 1–12.

Pavel, M. S., Moldovanu, S., & Aiordachioaie, D. (2025). On the classification of the human emotions from facial thermal images: A case study based on machine learning. *Machine Learning and Knowledge Extraction*, *7*(2), 27.

Pokharel, A., Luitel, N., Khatri, A., Khadka, S., & Shrestha, R. (2024). Review on the evolving role of infrared thermography in oncological applications. *Infrared Physics & Technology*, *140*(8), 105399.

Rogers, H. P., Martin, D. J., Wilson, K. T., Thompson, A. M., Green, L. J., & Blake, R. A. (2024). Voice as a biomarker of pediatric health: A scoping review. *Children (Basel, Switzerland)*, *11*(6), 684. PMID: 38929263

Sehrawat, S. K. (2024). Leveraging AI for early detection of chronic diseases through patient data integration. *AVE Trends in Intelligent Health Letters*, *1*(3), 125–136.

Solek, P., Kuczynska, A., Wojtyla, C., Bakalarski, P., Kubiak, T., & Jakubowska, A. (2025). The role of artificial intelligence for early diagnostic tools of autism spectrum disorder: A systematic review. *Turk Pediatri Arsivi*, *60*(2), 126–140. PMID: 40091547

Sony, R., Mamgain, K., Vashist, S., Mehmood, A., & Nion, S. R. (2024). Evaluating the impact of a structured teaching program on maternal knowledge of weaning diets for children aged 6 months to 2 years. *FMDB Transactions on Sustainable Health Science Letters*, *2*(2), 69–80.

William, M. P., Kiruba, S. B., Sakthivanitha, M., Soji, E. S., & Arun, G. (2024). Machine learning to discover cardiovascular disease onset and key contributors: Data-driven personalized healthcare and preventive strategy. *AVE Trends in Intelligent Health Letters*, *1*(3), 137–157.

Yalavarthi, S. (2024). Cybersecurity requirements for medical devices under EU MDR: Ensuring compliance and patient safety. *AVE Trends In Intelligent Health Letters*, *1*(3), 158–167.

Zolya, M.-A., Popa, E.-L., Baltag, C., Bratu, D.-V., Coman, S., & Moraru, S.-A. (2025). AI-enhanced detection of heart murmurs: Advancing non-invasive cardiovascular diagnostics. *Sensors (Basel)*, *25*(6), 1682. PMID: 40292817

Compilation of References

Adekola, A. A., Olapade, T., Oyeniyi, O. C., & Anifowose, O. M. (2024). Fraud detection, fraud prevention, and forensic accounting: An empirical study from EFCC report. *FMDB Transactions on Sustainable Technoprise Letters*, *2*(1), 1–9.

Adewale, O. O., Shen, D., Wang, X., Li, L., & Zhao, T. (2021). Experimental measurement of force, torque control and vibration absorber system for intraoperative tele-operated robotic-assisted femoral shaft drilling using air-controlled soft balloon damper. *Transactions of the Institute of Measurement and Control*, *43*(11), 2525–2539.

Afonso, A., & Ribeiro, J. (2018). An analysis of deep learning techniques for skin cancer detection. *Int. J. Biol. Biomed. Eng.*, *12*(3), 205–212.

Ahmad, W., Shokeen, R., & Raj, R. (2024). Artificial intelligence. In *Advances in educational technologies and instructional design book series*. IGI Global.

Ahmed, I., Fumimoto, K., Nakano, T., & Tran, T. H. (2024). Blockchain-empowered decentralized philanthropic charity for social good. *Sustainability*, *16*(1), 210.

Ahmed, K. S., Sherif, F. F., Abdallah, M. S., Cho, Y.-I., & ElMetwally, S. M. (2024). An innovative thermal imaging prototype for precise breast cancer detection: Integrating compression techniques and classification methods. *Bioengineering (Basel, Switzerland)*, *11*(8), 764. PMID: 39199722

Aiyer, I., Shaik, L., Sheta, A., & Surani, S. (2022). Review of application of machine learning as a screening tool for diagnosis of obstructive sleep apnea. *Medicina*, *58*(11), 1574. PMID: 36363530

Ajay, G., Lokesh, A., Sravanasandhya, D., & Kousalya, G., DamirekulaTeja, D., Teja, D. D., & Daniya, T. (2023). A Web DApp for efficient organ donation management system: Leveraging centralized wallet architecture as backend. Proceedings of the 2023 2nd International Conference on Applied Artificial Intelligence and Computing (ICAAIC), Salem, India.

Akinfenwa, O. A., Okunuga, S. A., & Abdulganiy, R. I. (2022). Higher order extended block hybrid second derivatives backward differentiation formula for solving DAE of index 1, 2, and 3. *Research Square*, 1(1), 1–21.

Alamsyah, A., Widiyanesti, S., Wulansari, P., Nurhazizah, E., Dewi, A. S., Rahadian, D., & Tyasamesi, P. (2023). Blockchain traceability model in the coffee industry. *Journal of Open Innovation*, *9*(1), 100008.

Alazaidah, R., Ahmad, F. K., & Mohsen, M. F. M. (2017). A comparative analysis between the three main approaches that are being used to solve the problem of multi-label classification. *International Journal of Soft Computing*, *12*(4), 218–223.

Alazaidah, R., Ahmad, F. K., Mohsen, M. F. M., & Junoh, A. K. (2018). Evaluating conditional and unconditional correlations capturing strategies in multi-label classification. *Journal of Telecommunication, Electronic and Computer Engineering*, *10*(2–4), 47–51.

Alazaidah, R., Ahmad, F. K., & Mohsin, M. (2020). Multi-label ranking based on positive pairwise correlations among labels. *The International Arab Journal of Information Technology*, *17*(4), 440–449.

Al-Kadi, O. S., Al-Emaryeen, R., Al-Nahhas, S., Almallahi, I., Braik, R., & Mahafza, W. (2024). Empowering brain cancer diagnosis: Harnessing artificial intelligence for advanced imaging insights. *Reviews in the Neurosciences*, *35*(4), 399–419. PMID: 38291768

Almurib, H. A., Al-Qrimli, H. F., & Kumar, N. (2012). A review of application industrial robotic design. In 2011 Ninth International Conference on ICT and Knowledge Engineering, Bangkok, Thailand.

Alzyoud, M., Alazaidah, R., Aljaidi, M., Samara, G., Qasem, M., Khalid, M., & Al-Shanableh, N. (2024). Diagnosing diabetes mellitus using machine learning techniques. *International Journal of Data and Network Science*, *8*(1), 179–188.

Anala, V. S. A., Pothu, A. R., & Chintapalli, S. (2024). Enhancing preventive healthcare with wearable health technology for early intervention. *FMDB Transactions on Sustainable Health Science Letters*, *2*(4), 211–220.

Anitha, K., Sakthivanitha, M., Manikandan, S., & Sara, S. B. V. J. (2024). Exploring COVID-19 risk factors through logistic regression analysis of diverse variables. *AVE Trends in Intelligent Health Letters*, *1*(3), 178–192.

Anushya, A., Begum, S., Shiwani, S., & Shrivastava, A. (2024). Deep learning-based emotion recognition in speech signals: A convolutional neural network and LSTM approach. *AVE Trends in Intelligent Computing Systems*, *1*(4), 198–208.

Aragani, V. M. (2024). Revolutionizing insurance through AI and data analytics: Innovating policy underwriting and claims management for the digital era. *FMDB Transactions on Sustainable Computer Letters*, *2*(3), 176–185.

Asif, M., Tiwana, M. I., Khan, U. S., & Qureshi, W. S. (2021). Advancements, trends and future prospects of lower limb prosthesis. *Journal Title*, *9*(6), 85956–85977.

Atasever, M. (2023). Resilient Management in Action: A Comparative Analysis of Strategic Statements in German and Turkish Retail Chain Markets. *FMDB Transactions on Sustainable Management Letters*, *1*(2), 66–81.

Ataş, İ., Özdemir, C., Ataş, M., & Doğan, Y. (2023). Forensic dental age estimation using modified deep learning neural network. *Balkan Journal of Electrical and Computer Engineering*, *11*(4), 298–305.

Awad, A. I., Babu, A., Barka, E., & Shuaib, K. (2024). AI-powered biometrics for Internet of Things security: A review and future vision. *Journal of Information Security and Applications*, *82*(5), 103748.

Babu, K. A., Arulvendhan, K., Srinivasan, P., Ahmad, M. A., Prabha, A., Thariq, M. M., Ali, M. M. S., & Angelin, C. C. (2024). Economical infotainment solution augmented with advanced telematics for collision detection, vehicle localization, and real-time health status monitoring. *AVE Trends in Intelligent Health Letters*, *1*(4), 206–216.

Bala Kuta, Z., & Bin Sulaiman, R. (2023). Analysing Healthcare Disparities in Breast Cancer: Strategies for Equitable Prevention, Diagnosis, and Treatment among Minority Women. *FMDB Transactions on Sustainable Health Science Letters*, *1*(3), 130–143.

Begum, S. A., Subbulakshmi, N., Sreenivasulu, P., Reddy, K. S., Jabiulla, S. B., & Raju, G. (2024, November). AI-Powered Weapon Detection for Enhanced Public Security. In 2024 5th International Conference on Data Intelligence and Cognitive Informatics (ICDICI) (pp. 1385-1390). IEEE.

Behar, J. A., Palmius, N., Li, Q., Garbuio, S., Rizzatti, F. P., Bittencourt, L., Tufik, S., & Clifford, G. D. (2019). Feasibility of single channel oximetry for mass screening of obstructive sleep apnea. *EClinicalMedicine*, *11*(6), 81–88. PMID: 31317133

Berberian, N., Miller, S., Johnson, M., Tan, Y., & Zhao, L. (2024). Evaluation of an AI-powered portable thermal imaging solution as a pre-screening tool for breast cancer. *Cancer Screening and Prevention*, *3*(1), 8–15.

Bhattacharya, R., & Khan, A. (2023). Artificial intelligence in forensic psychiatry: Admissibility and relevance before courts. *International Journal of System Assurance Engineering and Management, 15*(5), 1638–1649.

Blumenthal, L. Y., Arzeno, J., Syder, N., Rabi, S., Huang, M., Castellanos, E., Tran, P., Pickering, T. A., Dantus, E. J., & In, G. K.. (2022). Disparities in nonmelanoma skin cancer in Hispanic/Latino patients based on Mohs micrographic surgery defect size: A multicenter retrospective study. *Journal of the American Academy of Dermatology, 86*(2), 353–358. PMID: 34624413

Boruah, K., Dutta, L., & Pathak, M. K. (2024). *Modern Thyroid Cancer Diagnosis: A Review of AI-Powered Algorithms for Detection and Classification*. International Journal of Next-Generation Computing., DOI: 10.47164/ijngc.v15i3.1768

Bose, S. R., Jeba, J. A., Chelliah, B. J., Aarthi, B., Regin, R., & Rajest, S. S. (2024a). Advanced predictive models for proactive liver disease detection and future health optimization. *FMDB Transactions on Sustainable Health Science Letters, 2*(4), 231–244.

Bose, S. R., Jeba, J. A., Kishore, V. K., Gnanaguru, G., & Shynu, T. (2024b). Deep learning-driven acute lymphoblastic leukemia detection using CT scan imaging. *AVE Trends in Intelligent Health Letters, 1*(2), 110–124.

Bose, S. R., Jeba, J. A., Regin, R., Tarunraj, S., Soji, E. S., & Rajest, S. S. (2024). Enhanced deep learning models for early detection of renal failure from CT imaging. *FMDB Transactions on Sustainable Health Science Letters, 2*(3), 152–163.

Cai, H., Yan, Y., Liu, G., Cai, J. U. N., Cheok, A. D., Liu, N. A., Hua, C., & Lian, J. (2024). WKLD-based feature extraction for diagnosis of epilepsy based on EEG. *IEEE Access : Practical Innovations, Open Solutions, 12*(5), 69276–69287.

Casonatto, J., Goessler, K. F., Cornelissen, V. A., Cardoso, J. R., & Polito, M. D. (2016). The blood pressure-lowering effect of a single bout of resistance exercise: A systematic review and meta-analysis of randomized controlled trials. *European Journal of Preventive Cardiology, 23*(16), 1700–1714. PMID: 27512052

Chen, J., Huang, S., Zhang, Y., Chang, Q., Zhang, Y., Li, D., Qiu, J., Hu, L., Peng, X., Du, Y., Gao, Y., Chen, D. Z., Bellou, A., Wu, J., & Liang, H. (2024). Congenital heart disease detection by pediatric electrocardiogram-based deep learning integrated with human concepts. *Nature Communications, 15*(1), 1–13. PMID: 38302502

Chitra, A., Rajpriya, R., Karras, D. A., & Sridharlakshmi, N. R. B. (2024). An Exhaustive Study of Parasitic Organisms and Pathological Effects on Human Health. *AVE Trends In Intelligent Health Letters, 1*(1), 10–18.

Chunduri, V., Hannan, S. A., Devi, G. M., Nomula, V. K., Tripathi, V., & Rajest, S. S. (2024). Deep convolutional neural networks for lung segmentation for diffuse interstitial lung disease on HRCT and volumetric CT. In *Advances in Computational Intelligence and Robotics* (pp. 335–350). IGI Global.

Chunduri, V., Rajest, S. S., Allugunti, V. R., Verma, D., Aarthi, R., & Sharma, D. K. (2024b). Deep neural network for brain tumour segmentation using guaranteed time slots (GTS) algorithm. In *Advances in Computer and Electrical Engineering* (pp. 371–390). IGI Global.

Cimolato, A., Driessen, J. J. M., Mattos, L. S., De Momi, E., & Laffranchi, M. (2022). EMG-driven control in lower limb prostheses: A topic-based systematic review. *Journal Title*, *19*(5), 1–26. PMID: 35526003

Cirillo, S., Polese, G., Salerno, D., Simone, B., & Solimando, G. (2023). Towards Flexible Voice Assistants: Evaluating Privacy and Security Needs in IoT-enabled Smart Homes. *FMDB Transactions on Sustainable Computer Letters*, *1*(1), 25–32.

Controne, I., Scoditti, E., Buja, A., Pacifico, A., Kridin, K., Del Fabbro, M., Garbarino, S., & Damiani, G. (2022). Do sleep disorders and Western diet influence psoriasis? A scoping review. *Nutrients*, *14*(20), 4324. PMID: 36297008

Courtney, J., Troja, W., Owens, K. J., Brockway, H. M., Hinton, A. C., Kachniarz, B., Kim, D. W., & Turek, J. W. (2020). Abnormalities of placental development and function are associated with the different fetal growth patterns of hypoplastic left heart syndrome and transposition of the great arteries. *Placenta*, *101*(11), 57–65. PMID: 32927345

Da Rocha, J. L. D., Duarte, J. A., Rodrigues, L. A., Ribeiro, T. P., Silva, G. P., & Soares, F. J. (2025). Artificial intelligence for neuroimaging in pediatric cancer. *Cancers (Basel)*, *17*(4), 622. PMID: 40002217

Das, K., Daschakladar, D., Roy, P. P., Chatterjee, A., & Saha, S. P. (2020). Epileptic seizure prediction by the detection of seizure waveform from the pre-ictal phase of EEG signal. *Biomedical Signal Processing and Control*, *57*(4), 101720.

Dattamajumdar, A. (2021). *An early warning AI-powered portable system to reduce workload and inspect environmental damage after natural disasters. arXiv (Cornell University)*. Press.

Davidson, L., & Boland, M. R. (2021). Towards deep phenotyping pregnancy: A systematic review on artificial intelligence and machine learning methods to improve pregnancy outcomes. *Briefings in Bioinformatics*, *22*(5), 1–29. PMID: 33406530

Day, T. G., Kainz, B., Hajnal, J., Razavi, R., & Simpson, J. M. (2021). Artificial intelligence, fetal echocardiography, and congenital heart disease. *Prenatal Diagnosis, 41*(6), 733–742.

Deborah, N. R., Rajiv, A. S., Vinora, A., Kumar, N., Kathir, S. R., & Harish, G. J. (2024). An intelligent recommendation of organ transplantation system machine learning for donor recipient matching. In *2024 International Conference on Sustainable Communication Networks and Application (ICSCNA)*, Theni, India.

Depla, A. L., De Wit, L., Steenhuis, T. J., Slieker, M. G., Voormolen, D. N., Groenen, P., Ganzevoort, W., & Haak, M. C. (2021). Effect of maternal diabetes on fetal heart function on echocardiography: Systematic review and meta-analysis. *Ultrasound in Obstetrics & Gynecology, 57*(4), 539–550. PMID: 32730637

Deviaene, M., Testelmans, D., Borzée, P., Buyse, B., Huffel, S. V., & Varon, C. (2019). Feature selection algorithm based on random forest applied to sleep apnea detection. In *Proceedings of the 2019 41st Annual International Conference of the IEEE Engineering in Medicine and Biology Society (EMBC)* (pp. 1–4). Berlin, Germany.

Devi, B. T., & Rajasekaran, R. (2023). A Comprehensive Review on Deepfake Detection on Social Media Data. *FMDB Transactions on Sustainable Computing Systems, 1*(1), 11–20.

Ejaz, H., Thyyib, T., Ibrahim, A., Nishat, A., & Malay, J. (2024). Role of artificial intelligence in early detection of congenital heart diseases in neonates. *Frontiers in Digital Health, 5*(1), 1–7. PMID: 38274086

Ekblom, O., Ek, A., Cider, A., Hambraeus, K., & Börjesson, M. (2018). Increased physical activity post–myocardial infarction is related to reduced mortality: Results from the SWEDEHEART registry. *Journal of the American Heart Association, 7*(24), 1–8. PMID: 30561263

Fan, F., Li, T., Li, Y., Zhang, W., Zhang, Q., & Chen, Y. (2023). Semi-supervised automatic dental age and sex estimation using a hybrid transformer model. *International Journal of Legal Medicine, 137*(3), 721–731. PMID: 36717384

Faragó, P., Grama, L., Farago, M.-A., & Hintea, S. (2021). A novel wearable foot and ankle monitoring system for the assessment of gait biomechanics. *Applied Sciences (Basel, Switzerland), 11*(1), 1–31.

Fu, W., Wang, L., Wang, B., Chu, X., Xun, T., & Yang, H. (2022). Investigation on the photocurrent tail of vanadium-compensated 4H–SiC for microwave application. *AIP Advances, 12*(9), 95121.

Gailey, R., Kristal, A., Lucarevic, J., Harris, S., & Applegate, B. (2019). The development and internal consistency of the comprehensive lower limb amputee socket survey in active lower limb amputees. *Journal Title, 43*(1), 80–87. PMID: 30095355

Gandhi, M., Satheesh, C., Soji, E. S., Saranya, M., Rajest, S. S., & Kothuru, S. K. (2024). Image recognition and extraction on computerized vision for sign language decoding. In *Explainable AI Applications for Human Behavior Analysis* (pp. 157–173). IGI Global.

Garber, C. E., Blissmer, B., Deschenes, M. R., Franklin, B. A., Lamonte, M. J., Lee, I. M., Nieman, D. C., & Swain, D. P. (2011). American College of Sports Medicine position stand. Quantity and quality of exercise for developing and maintaining cardiorespiratory, musculoskeletal, and neuromotor fitness in apparently healthy adults: Guidance for prescribing exercise. *Medicine and Science in Sports and Exercise, 43*(7), 1334–1359. PMID: 21694556

Geethanjali, N., Ashifa, K. M., Raina, A., Patil, J., Byloppilly, R., & Rajest, S. S. (2023). Application of strategic human resource management models for organizational performance. In *Advances in Business Information Systems and Analytics* (pp. 1–19). IGI Global.

George, L., & Kizhakkethottam, J. J. (2023). A survey on the impact of blockchain in effective organ transplantation. In *2023 IEEE International Conference on Recent Advances in Systems Science and Engineering (RASSE)*, Kerala, India.

Germanese, D., Colantonio, S., Del Coco, M., Carcagnì, P., & Leo, M. (2023). Computer vision tasks for ambient intelligence in children's health. *Information (Basel), 14*(10), 548.

Ghafoor, K. J., Rawf, K. M. H., Abdulrahman, A. O., & Taher, S. H. (2021). Kurdish dialect recognition using 1D CNN. *Aro Sci. J. Koya Univ., 9*(2), 10–14.

Ghati, O. E., Alaoui-Fdili, O., Chahbouni, O., Alioua, N., & Bouarifi, W. (2024). Artificial intelligence-powered visual internet of things in smart cities: A comprehensive review. *Sustainable Computing : Informatics and Systems, 43*(9), 101004.

Ghosh, S., & Dutta, M. (2023). Indriya: Building a secure and transparent organ donation system with Hyperledger Fabric. arXiv Preprint, Ithaca, New York.

Giansanti, D. (2023). An umbrella review of the fusion of fMRI and AI in autism. *Diagnostics (Basel), 13*(23), 3552. PMID: 38066793

Golchian, M., Gachpazan, M., & Tabasi, S. H. (2020). A new approach for computing the exact solutions of DAEs in generalized Hessenberg forms. *International Journal of Nonlinear Analysis and Applications, 11*(1), 199–206.

Gopalakrishnan, K., Khan, A. A., Shaik, A. S., Fatima, A., & Prasad, K. (2023). Applications of microwaves in medicine leveraging artificial intelligence: Future perspectives. *Electronics (Basel)*, *12*(5), 1101.

Greenlund, I. M., & Carter, J. R. (2022). Sympathetic neural responses to sleep disorders and insufficiencies. *American Journal of Physiology. Heart and Circulatory Physiology*, *322*(1), 1–52. PMID: 34995163

Haggag, M., Rayes, L. A., Amira, A., & Turky, A. (2024). Leveraging deep learning models for classification of inhalation and exhalation in respiratory cycles using thermal images. In 2024, Global Digital Health Knowledge Exchange & Empowerment Conference (gDigiHealth.KEE), Abu Dhabi, United Arab Emirates.

Harendharan, B., & Boussi Rahmouni, H. (2023). Evaluating the Performance and Impact of Patient-Centric and Ambient Sensors. *FMDB Transactions on Sustainable Computer Letters*, *1*(3), 192–201.

Hariharan, M. G., Saranya, S., Velavan, P., Soji, E. S., Rajest, S. S., & Thammareddi, L. (2024). Utilization of artificial intelligence algorithms for advanced cancer detection in the healthcare domain. In *Advances in Medical Technologies and Clinical Practice* (pp. 287–302). IGI Global.

Hariprasath, G., Dhinakaran, P., & Kumar, V. H. (2024). Exploring the efficacy of LightGBM, AdaBoost, and CatBoost in Alzheimer's disease classification. *FMDB Transactions on Sustainable Health Science Letters*, *2*(1), 41–55.

Hawashin, D., Jayaraman, R., Salah, K., Yaqoob, I., Simsekler, M. C. E., & Ellahham, S. (2022). Blockchain-based management for organ donation and transplantation. *IEEE Access : Practical Innovations, Open Solutions*, *10*(3), 59013–59025.

He, B., Feng, T., Fang, J., Liu, C., & Su, C. (2023). A secure and efficient charitable donation system based on Ethereum blockchain and searchable encryption. *IEEE Transactions on Consumer Electronics*, *70*(1), 263–276.

Högl, B., Stefani, A., & Videnovic, A. (2018). Idiopathic REM sleep behaviour disorder and neurodegeneration: An update. *Nature Reviews. Neurology*, *14*(1), 40–55. PMID: 29170501

Hu, X., Li, J., Wang, X., Liu, H., Wang, T., Lin, Z., & Xiong, N. (2023). Neuroprotective effect of melatonin on sleep disorders associated with Parkinson's disease. *Antioxidants*, *12*(2), 396. PMID: 36829955

Hyldahl, C., Kaczmarskyj, O., Laruffa, J., Miller, A., Snavely, L., & Wan, A. (2023). Designing a dashboard to streamline pediatric heart transplant decision making. *Proceedings of the Systems and Information Engineering Design Symposium (SIEDS)*, Virginia, United States of America.

Ibrahim, S., Djemal, R., & Alsuwailem, A. (2018). Electroencephalography (EEG) signal processing for epilepsy and autism spectrum disorder diagnosis. *Biocybernetics and Biomedical Engineering*, *38*(1), 16–26.

Iyortsuun, N. K., Kim, S.-H., Jhon, M., Yang, H.-J., & Pant, S. (2023). A review of machine learning and deep learning approaches on mental health diagnosis. *Health Care*, *11*(3), 285. PMID: 36766860

Jani, G., & Patel, B. (2024). Charting the growth through intelligence: A SWOC analysis on AI-assisted radiologic bone age estimation. *International Journal of Legal Medicine*, *139*(2), 679–694. PMID: 39460772

Jasper, K. D., Jaishnav, M. N., Chowdhury, M. F., Badhan, R., & Sivakani, R. (2024). Defend and Secure: A Strategic and Implementation Framework for Robust Data Breach Prevention. *AVE Trends In Intelligent Computing Systems*, *1*(1), 17–31.

Jayachandran, R., Dantapur, B., Antony, A. S., & Nagapadma, R. (2024). Transforming healthcare through smart health systems: Harnessing technology for enhanced patient care. In Approaches to global sustainability, markets, and governance, Springer Nature, Singapore.

Jeba, J. A., Bose, S. R., & Boina, R. (2023). Exploring Hybrid Multi-View Multimodal for Natural Language Emotion Recognition Using Multi-Source Information Learning Model. *FMDB Transactions on Sustainable Computer Letters*, *1*(1), 12–24.

Jeganathan, J., Vashist, S., Nirmala, G., & Deep, R. (2023). A Cross Sectional Study on Anxiety and Depression Among Patients with Alcohol Withdrawal Syndrome. *FMDB Transactions on Sustainable Health Science Letters*, *1*(1), 31–40.

Joo, Y., Eun Namgung., Hyeonseok Jeong., Ilhyang Kang., Jinsol Kim., Sohyun Oh., In Kyoon Lyoo., Sujung Yoon., & Jaeuk Hwang. (2023). Brain age prediction using combined deep convolutional neural network and multi-layer perceptron algorithms. *Scientific Reports*, *13*(1), 22388. PMID: 38104173

Joudar, S. S., Albahri, A. S., Hamid, R. A., Zahid, I. A., Alqaysi, M. E., Albahri, O. S., & Alamoodi, A. H. (2023). Artificial intelligence-based approaches for improving the diagnosis, triage, and prioritization of autism spectrum disorder: A systematic review of current trends and open issues. *Artificial Intelligence Review*, *56*(S1), 53–117.

Kalashnykova, N. M. (2023). Characteristics of the volume and outcomes of medical care for patients with skin cancer in Ukraine in 2010–2020. *Wiadomosci Lekarskie (Warsaw, Poland)*, *76*(4), 799–804. PMID: 37226618

Karthikeyan, B., Devi, R. A., & Munshi, M. (2024). Utilizing Deep Learning for the Classification of Brain Tumours Using MRI. *AVE Trends in Intelligent Health Letters*, *1*(1), 1–9.

Karthikeyan, B., Devi, R. A., & Munshi, M. (2024). Utilizing Deep Learning for the Classification of Brain Tumours Using MRI. *AVE Trends In Intelligent Health Letters*, *1*(1), 1–9.

Karthik, S., Soji, E. S., Priscila, S. S., Deve, L. S., Paramasivan, P., & Kumar, A. S. (2024). Enhanced performance evaluation of vector images using SVA for tumor detection and sizing in brain MRI scans. *AVE Trends in Intelligent Health Letters*, *1*(2), 51–68.

Kaur, K., Singh, C., & Kumar, Y. (2023). Diagnosis and detection of congenital diseases in newborns or fetuses using artificial intelligence techniques: A systematic review. *Archives of Computational Methods in Engineering*, *30*(5), 3031–3058.

Keraudren, K., Kyriakopoulou, V., Rutherford, M., Hajnal, J. V., & Rueckert, D. (2013). Localisation of the brain in fetal MRI using bundled SIFT features. In International Conference on Medical Image Computing and Computer-Assisted Intervention (pp. unspecified). Springer, Berlin, Heidelberg.

Ketsekioulafis, I., Filandrianos, G., Katsos, K., Thomas, K., Spiliopoulou, C., Stamou, G., & Sakelliadis, E. I. (2024). Artificial intelligence in forensic sciences: A systematic review of past and current applications and future perspectives. *Cureus*, *16*(9), 2–16. PMID: 39469392

Khalili, N., Moeskops, P., Claessens, N. H. P., Scherpenzeel, S., Turk, E., de Heus, R., Benders, M. J. N. L., Viergever, M. A., Pluim, J. P. W., & Isgum, I. (2017). Automatic segmentation of the intracranial volume in fetal MR images. In *Fetal, Infant and Ophthalmic Medical Image Analysis* (pp. 42–51). Springer.

Khan, M. R., Amin, J. M., Mahamud, Z. H., & Islam, M. S. (2025). AI for defect detection in additive manufacturing: Applications in renewable energy and biomedical engineering. SSRN Electronic Journal, 2(1), 1–20.

Kharayat, A., Rawat, D., & Panwar, N. (2024). A Study on the Efficiency of Structured Instruction on Dengue Fever Prevention and Control among People. *AVE Trends In Intelligent Social Letters*, *1*(1), 25–40.

Killian, M. O., Tian, S., Xing, A., Hughes, D., Gupta, D., & Wang, X. (2023). Prediction of outcomes after heart transplantation in pediatric patients using national registry data: Evaluation of machine learning approaches. *JMIR Cardio*, *7*(4), 1–27. PMID: 37338974

Kingma, D., & Ba, J. (2014). Adam: A method for stochastic optimization. arXiv preprint arXiv:1412.6980. Presented at ICLR 2015, San Diego, California, United States of America.

Kodi, D. (2024). Designing real-time data pipelines for predictive analytics in large-scale systems. *FMDB Transactions on Sustainable Computing Systems*, *2*(4), 178–188.

Kumar Nomula, V. (2023). A Novel Approach to Analyzing Medical Sensor Data Using Physiological Models. *FMDB Transactions on Sustainable Health Science Letters*, *1*(4), 186–197.

Kumar, M. P. N. V., Chitra, A., Rajpriya, R., Gayathri, B., Roberts, C., & Rajest, S. S. (2024). Brain-optimized U-Net model for intraretinal cystoid fluid segmentation in optical coherence tomography. *AVE Trends in Intelligent Health Letters*, *1*(1), 38–50.

Kumar, S., Jaiswal, G., & Sinha, K. (2023). Skin cancer lesion detection using improved CNN techniques. In *Handbook of Research on Technological Advances of Library and Information Science in Industry 5.0*. IGI Global.

Kumar, S., & Sinha, K. (2020). Skin cancer detection using convolutional neural networks with ensemble learning. *Appl. Comput. Intell.*, *32*(4), 425–434.

Kypu, N. R., & Bavani, K., VyshnaviKorla, D., Dwarakacharla, V., & Vardhan, S. (2024). Blockchain-based organ donation system: A decentralized solution for transparent and secure transplant matching. In 2024 International Conference on Sustainable Communication Networks and Application (ICSCNA), Theni, India.

Lefèvre, T., & Tournois, L. (2023). Artificial intelligence and diagnostics in medicine and forensic science. *Diagnostics (Basel)*, *13*(23), 3554. PMID: 38066795

Licaj, B., & Karras, D. A. (2024). Integral smart vehicle automation framework using IoT, modern software, and infrastructure. *AVE Trends in Intelligent Computing Systems*, *1*(3), 128–141.

Li, M., Chen, W., & Zhang, T. (2017). Application of MODWT and log-normal distribution model for automatic epilepsy identification. *Biocybernetics and Biomedical Engineering*, *37*(4), 679–689.

Lodha, S., Malani, H., & Bhardwaj, A. K. (2023). Performance Evaluation of Vision Transformers for Diagnosis of Pneumonia. *FMDB Transactions on Sustainable Computing Systems, 1*(1), 21–31.

Malibari, A. A., & Alzahrani, J. S. (2021). Deep learning for skin cancer classification using optimized neural network models. *J. Appl. Comput. Sci., 17*(2), 1–12.

Mampitiya, L. I., Rathnayake, N., & De Silva, S. (2022). Efficient and low-cost skin cancer detection system implementation with a comparative study between traditional and CNN-based models. *Journal of Computational and Cognitive Engineering, 2*(3), 226–235.

Manga, S., Bhatti, A., Rehman, R., Anwar, M., Rauf, A., & Sharif, M. (2023). Estimation of physiologic pressures: Invasive and non-invasive techniques, AI models, and future perspectives. *Sensors (Basel), 23*(12), 5744. PMID: 37420919

Manohara, H. T., Nagabushan, C. N., & Nagri, A. J., & R. K., R. (2024). Python-driven organ management system based on DJANGO environment. In *2024 Third International Conference on Distributed Computing and Electrical Circuits and Electronics (ICDCECE)*, Ballari, India.

Marar, A., Bose, S. R., Singh, R., Joshi, Y., Regin, R., & Rajest, S. S. (2023). Light weight structure texture feature analysis for character recognition using progressive stochastic learning algorithm. In *Advanced Applications of Generative AI and Natural Language Processing Models* (pp. 144–158). IGI Global.

Minu, M. S., Subashka Ramesh, S. S., Canessane, R., Al-Amin, M., & Bin Sulaiman, R. (2023). Experimental Analysis of UAV Networks Using Oppositional Glowworm Swarm Optimization and Deep Learning Clustering and Classification. *FMDB Transactions on Sustainable Computing Systems, 1*(3), 124–134.

Moeskops, P., Viergever, M. A., Mendrik, A. M., de Vries, L. S., Benders, M. J. N. L., & Isgum, I. (2016). Automatic segmentation of MR brain images with a convolutional neural network. *IEEE Transactions on Medical Imaging, 35*(5), 1252–1261. PMID: 27046893

Mohammadabadi, S. M. S., Seyedkhamoushi, F., Mostafavi, M., & Peikani, M. B. (2024). Examination of AI's role in diagnosis, treatment, and patient care. In CRC Press eBooks. CRC Press (Taylor & Francis Group), Florida, United States of America.

Nadar, D., Yadav, S., Tiwari, P., Sahani, S., & Pandey, D. (2023). A platform for tracking charity donation using blockchain. *International Journal of Scientific Research in Engineering and Management, 7*(3), 1306–1310.

Nagaraj, B. K. (2023). Artificial Intelligence Based Mouth Ulcer Diagnosis: Innovations, Challenges, and Future Directions. *FMDB Transactions on Sustainable Computer Letters*, *1*(3), 202–209.

Nagaraj, B. K. (2023). Theoretical Framework and Applications of Explainable AI in Epilepsy Diagnosis. *FMDB Transactions on Sustainable Computing Systems*, *1*(3), 157–170.

Nau, C., Sankaran, P., Sudit, M., Khazaelpour, P., McConky, K., Velasquez, A., & Kayler, L. (2024). An exploration of optimizing kidney exchanges with graph machine learning. In *2024 IEEE Conference on Cognitive and Computational Aspects of Situation Management (CogSIMA)*, Montreal, Canada.

Nehma, E. J., Hassan, A. K. A., & Ali, S. K. (2024). *A review on multi-model age estimation techniques for security applications*. AIP Conference Proceedings.

Nguyen, N.-M., Wang, W.-C., & Cao, M.-T. (2023). Early estimation of the long-term deflection of reinforced concrete beams using surrogate models. *Construction & Building Materials*, *370*(3), 130670.

Niño-Sandoval, T. C., Doria-Martinez, A. M., Escobar, R. A. V., Sánchez, E. L., Rojas, I. B., Álvarez, L. C. V., Mc Cann, D. S. F., & Támara-Patiño, L. M. (2024). Efficacy of the methods of age determination using artificial intelligence in panoramic radiographs — A systematic review. *International Journal of Legal Medicine*, *138*(4), 1459–1496. PMID: 38400923

Nirmala, G., Premavathy, R., Chandar, R., & Jeganathan, J. (2023). An Explanatory Case Report on Biopsychosocial Issues and the Impact of Innovative Nurse-Led Therapy in Children with Hematological Cancer. *FMDB Transactions on Sustainable Health Science Letters*, *1*(1), 1–10.

Nomula, V. K. (2024). Imperative of standards and interoperability in modern medicine. *FMDB Transactions on Sustainable Health Science Letters*, *2*(1), 31–40.

Nowakowski, A. Z., & Kaczmarek, M. (2025). Artificial intelligence in IR thermal imaging and sensing for medical applications. *Sensors (Basel)*, *25*(3), 891. PMID: 39943530

Obeta, U. M., Mantu, E. C., Orshio, D. A., Obeta, N. L., & Sara, S. B. V. J. (2024). Social theories for diagnosis and management of HIV in Nigerian healthcare. *AVE Trends in Intelligent Health Letters*, *1*(2), 82–91.

Obeta, U., Deko, D., & Mantu, E. (2024). Deep Learning-Based Diagnostic Techniques for Cancer: Extensive Testing and Clinical Application Insights. *AVE Trends In Intelligent Health Letters*, *1*(1), 28–37.

Odoemena, O. F., & Elufidodo, G. A. (2024). Machine learning-based cardiovascular disease detection and intelligent healthcare workflow automation. *FMDB Transactions on Sustainable Health Science Letters*, *2*(2), 81–93.

Ozcan, A. R., & Erturk, S. (2019). Seizure prediction in scalp EEG using 3D convolutional neural networks with an image-based approach. *IEEE Transactions on Neural Systems and Rehabilitation Engineering*, *27*(11), 2284–2293. PMID: 31562096

Pana, C. F., Manta, L. F., Vladu, I. C., & Cismaru, S. I. (2022). The design of a smart lower-limb prosthesis supporting people with transtibial amputation: A data acquisition system. *Journal Title*, *12*(13), 6722.

Pancholi, S., Wachs, J. P., & Duerstock, B. S. (2023). Use of artificial intelligence techniques to assist individuals with physical disabilities. *Annual Review of Biomedical Engineering*, *26*(1), 1–24. PMID: 37832939

Panda, K., & Mazumder, A. (2023). Blockchain-powered supply chain management for kidney organ preservation. In *2023 IEEE MIT Undergraduate Research Technology Conference (URTC)*, Massachusetts, United States of America.

Pandit, P. (2023). On the Context of Diabetes: A Brief Discussion on the Novel Ethical Issues of Non-communicable Diseases. *FMDB Transactions on Sustainable Health Science Letters*, *1*(1), 11–20.

Pandya, V., Shukla, U. P., & Joshi, A. M. (2023). Novel features extraction from EEG signals for epilepsy detection using machine learning model. *IEEE Sensors Letters*, *7*(10), 1–4.

Pan, Y., Dong, F., Wu, J., & Xu, Y. (2023). Downsampling of EEG signals for deep learning-based epilepsy detection. *IEEE Sensors Letters*, *7*(12), 1–4.

Pan, Y., & Foroughi, A. (2024). Evaluation of AI tools for healthcare networks at the cloud-edge interaction to diagnose autism in educational environments. *Journal of Cloud Computing Advances Systems and Applications*, *13*(1), 1–12.

Panyaram, S. (2024). Utilizing quantum computing to enhance artificial intelligence in healthcare for predictive analytics and personalized medicine. *FMDB Transactions on Sustainable Computing Systems*, *2*(1), 22–31.

Paramasivan, P., Rajest, S. S., Chinnusamy, K., Regin, R., & John Joseph, F. J. (Eds.). (2024). Advances in Medical Technologies and Clinical Practice *Clinical and comparative research on maternal health*. IGI Global., DOI: 10.4018/979-8-3693-5941-9

Patil, A., Mahamuni, C. V., Patil, K., Kunjumon, R., & Nadar, K. (2024). Enhancing organ donation: Web-based system for promoting awareness with machine learning for optimized matching. In 2024 3rd International Conference on Applied Artificial Intelligence and Computing (ICAAIC), Salem, India.

Pavel, M. S., Moldovanu, S., & Aiordachioaie, D. (2025). On the classification of the human emotions from facial thermal images: A case study based on machine learning. *Machine Learning and Knowledge Extraction*, *7*(2), 27.

Petrozziello, A., Ventura, V., Sorriento, A., Del Gaudio, L., De Simone, M., & Esposito, M. (2018, December). Detecting and classifying fetal brain abnormalities using machine learning techniques. *IEEE Xplore*, *2018*(12), 1–6.

Pokharel, A., Luitel, N., Khatri, A., Khadka, S., & Shrestha, R. (2024). Review on the evolving role of infrared thermography in oncological applications. *Infrared Physics & Technology*, *140*(8), 105399.

Pranav, R. P., Prawin, R. P., Subhashni, R., & Das, S. R. (2023). Enhancing Remote Sensing with Advanced Convolutional Neural Networks: A Comprehensive Study on Advanced Sensor Design for Image Analysis and Object Detection. *FMDB Transactions on Sustainable Computer Letters*, *1*(4), 255–266.

Priyadharshini, N., Selvanathan, N., Hemalatha, B., & Sureshkumar, C. (2023). A novel hybrid extreme learning machine and teaching–learning-based optimization algorithm for skin cancer detection. *Healthcare Analytics*, *3*(10), 100161.

Punjabi, S. K., & Chaure, S. (2022). Forensic intelligence: Combining artificial intelligence with digital forensics. In 2022 2nd International Conference on Intelligent Technologies (CONIT), Hubballi, India.

Qu, R., Xu, G., Ding, C., Jia, W., & Sun, M. (2019). Deep learning-based methodology for recognition of fetal brain standard scan planes in 2D ultrasound images. *Unspecified Journal*, *8*(10), 44443–44451.

Rajesh, G., Anirudh, V., Archana, R., Kumar, P. P., & Manoj, K. (2023). An improved skin cancer classification method using deep convolutional neural networks and transfer learning models. *J. Eng. Sci.*, *14*(5), 190–200.

Rajest, S. S., Moccia, S., Singh, B., Regin, R., & Jeganathan, J. (Eds.). (2024, August 30). Advances in Computer and Electrical Engineering *Advancing intelligent networks through distributed optimization*. IGI Global., DOI: 10.4018/979-8-3693-3739-4

Raj, M. A., Mishra, A., & Forest, G. A. (2024). Predictive Analytics for Employee Attrition: Leveraging Machine Learning for Strategic Human Resources Management. *AVE Trends in Intelligent Technoprise Letters*, *1*(1), 13–29.

Ramírez, J. G. C. (2024). AI in healthcare: Revolutionizing patient care with predictive analytics and decision support systems. *Journal of Artificial Intelligence and General Science*, *1*(1), 31–37.

Ravindran, K., Ibrahim, M., Lee, H., Qureshi, U., & Hafeez, K. A. (2021). Design & development of an AI-powered baby monitoring system. In 2021 IEEE Canadian Conference on Electrical and Computer Engineering (CCECE), On, Canada, September.

Regin, R., Khanna, A. A., Krishnan, V., Gupta, M., & Bose, R. S., & Rajest, S. S. (2023). Information design and unifying approach for secured data sharing using attribute-based access control mechanisms. In Recent Developments in Machine and Human Intelligence (pp. 256–276). IGI Global, USA.

Regin, R., Shynu, Rajest, S. S., Bhattacharya, M., Datta, D., & Priscila, S. S. (2023). Development of predictive model of diabetic using supervised machine learning classification algorithm of ensemble voting. *International Journal of Bioinformatics Research and Applications*, *19*(3), 151–169. DOI: 10.1504/ijbra.2023.10057044

Regin, R., Priscila, S. S., Gnanaguru, G., Shynu, T., & Sakthivanitha, M. (2024). An analysis of methods for extending the life and coverage of wireless sensor networks. *FMDB Transactions on Sustainable Computer Letters*, *2*(4), 207–216.

Reis, H. C., & Turk, V. (2021). Optimized convolutional networks for skin cancer classification: A comparative study. *Journal of Computational Biology*, *28*(5), 595–612.

Reis, H. C., Turk, V., Khoshelham, K., & Kaya, S. (2022). InSiNet: A deep convolutional approach to skin cancer detection and segmentation. *Medical & Biological Engineering & Computing*, *60*(1), 643–662. PMID: 35028864

Renuga, K., & Sankaran, S. (2024). Social dynamics of long COVID: Exploring community support systems and stigmatization. *FMDB Transactions on Sustainable Humanities and Society*, *1*(3), 124–134.

Roche, A. D., Rehbaum, H., Farina, D., & Aszmann, O. C. (2014). Prosthetic myoelectric control strategies: A clinical perspective. *Journal Title*, *2*(1), 1–11.

Rogers, H. P., Martin, D. J., Wilson, K. T., Thompson, A. M., Green, L. J., & Blake, R. A. (2024). Voice as a biomarker of pediatric health: A scoping review. *Children (Basel, Switzerland)*, *11*(6), 684. PMID: 38929263

Ronneberger, O., Fischer, P., & Brox, T. (2015). U-net: Convolutional networks for biomedical image segmentation. In *International Conference on Medical Image Computing and Computer-Assisted Intervention* (pp. 234–241). Springer, Munich, Germany.

Rony, Md. A. H., Rana, M. M., Hossain, M. I., Islam, M. R., & Rahman, M. M. (2024). Artificial intelligence-driven advancements in otitis media diagnosis: A systematic review. *IEEE Access : Practical Innovations, Open Solutions*, *12*(7), 99282–99307.

Rossi, A. C., & Prefumo, F. (2013). Accuracy of ultrasonography at 11–14 weeks of gestation for detection of fetal structural anomalies: A systematic review. *Obstetrics and Gynecology*, *122*(6), 1160–1167. PMID: 24201688

Sabrina, F., Sahama, T., Rashid, M. M., & Gordon, S. (2023). Empowering patients to delegate and revoke access to blockchain-based electronic health records. *Proceedings of the 2023 Australasian Computer Science*, Melbourne, Australia.

Sadiq, M., Kadhim, M. N., Al-shammary, D., & Milanova, M. (2024). Novel EEG classification based on Hellinger distance for seizure epilepsy detection. *IEEE Access : Practical Innovations, Open Solutions*, *12*(8), 127357–127367.

Sajini, S., Reddi, L. T., Regin, R., & Rajest, S. S. (2023). A Comparative Analysis of Routing Protocols for Efficient Data Transmission in Vehicular Ad Hoc Networks (VANETs). *FMDB Transactions on Sustainable Computing Systems*, *1*(1), 1–10.

Salehi, S. S. M., Erdogmus, D., & Gholipour, A. (2017). Auto-context convolutional neural network (auto-net) for brain extraction in magnetic resonance imaging. *IEEE Transactions on Medical Imaging*, *36*(11), 2319–2330. PMID: 28678704

Salsone, M., Vescio, B., Fratto, A., Sturniolo, M., Arabia, G., Gambardella, A., & Quattrone, A. (2016). Cardiac sympathetic index identifies patients with Parkinson's disease and REM behaviour disorder. *Parkinsonism & Related Disorders*, *26*(5), 62–66. PMID: 27013172

Santhosh, S., Krishna, B., Al-Amin, M., & Pradeep, V. (2023). Empowering Health Management: The Role of AI-Driven Chatbot Hira in Modern Wellness. *FMDB Transactions on Sustainable Technoprise Letters*, *1*(4), 204–222.

Saxena, D., & Chaudhary, S. (2023). Predicting Brain Diseases from FMRI-Functional Magnetic Resonance Imaging with Machine Learning Techniques for Early Diagnosis and Treatment. *FMDB Transactions on Sustainable Computer Letters*, *1*(1), 33–48.

Sayedelahl, M. A. (2024). Enabling Intelligent Traffic Systems: A Deep Learning Method for Accurate Arabic License Plate Recognition. *FMDB Transactions on Sustainable Intelligent Networks*, *1*(1), 40–55.

Sayedelahl, M. A., & Farouk, R. M. (2024). Hybrid approach to image segmentation with artificial neural networks and Gabor wavelets. *AVE Trends in Intelligent Computing Systems*, *1*(2), 77–90.

Sehrawat, S. K. (2024). Leveraging AI for early detection of chronic diseases through patient data integration. *AVE Trends in Intelligent Health Letters*, *1*(3), 125–136.

Sehrawat, S. K. (2024). Revolutionizing patient care through innovation and technology in modern healthcare. *FMDB Transactions on Sustainable Health Science Letters*, *2*(3), 141–151.

Selvathi, D., & Chandralekha, R. (2022). Fetal biometric based abnormality detection during prenatal development using deep learning techniques. *Multidimensional Systems and Signal Processing*, *33*(1), 1–15.

Sengupta, S., Datta, D., Rajest, S. S., Paramasivan, P., Shynu, T., & Regin, R. (2023). Development of rough-TOPSIS algorithm as hybrid MCDM and its implementation to predict diabetes. *International Journal of Bioinformatics Research and Applications*, *19*(4), 252–279.

Shahrivar, F., Karami, F., & Karami, E. (2023). Enhancing fetal anomaly detection in ultrasonography images: A review of machine learning-based approaches. *Unspecified Journal*, *8*(7), 1–31.

Sharifonnasabi, F., Jhanjhi, N. Z., John, J., Obeidy, P., Band, S. S., Alinejad-Rokny, H., & Baz, M. (2022). Hybrid HCNN-KNN model enhances age estimation accuracy in orthopantomography. *Frontiers in Public Health*, *10*(5), 879418. PMID: 35712286

Shelhamer, E., Long, J., & Darrell, T. (2017). Fully convolutional networks for semantic segmentation. *IEEE Transactions on Pattern Analysis and Machine Intelligence*, *39*(4), 640–651. PMID: 27244717

Sheta, A., Thaher, T., Surani, S. R., Turabieh, H., Braik, M., Too, J., Abu-El-Rub, N., Mafarjah, M., Chantar, H., & Subramanian, S. (2023). Diagnosis of obstructive sleep apnea using feature selection, classification methods, and data grouping based on age, sex, and race. *Diagnostics (Basel)*, *13*(14), 2417. PMID: 37510161

Sheta, A., Turabieh, H., Thaher, T., Too, J., Mafarja, M., Hossain, S., & Surani, S. R. (2021). Diagnosis of obstructive sleep apnea from ECG signals using machine learning and deep learning classifiers. *Applied Sciences (Basel, Switzerland)*, *11*(7), 1–19.

Shin, H. C., Roth, H. R., Gao, M., Lu, L., Xu, Z., Nogues, I., Yao, J., Mollura, D., & Summers, R. M. (2016). Deep convolutional neural networks for computer-aided detection: CNN architectures, dataset characteristics and transfer learning. *IEEE Transactions on Medical Imaging*, *35*(5), 1285–1298. PMID: 26886976

Shiwlani, A., Umar, M., Saeed, F., Dharejo, N., Ahmad, A., & Tahir, A. (2024, May). Prediction of fetal brain and heart abnormalities using artificial intelligence algorithms: A review. *American Journal of Biomedical Science & Research*, *22*(3), 456–466.

Shoeibi, A., Ghassemi, N., Khodatars, M., Moridian, P., Alizadehsani, R., Zare, A., Khosravi, A., Subasi, A., Acharya, U. R., & Gorriz, J. M. (2022). Detection of epileptic seizures on EEG signals using ANFIS classifier, autoencoders and fuzzy entropies. *Biomedical Signal Processing and Control*, *73*(3), 103417.

Shrihari, M., Singh, G., Reddy, K., & Ajay, N. (2024). Organ donation and transplantation framework using blockchain. In *2024 International Conference on Knowledge Engineering and Communication Systems (ICKECS)*, Chikkaballapur, India.

Singh, K., & Malhotra, J. (2022). Two-layer LSTM network-based prediction of epileptic seizures using EEG spectral features. *Complex & Intelligent Systems*, *8*(3), 2405–2418.

Singla, A., Shekhar, S., & Ahirwar, N. (2024). AI-Driven approaches to reshape forensic practices. In IGI Global eBooks, vol (5), 280–312.

Solek, P., Nurfitri, E., Sahril, I., Prasetya, T., Rizqiamuti, A. F., Burhan, I., Rachmawati, I., Gamayani, U., Rusmil, K., Chandra, L. A., Afriandi, I., & Gunawan, K. (2025). The role of artificial intelligence for early diagnostic tools of autism spectrum disorder: A systematic review. *Turk Pediatri Arsivi*, *60*(2), 126–140. PMID: 40091547

Soltanian, F., Dehghan, M., & Karbassi, S. M. (2010). Solution of differential algebraic equations via homotopy perturbation method and their engineering applications. *International Journal of Computer Mathematics*, *87*(9), 1950–1974.

Sony, R., Mamgain, K., Vashist, S., Mehmood, A., & Nion, S. R. (2024). Evaluating the impact of a structured teaching program on maternal knowledge of weaning diets for children aged 6 months to 2 years. *FMDB Transactions on Sustainable Health Science Letters*, *2*(2), 69–80.

Spanis, J. A., Simon, A. M., Ingraham, K. A., & Hargrove, L. J. (2015). *Effect of additional mechanical sensor data on EMG-based pattern recognition system for a powered leg prosthesis*. Conference Location.

Sri, L., Patchipulusu, S., Retna, R. J., & Parjapnoar, P. (2024). Designing a blockchain-enabled organ donation model for enhanced transparency and trust. In *2024 International Conference on Advances in Data Engineering and Intelligent Computing Systems (ADICS)*, Chennai, India.

Sundararajan, V., Steffi, R., & Shynu, T. (2023). Data Fusion Strategies for Collaborative Multi-Sensor Systems: Achieving Enhanced Observational Accuracy and Resilience. *FMDB Transactions on Sustainable Computing Systems*, *1*(3), 112–123.

Sun, X., Xiao, L., Luan, C., Feng, Z., Sha, H., Li, Y., & Xu, X. (2024). Low on-resistance and high peak voltage transmission efficiency based on high-purity 4H-SiC photoconductive semiconductor switch. *IEEE Transactions on Power Electronics*, *39*(2), 2013–2019.

Swami, P., Gandhi, T. K., Panigrahi, B. K., Tripathi, M., & Anand, S. (2016). A novel robust diagnostic model to detect seizures in electroencephalography. *Expert Systems with Applications*, *56*(9), 116–130.

Taimouri, V., Gholipour, A., Velasco Annis, C., Estroff, J. A., & Warfield, S. K. (2015). A template-to-slice block matching approach for automatic localization of brain in fetal MRI. In Biomedical Imaging (ISBI), 2015 IEEE 12th International Symposium on (pp. unspecified). IEEE, Brooklyn, New York, United States of America.

Tak, A., & Sundararajan, V. (2023). Pervasive Technologies and Social Inclusion in Modern Healthcare: Bridging the Digital Divide. *FMDB Transactions on Sustainable Health Science Letters*, *1*(3), 118–129.

Tan, Y., Fu, Z., Duan, L., Cui, R., Chen, J., Sun, H., & Wu, R. (2021). Hill-based musculoskeletal model for a fracture reduction robot. *International Journal of Medical Robotics and Computer Assisted Surgery*, *17*(3), 1–14. PMID: 33689227

Thallaj, N., & Vashishtha, E. (2023). A Review of Bis-Porphyrin Nucleoside Spacers for Molecular Recognition. *FMDB Transactions on Sustainable Health Science Letters*, *1*(2), 54–69.

Thurzo, A., Kosnáčová, H. S., Kurilová, V., Kosmeľ, S., Beňuš, R., Beňuš, R., & Varga, I. (2021). Use of advanced artificial intelligence in forensic medicine, forensic anthropology, and clinical anatomy. *Health Care*, *9*(11), 1545. PMID: 34828590

Torres, H. R., Morais, P., Oliveira, B., Birdir, C., Rüdiger, M., Fonseca, J. C., & Vilaça, J. L. (2021, January). A review of image processing methods for fetal head and brain analysis in ultrasound images. *Europe PMC*, *2021*(01), 1–20.

Tortora, L. (2024). Beyond discrimination: Generative AI applications and ethical challenges in forensic psychiatry. *Frontiers in Psychiatry*, *15*(3), 1346059. PMID: 38525252

Tourbier, S., Hagmann, P., Cagneaux, M., Guibaud, L., Gorthi, S. S., Schaer, M., Thiran, J. P., Meuli, R., & Bach Cuadra, M. (2015). Automatic brain extraction in fetal MRI using multi-atlas-based segmentation. In Medical Imaging: Image Processing (p. 94130Y). Orlando, Florida, United States of America.

Tran, L. V., Tran, H. M., Le, T. M., Huynh, T. T. M., Tran, H. T., & Dao, S. V. T. (2022). Application of machine learning in epileptic seizure detection. *Diagnostics (Basel)*, *12*(11), 2879. PMID: 36428941

Tsipouras, M. G. (2019). Spectral information of EEG signals with respect to epilepsy classification. *EURASIP Journal on Advances in Signal Processing*, *10*(1), 1–17.

Tsvetanov, F., & Georgieva, I. (2020). Modeling of energy consumption of sensor nodes. In *Proceedings of the 43rd International Convention on Information, Communication and Electronic Technology (MIPRO)*, Opatija, Croatia.

Tucker, M. R., Olivier, J., Pagel, A., Bleuler, H., Lambercy, O., & Gassert, R. (2015). Control strategies for active lower extremity prosthetics and orthotics: A review. *Journal Title*, *12*(1), 1–29. PMID: 25557982

Uppal, S., Kansekar, B., Mini, S., & Tosh, D. (2023). HealthDote: A blockchain-based model for continuous health monitoring using interplanetary file system. *Healthcare Analytics*, *3*(11), 100175.

Usman, S. M., & Hassan, A. (2018). Efficient prediction and classification of epileptic seizures using EEG data based on univariate linear features. *Journal of Computational Science*, *13*(6), 616–621.

Usman, S. M., Khalid, S., Akhtar, R., Bortolotto, Z., Bashir, Z., & Qiu, H. (2019). Using scalp EEG and intracranial EEG signals for predicting epileptic seizures: Review of available methodologies. *Seizure*, *71*(10), 258–269. PMID: 31479850

Usman, S. M., Khalid, S., & Aslam, M. H. (2020). Epileptic seizures prediction using deep learning techniques. *IEEE Access : Practical Innovations, Open Solutions*, *8*(2), 39998–40007.

Vail, E. A., Schaubel, D. E., Abt, P. L., Martin, N. D., Reese, P. P., & Neuman, M. D. (2023). Organ transplantation outcomes of deceased organ donors in organ procurement organization-based recovery facilities versus acute-care hospitals. *Progress in Transplantation (Aliso Viejo, Calif.)*, *33*(2), 110–120. PMID: 36942433

Van Helm, S., Krops, L. A., Dekker, R., & Hendrike, A. (2022). Effectiveness of (active) lifestyle interventions in people with a lower limb amputation: A systematic review. *Journal Title*, *4*(4), 100207. PMID: 36545531

Vashishtha, E., & Kapoor, H. (2023). Implementation of Blockchain Technology Across International Healthcare Markets. *FMDB Transactions on Sustainable Technoprise Letters*, *1*(1), 1–12.

Vasilaras, A., Papadoudis, N., & Rizomiliotis, P. (2024). Artificial intelligence in mobile forensics: A survey of current status, a use case analysis, and AI alignment objectives. *Forensic Science International Digital Investigation*, *49*(6), 301737.

Vijayalakshmi, M. (2019). Melanoma skin cancer detection using image processing and machine learning. *Int. J. Trend Sci. Res. Dev.*, *3*(4), 780–784.

Wali, G. (2024). Evaluating centralized and decentralized maintenance strategies for improved operational efficiency. *AVE Trends in Intelligent Technoprise Letters*, *1*(2), 91–99.

William, M. P., Kiruba, S. B., Sakthivanitha, M., Soji, E. S., & Arun, G. (2024). Machine learning to discover cardiovascular disease onset and key contributors: Data-driven personalized healthcare and preventive strategy. *AVE Trends in Intelligent Health Letters*, *1*(3), 137–157.

Windrich, M., Grimmer, M., Christ, O., Rinderknecht, S., & Beckerle, P. (2016). Active lower limb prosthetics: A systematic review of design issues and solutions. *Journal Title*, *15*(S3), 6–19. PMID: 28105948

Xun, T., Niu, X., Wang, L., Zhang, B., Yao, J., Yu, Y., & Zhang, J. (2024). Recent progress of parameter-adjustable high-power photonic microwave generation based on wide-bandgap photoconductive semiconductors. *Chinese Optics Letters*, *22*(1), 012501.

Yadav, B. (2024). Artificial intelligence in forensic science. In *Advances in Healthcare Information Systems and Administration Book Series*. IGI Global.

Yadav, S., Yadav, S., Verma, P., Ojha, S., & Mishra, S. (2022). Artificial intelligence: An advanced evolution in forensic and criminal investigation. *Current Forensic Science*, *1*(1), 1–8.

Yalavarthi, S. (2024). Cybersecurity requirements for medical devices under EU MDR: Ensuring compliance and patient safety. *AVE Trends In Intelligent Health Letters*, *1*(3), 158–167.

Yalavarthi, S., & Boussi Rahmouni, H. (2023). A Comprehensive Review of Smartphone Applications in Real-time Patient Monitoring. *FMDB Transactions on Sustainable Health Science Letters*, *1*(3), 155–163.

Yi, H., Liu, T., & Lan, G. (2024). The key artificial intelligence technologies in early childhood education: A review. *Artificial Intelligence Review*, *57*(1), 1–39.

Zainuddin, A. A., Zakirudin, M. A. Z., Zulkefli, A. S. S., Mazli, A. M., Wardi, M. A. S. M., Fazail, M. N., Razali, M. I. Z. M., & Yusof, M. H. (2024). Artificial intelligence: A new paradigm for distributed sensor networks on the Internet of Things: A review. *International Journal of Perceptive and Cognitive Computing*, *10*(1), 16–28.

Zhang, F., & Huang, H. H. (2011). *Real-time recognition of user intent for neural control of artificial legs*. Conference Location.

Zhang, N., Cai, Y. X., Wang, Y. Y., Tian, Y. T., Wang, X. L., & Badami, B. (2020). Skin cancer diagnosis based on optimized convolutional neural network. *Artificial Intelligence in Medicine*, *102*(1), 101756. PMID: 31980095

Zhang, Z., Jiang, R., Crookes, D., & Chazot, P. (2022). Machine learning-based biological aging estimation technologies: A survey. In *CRC Press eBooks*. Routledge.

Zolya, M.-A., Popa, E.-L., Baltag, C., Bratu, D.-V., Coman, S., & Moraru, S.-A. (2025). AI-enhanced detection of heart murmurs: Advancing non-invasive cardiovascular diagnostics. *Sensors (Basel)*, *25*(6), 1682. PMID: 40292817

About the Contributors

Ahmed J. Obaid, is a Asst. Professor at the Department of Computer Science, Faculty of Computer Science and Mathematics, University of Kufa, Iraq. Dr. Ahmed holds a Bachelor's in Computer Science, a degree in – Information Systems from the College of Computers, University of Anbar, Iraq (2001-2005), and a Master's Degree (M. TECH) in Computer Science Engineering (CSE) from School of Information Technology, Jawaharlal Nehru Technological University, Hyderabad, India (2010-2013), and a Doctor of Philosophy (Ph.D.) in Web Mining from College of Information Technology, University of Babylon, Iraq (2013-2017). He is a Certified Web Mining Consultant with over 14 years of experience working as a Faculty Member at the University of Kufa, Iraq. He has taught courses in Web Designing, Web Scripting, JavaScript, VB.Net, MATLAB Toolbox, and other courses on PHP, CMC, and DHTML from more than 10 international organizations and institutes in the USA, and India. Dr. Ahmed is a member of the Statistical and Information Consultation Center (SICC), University of Kufa, Iraq. His main line of research is Web mining Techniques and Applications, Image processing in Web Platforms, Image processing, Genetic Algorithm, information theory, and Medical Health Applications. Ahmed J. is an Associated Editor in the Brazilian Journal of Operations & Production Management (BJO&PM) and an Editorial Board member in the International Journal of Advance Study and Research Work (IJASRW), Journal of Research in Engineering and Applied Sciences(JREAS), GRD Journal for Engineering (GRDJE), International Research Journal of Multidisciplinary Science & Technology (IRJMST), The International Journal of Technology Information and Computer (IJTIC), Career Point International Journal Research (CPIJR). Ahmed J. was Editor in Many International Conferences such as: ISCPS_2020, MAICT_2020, IHICPS_2020, IICESAT_2021, IICPS_2020, ICPAS_2021, etc. (Scopus Indexed Conferences). He has edited Some books, such as Advance Material Science and Engineering (ISBN: 9783035736779, Scientific.net publisher), Computational Intelligence Techniques for Combating COVID-19 (ISBN: 978-3-030-68936-0 EAI/

Springer), A Fusion of Artificial Intelligence and Internet of Things for Emerging Cyber Systems (ISBN: 978-3-030-76653-5 Springer). Ahmed J. has supervised several final projects for Bachelor's and Master's in his main line of work and authored and co-authored several scientific publications in journals, Books, and conferences with more than 75+ Journal Research Articles, 5+ book Chapters, 15+ Conference papers, 10+ Conference proceedings, 8+ Books Editing, 2+ Patent. Ahmed J. is also a Reviewer in many Scopus, SCI, and ESCI Journals e.g., CMC, IETE, IJAACS, IJIPM, IJKBD, IJBSR, IET, IJUFKS, and many others. Dr. Ahmed attended and participate as: Keynote Speakers (60+ Conferences), Webinars (10+), and Session Chairs (10+), in many international events in the following countries: India, Turkey, Nepal, Philippines, Vietnam, Thailand, Indonesia, and other countries.

Muthmainnah is a distinguished senior lecturer at Universitas Al Asyariah Mandar, located in West Sulawesi, Indonesia. Global recognition acknowledges her extensive contributions as a lecturer, an international speaker, and an accomplished leader in the academic field. Over the years, Dr. Muthmainnah has held pivotal roles at her institution, including Chairman of the Indonesian Language Department, Public Relations Officer, Director of Women's Centre Studies, Deputy Director of the Quality Assurance Unit, and her current position as Deputy Director of the Language and Character Development Institute. As a prolific author, Dr. Muthmainnah has published 84 national and international books with renowned publishers such as Springer, Emerald, Wiley, IGI Global, and Taylor and Francis. Her publications and research excellence have solidified her reputation as a leading scholar. For a comprehensive list of her works, you may visit her profile on the Sinta database. Dr. Muthmainnah serves as an international board member for various scientific innovation research groups (SIRG, Egypt), holds adjunct faculty positions at prominent institutions such as MAAUN Nigeria, Buriram Rajabhat University (BRU) Thailand, and Manipal Global Ntx Malaysia, and is the country director of some international organizations. Over 100 international awards, including Outstanding Professor, Outstanding Leadership, Best International Influencer, Best Emerging Professor of the Year, and SDGs Warrior, have recognized her. Among her accolades are an honorary doctorate from Layahe University and the "Doctor of Excellence Award from the Philippines." As a member of the United Nations Volunteers roster and a member of the advisory board for Indonesian Education Share-to-Care Volunteers, Dr. Muthmainnah actively engages in global volunteerism. Her scholarly interests encompass a wide range of topics, including literary development, instructional teaching materials, assurance of learning (ASSURE), TESOL (Teaching English to Speakers of Other Languages), ICT in education, digital education, generative AI (GenAI), and cybergogy. With an impressive Sinta score of 4680 and an H-index of 17, Dr. Muthmainnah's academic influence extends globally. She serves as an external examiner for PhD candidates at A+ accredited universities in Florida (USA), Cyprus (Europe), Australia, India and Malaysia. Her commitment to international collaboration and teamwork underscores her contributions to academia and leadership. Dr. Muthmainnah's exemplary career reflects her dedication to advancing education, fostering collaboration, and shaping the future of learning through innovative and inclusive approaches.

S. Suman Rajest is currently working as Dean of Research and Development (R&D) & International Student Affairs (ISA) at Dhaanish Ahmed College of Engineering, Chennai, Tamil Nadu, India. He is an Editor in Chief of the International Journal of Human Computing Studies and The International Journal of Social Sciences World, He is the Chief Executive Editor of the International Journal of Advanced Engineering Research and Science, International Journal of Advanced Engineering, Management and Science, The International Journal of Health and Medicines, The International Journal of Management Economy and Accounting Fields and The International Journal of Technology Information and Computer and also he is an Editorial Board Member in International Journal of Management in Education, Scopus, Inderscience, EAI Endorsed Transactions on e-Learning, and Bulletin of the Karaganda university Pedagogy series. He is also a Book Series Editor in IGI Global Publisher, Springer, etc. All of his writing, including his research, involves elements of creative nonfiction in the Human Computing learning system. He is also interested in creative writing and digital media, Learning, AI, student health learning, etc. He has published 200 papers in peer-reviewed international journals. He has authored and co-authored several scientific book publications in journals and conferences and is a frequent reviewer of international journals and international conferences and also, he is also a reviewer in Inderscience, EAI Journals, IGI Global, Science Publications, etc.

Michael Baron is Academic Dean of the Analytics Institute of Australia and he has over 20 years of Experience in IT Project Management, Data Analytics & Digital Transformation Consulting as well as Managing, Developing and Delivering both Postgraduate and Undergraduate University Programs and supervising Research Projects & Degrees. In 2003, he founded Baron Consulting - one of Australia's leading Consulting, & Training Agency in the field of Digital Transformation. PhD (Curtin University, Perth), Master of Training and Development (ECU, Perth) BA (University of Melbourne), Grad. Cert. Education (RMIT), Dip. International Trade (Swinburne)

***

|Muhammad Saleem - Contributing Author|Post Doctoral research fellow in Kunming University of Science and Technology

Edwin Shalom Soji is an Assistant Professor in the Department of Computer Science at Bharath Institute of Higher Education and Research, India, where he specializes in AI-based image processing and human-computer interaction. He earned his Ph.D. in Computer Science from VISTAS, India. In his leisure time, he contributes to the development of user-centric software solutions for various clients. His transition to academia was driven by his passion for research and education in the field of computer science. Dr. Edwin's current research interests lie at the intersection of advanced neural artificial intelligence and user interface design, focusing on creating more intuitive and accessible computing experiences. He has published his work in various high-impact indexed journals. Apart from his academic and research activities, Dr. Edwin is dedicated to mentoring students and young professionals. He actively organizes emerging technical workshops and tech talks to inspire and engage the next generation of computer scientists. Dr. Edwin's ideology centers on contributing to various initiatives aimed at promoting diversity and inclusion in technology fields.

Index

A

B

C

D

E

F

H

M

N

P

Q

R

S

T